Immunology for Dentistry

Immunology for Dentistry

Edited by

Mohammad Tariqur Rahman
University of Malaya, Kuala Lumpur, Malaysia

Wim Teughels
KU Leuven, Leuven, Belgium

Richard J. Lamont
University of Louisville, Louisville, USA

WILEY Blackwell

Registered Offices
John Wiley & Sons, Inc., 111 River Street, Hoboken, NJ 07030, USA
John Wiley & Sons Ltd, The Atrium, Southern Gate, Chichester, West Sussex, PO19 8SQ, UK

For details of our global editorial offices, customer services, and more information about Wiley products visit us at www.wiley.com.

Wiley also publishes its books in a variety of electronic formats and by print-on-demand. Some content that appears in standard print versions of this book may not be available in other formats.

Library of Congress Cataloging-in-Publication Data
Names: Rahman, Mohammad Tariqur, editor. | Teughels, Wim, editor. | Lamont, Richard J., 1961– editor.
Title: Immunology for dentistry / edited by Mohammad Tariqur Rahman, Wim Teughels, Richard J. Lamont.
Description: Hoboken, NJ : Wiley-Blackwell, 2023. | Includes index.
Identifiers: LCCN 2022059914 (print) | LCCN 2022059915 (ebook) | ISBN 9781119893004 (paperback) | ISBN 9781119893011 (adobe pdf) | ISBN 9781119893028 (epub)
Subjects: MESH: Stomatognathic Diseases–microbiology | Stomatognathic Diseases–immunology | Dentistry–methods
Classification: LCC RK301 (print) | LCC RK301 (ebook) | NLM WU 140 | DDC 617.5/22–dc23/eng/20230518
LC record available at https://lccn.loc.gov/2022059914
LC ebook record available at https://lccn.loc.gov/2022059915

Cover Design: Wiley
Cover Image: Courtesy of Wannes Van Holm & Merve Kübra Aktan

Set in 9.5/12.5pt STIXTwoText by Straive, Pondicherry, India
Printed and bound by CPI Group (UK) Ltd, Croydon, CR0 4YY

C9781119893004_310523

Contents

List of Contributors

Maha Abdullah
Universiti Putra Malaysia,
Serdang, Malaysia

Nazmul Ahsan
University of Dhaka,
Dhaka, Bangladesh

Anwarul Azim Akhand
University of Dhaka,
Dhaka, Bangladesh

Shelly Arora
University of Otago,
Dunedin, New Zealand

Nor Adinar Baharuddin
University of Malaya,
Kuala Lumpur, Malaysia

Siew Wui Chan
University of Malaya,
Kuala Lumpur, Malaysia

Chia Wei Cheah
University of Malaya,
Kuala Lumpur, Malaysia

Paul R. Cooper
University of Otago,
Dunedin, New Zealand

Firdaus Hariri
University of Malaya,
Kuala Lumpur, Malaysia

Wan Nurazreena Wan Hassan
Universiti Malaya,
Kuala Lumpur, Malaysia

Haizal M. Hussaini
University of Otago,
Dunedin, New Zealand

Wan Izlina Wan-Ibrahim
University of Malaya,
Kuala Lumpur, Malaysia

Reezal Ishak
Universiti of Kuala Lumpur,
Kuala Lumpur, Malaysia

Muhammad Manjurul Karim
University of Dhaka,
Dhaka, Bangladesh

Noor Lide Abu Kassim
International Islamic University Malaysia,
Kuala Lumpur, Malaysia

Cornelis J. Kleverlaan
Academic Centre for Dentistry Amsterdam (ACTA),
Amsterdam, The Netherlands

Norhafizah Mohtarrudin
Universiti Putra Malaysia,
Serdang, Malaysia

Sabri Musa
University of Malaya,
Kuala Lumpur, Malaysia

Ngui Romano
University of Malaya,
Kuala Lumpur, Malaysia

Irosha Perera
National Dental Hospital (Teaching),
Colombo, Sri Lanka

Manosha Perera
General Sir John Kotelawala Defence University,
Dehiwala-Mount Lavinia, Sri Lanka

Dessy Rachmawati
University of Jember,
Jember, Indonesia

Zamri Radzi
University of Malaya,
Kuala Lumpur, Malaysia

Mohammad Tariqur Rahman
University of Malaya,
Kuala Lumpur, Malaysia

Srinivas Sulugodu Ramachandra
Gulf Medical University,
Ajman, United Arab Emirates

Aruni Tilakaratne
University of Peradeniya, Sri Lanka;
University of Malaya,
Kuala Lumpur, Malaysia

W.M. Tilakaratne
University of Malaya,
Kuala Lumpur, Malaysia

Wei Seong Toh
National University of Singapore,
Singapore

Rathna Devi Vaithilingam
University of Malaya,
Kuala Lumpur, Malaysia

Rachel J. Waddington
Cardiff University,
Cardiff, UK

Noor Azlin Yahya
University of Malaya,
Kuala Lumpur, Malaysia

Preface

Immunology has been an independent discipline since the beginning of the twentieth century, although it remains an integral part of tertiary education for health and medical sciences. Nevertheless, the ever expanding insights of theoretical immunology and its clinical relevance and exercise in dentistry have driven the emergence of oral immunology. Hence, this book *Immunology in Dentistry*.

The first three chapters deal with the fundamental aspects of immunology such as cells and organs of the immune system, the oral immune system and mechanisms of immunity. These introductory chapters will be useful for undergraduate dental students in the beginning years of their education. Chapters on the in-depth clinical relevance of immunology in various disciplines of dentistry such as orthodontics, endodontics, oral cancer, periodontology and oral surgery will be useful towards the end of dental education in the final years. This book also contains a chapter that will allow both undergraduate and postgraduate dentistry students to understand the basic principles and applications of various immunological techniques that are commonly used for research and diagnostic purposes. Additionally, Chapter 16 explains how to define and select control subjects (or participants) in immunological research. Each chapter is enhanced with relevant illustrations and schematic presentations.

The internationally renowned authors, the majority of whom are dentists in academia, have extensively updated all aspects of the book. I am happy to be guided by two co-editors, Wim Teughels (KU Leuven) and Richard J. Lamont (University of Louisville), in the editing of this book.

Mohammad Tariqur Rahman
Editor

Acknowledgements

The editors wish to acknowledge the contribution and support from all authors to make this dream come true and this book *Immunology for Dentistry* is now a reality. We are indebted to the Faculty of Dentistry, University of Malaya, for invaluable support and encouragement. Thank you also to all those at John Wiley & Sons Ltd for a job well done.

1

Cells and Organs of the Immune System

Anwarul Azim Akhand and Nazmul Ahsan

Department of Genetic Engineering and Biotechnology, University of Dhaka, Dhaka, Bangladesh

1.1 Introduction

Living animals grow in an environment that is heavily populated with both pathogenic and non-pathogenic micro-organisms. These micro-organisms contain a vast array of toxic or allergenic substances that may be life-threatening. Pathogenic microbes possess a variety of mechanisms by which they replicate, spread and threaten host functions. To counteract this array of threats, the immune system has evolved functional responses using specialised cells and molecules. The immune system is, therefore, a system of cells, organs and their soluble products that recognises, attacks and destroys any sort of threatening entity. By doing so, the immune system primarily protects us from various toxic substances and pathogens. At the same time, it essentially distinguishes dangerous substances from harmless ones. Infiltration with bacterial or viral molecules, for example, can be a dangerous attack on an organism, whereas inhalation of odorant or infiltration of food antigen into the bloodstream is harmless. The destruction of malignant cells is desirable but unnecessary attacks against host tissues are undesirable. Therefore, the cells of the immune system must be capable of distinguishing self from non-self and, furthermore, discriminating between non-self molecules which are harmful or innocuous (e.g. foods).

Two overlapping mechanisms are employed by the immune system to destroy pathogens: the innate immune response and the adaptive immune response. The first is relatively rapid but non-specific and therefore not always effective. The second is slower; it requires time to develop while the initial infection is going on. Although slower, this response is highly specific and effective at attacking a wide variety of microbial pathogens. The detailed mechanism of immune responses is discussed in Chapter 3.

The innate immune system has several first-line barriers that mostly act to limit entry and growth of microbial pathogens. These include physical barriers such as the skin, mucosal epithelia and bronchial cilia. Chemical and biochemical barriers include acidic pH of the stomach and sebaceous gland secretions containing fatty acids, lysozyme and beta-defensins. Once a pathogen overcomes these barriers and gains access to the body, cellular components must come forward to combat the invading organisms.

The immune response to a pathogen depends on sequential and integrated interactions among diverse innate and adaptive immune cells. Innate immune cells mount a first line of defence against pathogens, as antigen-presenting cells communicate the infection to lymphoid cells, which then co-ordinate the adaptive response and generate memory cells that help to prevent future infections. The cells of the innate and adaptive immune response normally circulate in the blood and lymph, and are also scattered throughout tissues and lymphoid organs. The primary lymphoid organs, including the bone marrow and thymus, regulate the development of immune cells from immature precursors. The secondary lymphoid organs – including the spleen, lymph nodes and specialised sites in the gut and other mucosal tissues – co-ordinate the antigen encounter with antigen-specific lymphocytes and their development into effector and memory cells. Blood vessels and lymphatic systems connect these organs, uniting them into a functional whole.

Immunology for Dentistry, First Edition. Edited by Mohammad Tariqur Rahman, Wim Teughels and Richard J. Lamont.
© 2023 John Wiley & Sons Ltd. Published 2023 by John Wiley & Sons Ltd.

1.2   Hematopoietic Stem Cells: Origin of Immune Cells

Most immune system cells arise from hematopoietic stem cells (HSCs) in the fetal liver and postnatal bone marrow. HSCs are pluripotent cells, i.e. they have the potential to produce all blood cell types. They also have self-renewal capability. Remarkably, all functionally specialised, mature blood cells (erythrocytes, granulocytes, macrophages, dendritic cells and lymphocytes) arise from a single HSC type (Figure 1.1). The process by which HSCs differentiate into mature blood cells is called haematopoiesis. The differentiation of HSCs into various types of immune cells occurs under the influence of cytokines. Two primary lymphoid organs are responsible for the differentiation of stem cells into mature immune cells: the bone marrow, where HSCs reside and give rise to all cell types; and the thymus, where T cells complete their maturation. First, let us focus on the structural features and function of each cell type that arises from HSCs.

1.3   Cells of the Immune System

The immune system may seem like a less substantial entity than the heart or liver; however, immunity collectively consumes enormous resources, producing a large number of cells that it engages for successful function. After being produced from the bone marrow, the immune cells undergo significant secondary education before they are released to patrol the body. Many immune cell types have been identified and extensively studied. Among them, blood leucocytes provide either innate or specific adaptive immunity. They are derived from myeloid or lymphoid lineages. The myeloid lineage produces highly phagocytic cells, including polymorphonuclear neutrophils (PMN), monocytes and macrophages that provide a first line of defence against most pathogens (Table 1.1; see also Figure 1.1). The other myeloid cells include polymorphonuclear eosinophils, basophils and their tissue counterparts – mast cells. They are involved in defence against parasites and in

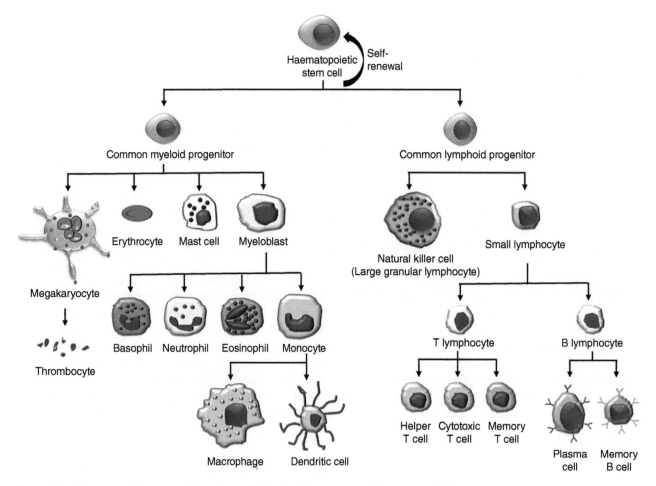

Figure 1.1   Haematopoietic stem cells produce all blood cells by a process of haematopoiesis.

Table 1.1 Myeloid cells and their properties.

Cell	Morphology	Count/L	Function
Neutrophil	PMN granulocyte	2 to 7.5×10^9	Phagocytosis and killing of microbes
Eosinophil	PMN granulocyte	0.04 to 0.44×10^9	Allergic reactions, defence against parasites
Basophil	PMN granulocyte	0 to 0.1×10^9	Allergic reactions
Mast cell	PMN granulocyte	Tissue specific	Allergic reactions
Monocyte	Monocytic	0.2 to $0.8 \, 10^9$	Phagocytosis and antigen presentation. Mature as macrophages in the tissue
Macrophage	Tissue specific	Tissue specific	Phagocytosis and antigen presentation
Dendritic cell	Monocytic	Tissue specific	Antigen presentation, initiation of adaptive responses

PMN, polymorphonuclear neutrophils.

allergic reactions. The lymphoid lineage produces cells that are mainly responsible for humoral immunity (B lymphocytes) and cell-mediated immunity (T lymphocytes).

1.4 Cells of the Myeloid Lineage: First Line of Defence

Myeloid cells are the front-line attacking cells during an immune response. Cells that arise from a common myeloid progenitor include erythroid cells such as red blood cells (RBCs) and myeloid cells such as white blood cells (granulocytes, monocytes, macrophages and some dendritic cells). Granulocytes are identified by characteristic staining patterns of 'granules' that are released in contact with pathogens. Granulocytes mainly include neutrophils, basophils and eosinophils.

1.4.1 Neutrophils

Neutrophils are the most abundant of the leucocytes, normally accounting for 50–70% of circulating leucocytes. They have a short life span. They circulate in the blood for 7–10 hours and then migrate to the tissue spaces, where they live only for a few days and do not multiply. During an active infection, the number of circulating neutrophils may increase two- to three-fold. Some neutrophils may remain attached to the endothelial lining of large veins and can be mobilised during inflammation. Neutrophils are about 10–20 μm in diameter and their nucleus is segmented into 3–5 connected lobes; hence they are called polymorphonuclear leucocytes. These cells are highly motile which allows them to move quickly in and out of the tissue during infection. They use their granules to ingest, kill and digest pathogenic micro-organisms. The primary granules include cationic defensins and myeloperoxidase. The secondary granules mostly include iron chelators, lactoferrin and various proteolytic enzymes such as lysozyme, collagenase and elastase. They do not stain with either acidic or basic dyes. The azurophilic granules are mostly lysosomes. Neutrophils dying at the site of infection contribute to the formation of the whitish exudate called pus.

1.4.2 Basophils

Basophils are a type of bone marrow-derived circulating leucocyte. They are also highly granular but with mononuclear appearance and are 12–15 μm in diameter. They account for less than 0.2% of leucocytes, and are therefore difficult to find in normal blood smears. They contain histamine, do not participate in phagocytosis and share many similarities with mast cells. In addition to histamine, basophilic granules also contain various other mediators of inflammation, including platelet-activating factor, eosinophil chemotactic factor and the enzyme phospholipase A. Basophils play roles in the body's response to allergens. They can be activated by antigen/allergen cross-linking of FcεRI receptor-bound IgE. This activation can cause them to release histamine, which is partially responsible for inflammation during an allergic reaction.

1.4.3 Mast Cells

Mast cells are not found in the circulation but exist in a wide variety of tissues, including the skin, connective tissues of various organs and mucosal epithelial tissue of the respiratory, genitourinary and digestive tracts. These cells are mostly indistinguishable from the basophil, but display some distinctive morphological features. They also have large numbers of cytoplasmic granules that contain histamine and other pharmacologically active substances. Mast cells also play an important role in many inflammatory settings including host defence against parasitic infection and in allergic reactions. When activated by allergens or pathogens, these cells can release wide varieties of inflammatory mediators that take part in inflammatory reactions.

1.4.4 Eosinophils

Eosinophils are polymorphonuclear granulocytes that play roles in host defence against parasites and participate in hypersensitivity reactions. Eosinophil accumulation and inappropriate activation cause pathological asthmatic allergy. Eosinophils make up approximately 2–5% of blood leucocytes in normal individuals and are about 15 μm in diameter, larger than other blood cells like erythrocytes, lymphocytes and basophils. Eosinophils usually have a bilobed nucleus and contain many cytoplasmic granules that are stained with acidic dyes such as eosin. Eosinophil counts may often be raised in people with allergic symptoms as well as in those exposed to parasitic worms. They possess phagocytic activity and destroy ingested microbes.

1.4.5 Mononuclear Phagocytes

Mononuclear phagocytes, which mainly include monocytes, macrophages and dendritic cells, play important roles in both innate and adaptive immunity. Cells of the mononuclear phagocytic system are found in virtually all organs of the body where the local microenvironment determines their morphology and functional characteristics. After development from precursor cells, some monocytes and dendritic cells remain in the circulation, but most enter body tissues. Monocytes are relatively large (10–18 μm diameter), have horseshoe-shaped nuclei with finely granular cytoplasm and a half-life of three days in circulation. They normally make up 5–8% of leucocytes. In tissues, monocytes develop into much larger phagocytic cells known as macrophages, which may differ in appearance and name on the basis of their existing tissue locations. For example, specialised macrophages include Kupffer cells in the liver, Langerhans cells in the skin, glial cells in the central nervous system, alveolar macrophages in the lung and mesangial cells in the kidney (Table 1.2).

The main role of the mononuclear phagocytes is to destroy and remove infectious foreign microbes or dead self-cells (erythrocytes) through phagocytosis (see below). Macrophages are also involved in killing and removing infected cells/tumour cells, secretion of immunomodulatory cytokines and antigen processing and presentation to T cells. Macrophages usually respond to infections as quickly as neutrophils but persist much longer; hence they are more dominant effector cells.

1.4.5.1 The Process of Phagocytosis

Phagocytosis is a type of endocytosis in which a phagocytic cell engulfs a particle to form an internal compartment called a *phagosome*. The cell rearranges its membrane to surround the particle with the ultimate aim of digestion and

Table 1.2 Tissue-specific macrophages and their functions.

Macrophage type	Specific location	Function
Kupffer cells	Liver	Phagocytosis, killing of microbes, hepatic clearance
Langerhans cells	Skin	Participate in immune responses against microbes that invade skin
Glial cells	CNS	Interact with neurons, participate in defence and immune functions
Alveolar macrophages	Lung	Phagocytosis, particle clearance
Mesangial cells	Kidneys	Phagocytosis, cytokine release
Macrophage	Tissue specific	Phagocytosis, interaction with other cells, receptor-mediated endocytosis, release cytokines
Osteoclasts	Bone	Bone remodelling, modulation of immune responses
Splenic macrophages	Spleen	Blood-borne pathogen filtering, culling and pitting of RBCs
Cardiac macrophages	Heart	Regulate cardiomyocyte electrical activity

CNS, central nervous system; RBC, red blood cell.

destruction. The formation of the phagosome triggers acquisition of lysosomes. Phagosomes mobilise and fuse with lysosomes to form phagolysosomes. Within these phagolysosomes, the particles are degraded, destroyed and eventually eliminated in a process called exocytosis. The immune system utilises this process as a major mechanism to remove potentially pathogenic material. A simplified flow chart of the process of phagocytosis is shown in Figure 1.2.

1.4.6 Dendritic Cells

Dendritic cells (DCs) are covered with long membranous extensions that resemble the dendrites of nerve cells. These dendrites extend and retract dynamically to increase the surface area available for browsing lymphocytes and other immune cells. The main function of DCs is to capture antigens in one location and present them to adaptive immune cells in another location. DCs are therefore capable of bridging between innate and adaptive immunity, and are considered excellent antigen-presenting cells (APC). Outside lymph nodes, immature DCs monitor the body for signs of invasion by pathogens and capture invading foreign antigens. They process these antigens intracellularly, migrate to lymph nodes and present the antigen to naive T cells, thus initiating the adaptive immune response. Another category of DCs, known as follicular DCs, also play roles in the maintenance of B-cell function and immune memory.

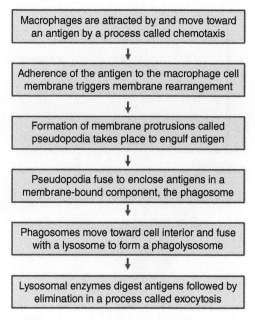

Figure 1.2 Major steps in phagocytosis.

1.4.7 Erythrocytes and Platelets

Erythrocytes (red blood cells, RBCs) and platelets arise from myeloid megakaryocyte precursors in the bone marrow. RBCs are anucleate biconcave cells in the circulation, which contain haemoglobin and transport body's oxygen and carbon dioxide. They survive around 100–120 days in the bloodstream. Dead RBCs are recycled by the macrophages of the reticuloendothelial system. Although mostly known as oxygen carriers, RBCs are emerging as important modulators of the innate immune response. Haem, the non-protein component of haemoglobin, is capable of generating antimicrobial reactive oxygen species to defend against invading hemolytic microbes. RBCs can also bind and scavenge chemokines, nucleic acids and pathogens in the circulation.

Platelets, also called thrombocytes, are small, colourless cell fragments in the blood that form clots and stop or prevent bleeding. Clot formation is helped by the platelet contents such as granules, microtubules and actin/myosin filaments. Platelets also release inflammatory mediators, thereby participating in immune responses, especially in inflammation. The adult human produces 10^{11} platelets each day. About 30% of platelets are stored in the spleen but may be released when required.

1.4.8 Blood Clotting (Coagulation)

Blood clots are formed by a cascade of complex reactions (Figure 1.3). This process is stimulated by various clotting factors released from the damaged cells (extrinsic pathway) and platelets (intrinsic pathway). Following injury to endothelial cells, platelets adhere to and aggregate at the damaged endothelial surface. Clotting factors cause platelets to become sticky and adhere to the damaged region, forming a solid plug. Release of platelet granule contents results in increased capillary permeability, activation of complement, attraction of leucocytes and bonding between fibrin fibres. Additionally, clotting factors trigger conversion of the inactive zymogen prothrombin to the activated enzyme thrombin. Thrombin in turn catalyses the conversion of the soluble plasma protein fibrinogen into an insoluble fibrous form called fibrin. The fibrin strands form a mesh of fibres around the platelet plug and trap blood cells to form a temporary clot. After the damaged region is completely repaired, the clot is dissolved by an enzyme called plasmin. Clot formation within small blood vessels may also help to fight against pathogenic microbes.

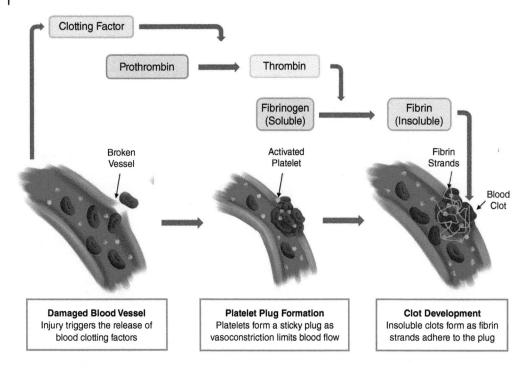

Figure 1.3 Blood coagulation cascade.

1.5 Cells of the Lymphoid Lineage: Specific and Long-lasting Immunity

Lymphoid organs are scattered throughout the body and are mainly concerned with the growth and deployment of lymphocytes. The diverse lymphoid organs and tissues that differ in their structure and function are interconnected by the blood vessels and lymphatic vessels through which lymphocytes circulate. Both the primary (central) lymphoid organs and secondary (peripheral) lymphoid organs are involved in specific as well as non-specific immunity. The blood and lymphatic vessels that carry lymphocytes to and from the other structures can also be considered lymphoid organs. It is also known that the liver can be a haematopoietic organ in the fetus, giving rise to all leucocyte lineages.

Large numbers of lymphocytes are produced daily in the primary lymphoid organs such as the thymus and bone marrow. Some cells then migrate via the circulation into the secondary lymphoid tissues such as the spleen, lymph nodes and mucosa-associated lymphoid tissue (MALT). Lymphocytes represent 20–40% of circulating leucocytes and 99% of cells in the lymph. A healthy human adult has about 2×10^{12} lymphoid cells, and lymphoid tissue as a whole represents about 2% of total body weight.

Lymphocytes differentiate into three major populations based on functional differences: T lymphocytes (T cells) that operate in cellular and humoral immunity; B lymphocytes (B cells) that differentiate into plasma cells to secrete antibodies; and natural killer (NK) cells that can destroy infected target cells. T and B lymphocytes produce and express specific receptors for antigens whereas NK cells do not. In addition, another small group of cells exists, called NKT cells, which are T cells with NK markers (Table 1.3).

1.5.1 T Cells

T cells, responsible mainly for cellular immunity, arise from a lymphoid progenitor cell in the bone marrow. Later, these cells move to the thymus for maturation. The name *T cell* is based on the cell's **T**hymus-dependent development. T cells express a unique antigen-binding receptor called the T-cell antigen receptor (TCR). Cells are selected for maturation in the thymus only if their TCRs do not interact with self-peptides bound to the major histocompatibility complex (MHC) molecules on APCs. Most T cells (90–95%) express the αβ TCR and the rest express γδ TCR. T cells that survive thymic selection become mature and circulate through the peripheral lymphoid organs. Each of these T cells is ready to encounter a specific antigen and thereby become activated. Once activated, the T cells proliferate and differentiate into effector T cells. Some also remain for a longer time as memory T cells.

Table 1.3 Lymphoid cells and their properties.

Lymphocytes	Morphology	Percentage in blood	Function
T cell	Monocytic	70–80	Cell-mediated immunity, immune regulation
B cell	Monocytic	10–15	Antibody production, humoral immunity
NK cell	Monocytic	10–15	Innate response to microbial or viral infection
NKT cell	Monocytic	0.01–0.1	Cell-mediated immunity (glycolipids)

T lymphocytes are divided into two major cell types – T helper (T_H) cells and T cytotoxic (T_C) cells – that can be distinguished from one another by the presence of either CD4 or CD8 molecules on their cell surfaces. These are accessory membrane glycoproteins capable of working as co-receptors. Every T cell also expresses CD3, a multi-subunit cell signalling complex that is non-covalently associated with the TCR. This TCR/CD3 complex specifically recognises antigens associated with the MHC molecules on APCs or infected target cells. In addition to T_H and T_C cells, there is another small group of cells called T regulatory (T_{REG}) cells.

1.5.1.1 T_H Cells (CD4 T Cells)

T_H cells have a wider range of effector functions than T_C cells and can differentiate into many different subtypes, such as T_H1, T_H2 and regulatory T cells. APCs, which express MHC class II molecules on their surfaces, present peptide antigen to T_H cells and thereby these cells become activated. The T_H cells may activate various other immune cells, release *cytokines* and assist B cells to produce antibodies. In this way, they help to activate, shape up and regulate the adaptive immune response.

1.5.1.2 T_C Cells (CD8 T Cells)

T_C cells, on the other hand, kill the infected target cells by releasing their cytotoxic granules. Cytotoxic T cells recognise specific antigens, such as viral fragments presented by *MHC class I* molecules on APCs. In this regard, CD8 co-receptor molecules on the T_C cells help to interact with APCs through their MHC class I molecules. T_C cells require several signals from other cells such as DCs and T_H cells to become activated. T_C cells mainly kill virally infected cells, but are also capable of killing tumour cells and bacteria-infected cells.

1.5.1.3 T_{REG} Cells

T_{REG}s are T cells which have a unique role in regulating or inhibiting other cells in the immune system. These regulatory cells may arise during T-cell maturation in the thymus (natural T_{REG}), but can also be induced during an immune response in an antigen-dependent manner (induced T_{REG}). T_{REG}s control the immune response to self and foreign antigens and help prevent autoimmune disease. T_{REG} cells are also capable of playing a role in limiting our normal T-cell response to pathogens.

1.5.1.4 Memory T Cells

Memory T cells are formed following an infection. These cells are antigen specific and long-lived; they may survive in a functionally quiescent state for months or years presumably after the antigen is eliminated. This survival basically does not need any antigen stimulation. As the memory T cells underwent training previously to recognise a specific antigen, they trigger a faster and stronger immune response soon after encountering it. Memory T cells may either be CD4$^+$ or CD8$^+$. They can be identified by their expression of surface proteins that distinguish them from naive and recently activated effector lymphocytes. Understanding the origins and functions of memory T cells may help in designing and developing vaccines.

1.5.2 Natural Killer Cells

Natural killer (NK) cells are lymphocytes that are closely related to B and T cells. NK cells constitute 5–10% of lymphocytes in human peripheral blood. They do not express antigen-specific receptors such as the TCR/CD3 complex. Instead, they express a variety of killer immunoglobulin-like receptors that are capable of binding MHC class I molecules as well as stress molecules on target cells. After binding, either a positive or a negative signal is generated for NK cell activation. NK cells are best known for killing virally infected cells as well as detecting and controlling early signs of cancer. NK cells induce death of the infected cells via delivery of apoptotic signals mediated by perforins, granzymes and tumour necrosis factor alpha.

1.5.2.1 Natural Killer T Cells

Natural killer T (NKT) cells belong to T lineage cells that share morphological and functional characteristics with both T cells and NK cells. Characteristically, these cells express CD3 and have a unique $\alpha\beta$ TCR. NKT cells are found in low numbers in every tissue where NK and T cells are found. Following activation, NKT cells can release cytotoxic granules that kill targets. They can also immediately release large quantities of cytokines that can both enhance and suppress the immune response. The rapidity of their response makes NKT cells important players in the very first lines of innate defence against some types of bacterial and viral infections. These cells appear to have roles in inhibiting the clinical symptoms of asthma, but also may inhibit the development of autoimmunity and cancer.

1.5.3 B Cells

B cells are considered one of the most important immune cells of the body. Their letter designation (B cell) came from their site of maturation – in the **B**ursa of Fabricius in birds and in **B**one marrow in most mammals. These cells express immunoglobulins on the cell surfaces, where the embedded immunoglobulins act as specific B cell antigen receptors (BCR). B cells constitute about 10–15% of the circulating lymphoid pool. They play a vital role in the adaptive immune response by producing antibodies and presenting antigens to T cells. The activation of B cells is mostly dependent on antigen exposure. Mature B cells can have $1–1.5 \times 10^5$ immunoglobulin receptors for interacting with antigens. Once specific antigens bind to the BCR, the B cells become activated and differentiated into plasma cells that produce and secrete antibodies. Some of the activated cells remain as memory B cells.

1.5.3.1 Plasma Cells

When activated, B cells differentiate into plasma cells which are important for their extended lifespan as well as their ability to secrete large amounts of antibodies. Specific antibodies against an antigen continue to be produced until the infection is controlled. Plasma cells are relatively larger in size and have vast quantities of RNA, which is used for antibody synthesis. Antibodies produced by a plasma cell are of single specificity and immunoglobulin class. Plasma cells are infrequent in the blood, comprising less than 0.1% of circulating lymphocytes, but they are relatively abundant in the secondary lymphoid organs and tissues as well as the bone marrow.

1.5.3.2 Memory B Cells

When activated, some B cells may also differentiate into memory B cells. These usually remain within the body to respond more rapidly in the event of a subsequent infection. Memory B cells are a classic example of immune memory that shows its vigorous antibody response after rechallenge with the same infectious agent. During this type of recall response, reactivated memory B cells can differentiate into antibody-secreting plasma cells which then produce a faster, larger and higher-avidity antibody response. Memory B cell survival is independent of the presence of cognate antigen. The life span of memory B cells may vary. Some human memory B cells can be detected for decades, as in the case of smallpox-specific memory cells. However, in other cases such as in B cell memory response to influenza virus, the memory cell population declines quickly after infection.

1.6 Lymphoid Tissues and Organs

The immune cells are organised into tissues and organs in order to perform their functions most effectively. The structurally and functionally diverse lymphoid tissue and organs are interconnected by blood vessels and lymphatic vessels through which lymphocytes circulate. As mentioned earlier, lymphoid organs are divided broadly into central or primary lymphoid organs and peripheral or secondary lymphoid organs. Lymphocytes develop within the primary organs such as the thymus and bone marrow (Figure 1.4). The secondary lymphoid organs such as spleen, lymph nodes and related lymphoid tissues trap and concentrate antigens. These sites then provide opportunities for the circulating immune cells to contact with the antigens to initiate specific immune reactions.

1.6.1 Primary Lymphoid Organs

Primary lymphoid organs are the major sites for lymphopoiesis. Lymphocyte differentiation, proliferation and maturation take place in these organs. T cells mature in the thymus and B cells in the bone marrow. During maturation in the primary lymphoid organs, the lymphocytes acquire antigen receptors to recognise and fight against invading antigens.

1.6.1.1 Bone Marrow
Bone marrow is a soft, spongy substance found inside the hard cover of the bones. This spongy marrow is packed full of cells. All the cells of the immune system are initially derived from the bone marrow through haematopoiesis. During fetal development, haematopoiesis occurs initially in the yolk sac and later in the liver. However, after birth this function is gradually taken over by the bone marrow. The adult bone marrow gives rise to granulocytes, NK cells, DCs, B cells, precursor T cells, RBCs and platelets. Various cytokines play roles in the process of differentiation, proliferation and maturation of the cells. Once mature, the cells proceed through the sinusoidal passage from the bone marrow into the blood circulation and other tissues (Figure 1.5). Although the bone marrow is considered a primary lymphoid organ, facilitated entry of circulating leucocytes from peripheral tissue enables it to serve as a secondary lymphoid organ as well.

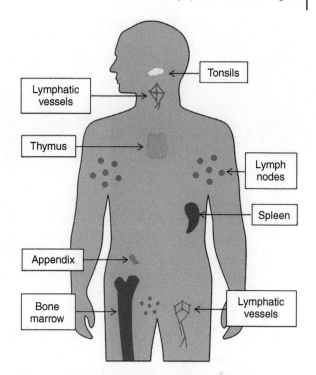

Figure 1.4 Organs and tissues of the immune system.

1.6.1.2 Thymus
The thymus is a lymphocyte-rich, bilobed, encapsulated organ located above and in front of the heart. The size and activity of the thymus are maximal in the fetus and in early childhood. It then undergoes atrophy at puberty although it never totally disappears.

The two thymic lobes are surrounded by a thin connective tissue capsule. Connective tissues around the thymus, called *trabeculae*, divide thymus into lobules containing cortex and medulla regions (Figure 1.6). Hassall's corpuscles are a characteristic morphological feature located within the medullary region of the thymus. There is a network of epithelial cells throughout the lobules, which plays a role in the differentiation process from stem cells to mature T lymphocytes. Precursor T lymphocytes differentiate to express specific receptors for antigen. The cortex contains immature lymphocytes, and more mature lymphocytes pass through the medulla, implying a differentiation gradient from the cortex to the medulla.

The principal function of the thymus gland is to educate T lymphocytes to differentiate between self and non-self antigens. After immature T cell precursors reach the thymus from the bone marrow, they gradually generate antigen specificity, undergo thymic education and then migrate to the peripheral lymphoid tissues as mature T cells.

1.6.2 Secondary Lymphoid Organs

The secondary or peripheral lymphoid organs provide localised environments where lymphocytes recognise foreign antigen and mount a response against it. The spleen and lymph nodes are the major secondary lymphoid organs. Additional secondary lymphoid organs include the mucosa-associated lymphoid tissue (MALT). Examples of MALT include tonsils and Peyer's patches. All secondary or lymphoid organs serve to generate immune responses and tolerance.

1.6.2.1 Spleen
The spleen is situated in the upper left quadrant of the abdominal cavity behind the stomach and close to the diaphragm. It is a large, ovoid secondary lymphoid organ that plays a key role in mounting immune responses against antigens. The spleen functions as a filter for blood, and the filtration is aided by two main microenvironmental compartments in splenic

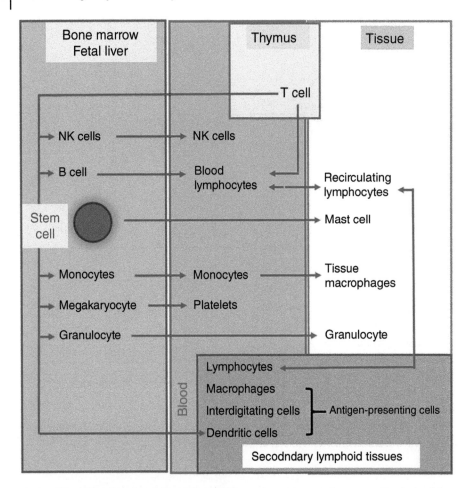

Figure 1.5 Migration of immune cells to different tissues/organs. Immune cells, derived from stem cells in the bone marrow, migrate to different tissues and organs. B cells mature in the bone marrow in adults, whereas T cells mature in the thymus. Lymphocytes recirculate through secondary lymphoid tissues. Tissues/organs are shown in different shading.

Figure 1.6 Schematic illustration of the thymus.

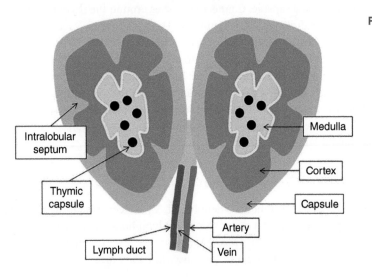

tissue: the red pulp and the white pulp (Figure 1.7). The red pulp is made up of a network of sinusoids containing large numbers of macrophages, RBCs and some lymphocytes. It is actively involved in the removal of dead RBCs and infectious agents. The white pulp consists of periarteriolar sheaths of lymphatic tissue, and is composed of T- and B-cell areas and follicles containing germinal centres. These follicles are the centre of lymphocyte production, composed mainly of follicular dendritic cells (FDC) and B cells. The germinal centres are where B cells are stimulated by antigens to become plasma cells that produce and secrete specific antibodies. Every day, approximately half of the total blood gets filtered through the spleen where lymphocytes, DCs and macrophages survey for evidence of infectious agents. The spleen thus serves as a critical line of defence against blood-borne pathogens.

1.6.2.2 Lymph Node

Lymph nodes are small solid structures situated at strategic positions throughout the body along the lymphatic system. They are found clustered in strategically important places such as the neck, axillae, groin, mediastinum and abdominal cavity. Human lymph nodes are 2–10 μm in diameter, spherical in shape and encapsulated (Figure 1.8). Each lymph node is surrounded by a fibrous capsule, which extends inside the node to form trabeculae. Lymph enters a node through numerous afferent

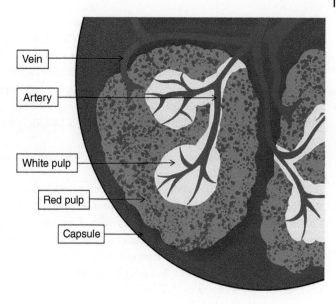

Figure 1.7 Schematic illustration of a portion of the spleen.

lymphatic vessels that drain lymph into the marginal sinus. The lymph flows through the medullary sinus and leaves through efferent lymphatics. The lymph nodes filter antigens from the lymph during its passage from the periphery to the thoracic duct. Each lymph node is divided into an outer cortex, inner medulla and intervening paracortical region. The lymph nodes contain both T and B lymphocytes and are primarily responsible for mounting immune responses against foreign antigens. The lymph nodes may be enlarged following antigenic stimulation.

1.6.2.3 Mucosa-Associated Lymphoid Tissue

Mucosa-associated lymphoid tissue (MALT) is scattered along the mucosal linings and constitutes the most extensive component of human lymphoid tissue. More than half of the total lymphoid tissue in the body is found associated with the mucosal system. These surfaces are therefore capable of protecting the body from an enormous variety and quantity of antigens.

The most common examples of MALT are the tonsils, Peyer's patches within the small intestine and the vermi-

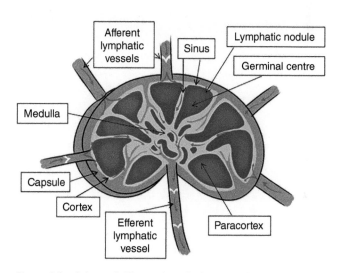

Figure 1.8 Schematic illustration of a lymph node.

form appendix. Location-wise, MALT can be referred to more specifically as gut-associated lymphoid tissue (GALT), bronchial/tracheal-associated lymphoid tissue (BALT) and nose-associated lymphoid tissue (NALT). Tonsils are clusters of lymphatic tissue under the mucous membrane lining of the nose, mouth and throat. Lymphocytes and macrophages in the tonsils provide protection against pathogens that enter the body through the respiratory tract. Similar to tonsils, some non-encapsulated lymphoid nodules are present in the ileum of the small intestine, called Peyer's patches. They play an important role in defending against pathogenic substances that enter the gastrointestinal system.

Further Reading

Male, D., Brostoff, J., Roth, D. and Roitt. I. (2006). *Immunology*, 7e. St Louis, MO: Elsevier.

Abbas, A.K., Lichtman, A.H. and Pillai, S. (2019). *Basic Immunology: Functions and Disorders of the Immune System*. Amsterdam: Elsevier.

Actor, J.K. (2012). *Elsevier's Integrated Review Immunology and Microbiology*, 2e. St Louis, MO: Elsevier.

Punt, J., Stranford, S.A., Jones, P.P. and Owen, J.A. (2019). *Kuby Immunology*, 8e. New York: W.H. Freeman.

Mohanty, S. and Leela, K.S. (2014). *Text book of Immunology*, 2e. New Delhi: Jaypee Brothers.

Abbas, A.K., Lichtman, A.H. and Pillai, S. (2018). *Cellular and Molecular Immunology*, 9e. St Louis, MO: Elsevier.

Bernareggi, D., Pouyanfard, S. and Kaufman, D.S. (2019). Development of innate immune cells from human pluripotent stem cells. *Exp. Hematol.* 71: 13–23.

Anderson, H.L., Brodsky, I.E. and Mangalmurti, N.S. (2018). The evolving erythrocyte: red blood cells as modulators of innate immunity. *J. Immunol.* 201: 1343–1351.

Minai-Fleminger, Y. and Levi-Schaffer, F. (2009). Mast cells and eosinophils: the two key effector cells in allergic inflammation. *Inflamm. Res.* 58: 631–638.

Schroeder, J.T. (2009). Basophils: beyond effector cells of allergic inflammation. *Adv. Immunol.* 101: 123–161.

Parkin, J. and Cohen, B. (2001). An overview of the immune system. *Lancet* 357: 1777–1789.

Calder, P.C. (2013). Feeding the immune system. *Proc. Nutr. Soc.* 72 (3): 299–309.

Mellman, I. (2013). Dendritic cells: master regulators of the immune response. *Cancer Immunol. Res.* 1: 145–149.

Parker, G.A. (2017). Cells of the immune system. In: *Immunopathology in Toxicology and Drug Development. Molecular and Integrative Toxicology* (ed. G. Parker). Cham: Humana Press.

Gordon, S. and Plüddemann, A. (2017). Tissue macrophages: heterogeneity and functions. *BMC Biol.* 15: 53.

2

Oral Immune System

Maha Abdullah and Norhafizah Mohtarrudin

Universiti Putra Malaysia, Serdang, Malaysia

2.1 Introduction

The oral cavity is the gateway to the gastrointestinal and respiratory systems. It is also the inlet to microbes, allergens and foreign substances which may pose danger to the body. An array of immune surveillance mechanisms provided by different types of cells, organs and their secretory products in the oral cavity ensures the maintenance of a healthy ecosystem.

Soft and pliable areas such as the ventral tongue, cheeks and lips are non-keratinised areas of the mucosa made up of an overlying epithelium and underlying connective tissue rich in salivary glands and lymphoid tissues. The cornified dorsal tongue contributes further protective specialised structures in the mucosa (Cooke et al. 2017).

Mucosal layers play a critical role in immunosurveillance using the epithelial cells and antigen-presenting cells (APCs) that are present therein. These cells also send signals from the mucosal surface to the nearest lymph node and subsequently to the rest of the body.

The hard tissues and teeth in the oral cavity bridge systemic immune factors stimulated at distal sites into the cavity through crevicular fluid, discharged from cells and serum to protect the teeth and gingiva. Saliva, the most important body fluid, is composed of a number of immune factors that also contribute to the removal of invading microbes. The presence of both local secretory and systemic components of immune defence in the mouth is a unique immunological identity compared to other physiological mucosal immune systems (Challacombe et al. 2015).

The mouth also encounters many innocuous antigens brought in with the air as well as food products which do not cause harm but as antigens are able to activate a response. Here, a state of oral tolerance is induced which allows the immune system to ignore their presence. This state of acceptance is also extended to the microbiome in the oral cavity.

As food exits the oral cavity and enters the rest of the gastrointestinal system, it encounters a circle of mucosa-associated lymphoid tissue called Waldeyer's ring which is an additional surveillance layer. Here, antigens are picked up from the mucosa surface and brought to lymphoid follicles where activation of local and systemic immune responses takes place to remove pathogenic particles.

A breakdown in any of these barriers increases the risk of spreading potential contaminants into the body, not only causing infections but increasing susceptibility to chronic inflammatory diseases.

2.2 Mucosa

The enormous amount and variety of foreign entities brought into the oral cavity from consumption of food and drinks as well as breathing in air require that the mucosal immune system be able to distinguish and balance between mounting immunity and inducing tolerance in response to harmful or beneficial micro-organisms. It is also important that the immune system maintain homeostasis to fight infections or activate the healing process. The mucosa is constructed with some degree of complexity and properties in achieving these tasks.

Immunology for Dentistry, First Edition. Edited by Mohammad Tariqur Rahman, Wim Teughels and Richard J. Lamont.
© 2023 John Wiley & Sons Ltd. Published 2023 by John Wiley & Sons Ltd.

(a)

(b)

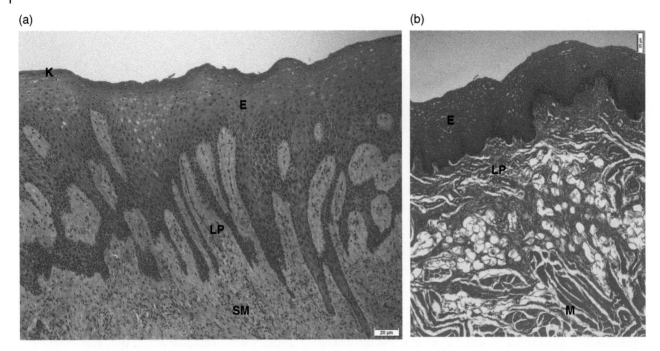

Figure 2.1 Types of oral membrane. (a) Lining mucosa and (b) specialised mucosa (dorsum of tongue) and compartments. Note the absence of submucosa in the tongue. Mucosa firmly adheres to underlying muscle by dense collagenous lamina propria. Stratified squamous epithelium (E), keratin layer (K), lamina propria (LP), submucosa (SM), muscle (M).

Mucosa or mucous membrane is a moist coating inside the oral cavity and other parts of the gastrointestinal, respiratory and genitourinary tracts that communicate to the outside. Mucosa consists of an outer layer of epithelium and an inner layer, the lamina propria. A basement membrane separates the epithelium from the underlying lamina propria. The oral mucosa has no muscularis mucosae (Squier and Brogden 2011). The lamina propria is loose connective tissue which contains mucosal lymphoid tissue and fenestrated capillaries (Figure 2.1).

Epithelium is a continuous sheet of tightly packed cells over the internal surfaces of the body. This acts as a barrier that protects internal tissues from onslaught from the exterior environment. The oral epithelium consists of stratified squamous epithelium, which may or may not be keratinised. The unique functions in the mouth have resulted in histological differences in the mucosa. The practical function of the oral mucosa is organised into three groups: (i) masticatory mucosa comprising 25% of the total mucosa; (ii) lining mucosa covers about 60%; and (iii) specialised mucosa makes up 15% (Squier and Kremer 2001).

Masticatory mucosa, which covers the gingiva and hard palate and tissue, has an additional non-living tough layer of keratinising epithelium.

Lining mucosa forms the floor of the mouth, ventral (underside) tongue, cheeks, lips and soft palate. The epithelium of the lining mucosa is non-keratinised multilayered stratified squamous epithelium in contrast to the mainly single-layered columnar epithelium of the small intestine, nasal cavity, trachea and bronchi (Kraan et al. 2014). The differences in structure of mucosa in the mouth and gut suggest that findings from the gut do not necessarily apply to the mouth (Challacombe et al. 2015).

Junctional epithelium (JE) is a non-keratinised layer of flattened cells that is part of the gingiva that attaches the connective tissue to the tooth surface.

2.2.1 Microbiome of the Oral Cavity

Oral mucosa nurtures a rich flora of the oral microbiome which has the potential of causing harm to the body. Throughout the length of mucosa are barriers set up for immunosurveillance, in order to perceive, react and eliminate and sound the alert to other components of the immune system. The microbiome also has a critical role in maintaining the homeostatic state in the oral cavity by interacting with the immunobiome.

Hard tissue surfaces, unlike soft mucosa, support development of biofilm, an aggregate of heterogeneous bacteria and their essential metabolites. Biofilms are just as important as local infections from whence oral microbes can gain access to the gastrointestinal tract or the circulation, causing infections at distal locations. Micro-organisms and microbial by-products can pass through the highly permeable junctional epithelium and enter the lamina propria. These attract T cells from the blood through activation of adhesion molecules (Squier and Brogden 2011).

Oral pathogens have been implicated in contributing at distant sites to disease pathology including atherosclerotic plaques, rheumatoid arthritis and colorectal cancer lesions (Park and Lee 2018).

2.2.2   Mucosal Immunity at the Epithelium

The epithelium's rigid physical structure provides a crucial first-line barrier to keep out exogenous antigens, allergens and invading pathogens. The tough non-keratinised epithelium that protects from the shearing forces of mastication is also impervious to bacterial invasion.

Structural integrity of the oral mucosa, including mucins produced by goblet cells as well as continual shedding by exfoliation of epithelial squamous cells, all helps to prevent microbial colonisation at the surface of the oral cavity. Other innate immune components of the oral mucosa include lysozyme, lactoferrin and lactoperoxidase produced in saliva, as well as antimicrobial peptides such as histatins, beta-defensins and protease inhibitors released onto mucosal surfaces to participate in ridding the oral cavity of harmful agents (Challacombe et al. 2015).

Epithelial cells (keratinocytes) themselves are responsive and express an assortment of receptors, including Toll-like receptors (TLR), and produce different cytokines upon activation by foreign antigens. In intestinal epithelial cells, TLR4 mediates signalling through other pathways to induce inflammatory cytokines (Abreu et al. 2005). Epithelial cells can create and send signals between micro-organisms and cells in the mucosa to provide the necessary cell-to-cell communication and upkeep of homeostasis between the host's inner milieu and the outside condition (Kagnoff and Eckmann 1997).

2.2.3   Immune Cells in the Epithelium

Immune surveillance is an important function of antigen-presenting cells. In murine models, different subsets of dendritic cells (DC) and Langerhans cells (LC) are found in the epithelium of buccal, sublingual and gingival mucosa (Wu et al. 2014). DC processes are extended in between the cells, to capture bacteria for direct uptake. Goblet cells provide a conduit for small molecular weight soluble proteins to pass across the epithelial barrier. After antigen uptake, DCs, macrophages and LCs residing in the epithelium migrate into mucosa-associated lymphoid tissue (MALT) and draining lymph nodes and initiate the adaptive immune responses by inducing T-cell proliferation and differentiation. Distribution of neutrophils in the mucosa is shown in Figure 2.2.

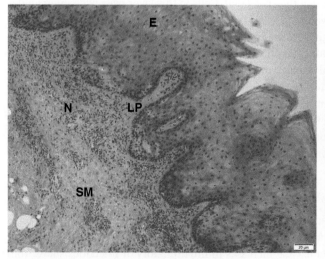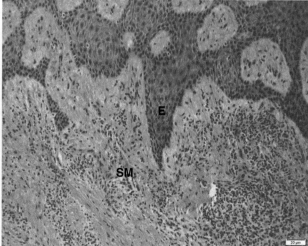

Figure 2.2   Infiltration of neutrophils and other immune cells in the oral mucosa. Stratified squamous epithelium (E), keratin layer (K), lamina propria (LP), submucosa (SM), neutrophils (N).

Unlike LCs in the skin which originate from embryonic precursors and are maintained independently in the epidermis, LCs in the mucosa are continually replenished by circulating precursors and recruited from LC precursors from the adult bone marrow (BM), predendritic cells (pre-DCs) and monocytes (Wu et al. 2014).

Another cell type providing luminal surveillance is the specialised epithelial M cell found overlying organised mucosa-associated lymphoid tissues (MALT). MALTs in the oral cavity include the tonsils of Waldeyer's ring found at the back of the mouth. M cells recruit novel cellular mechanisms to capture and transport selected microbial particles of interest across the mucosal barrier into the lamina propria. This process is known as *transcytosis* which effectively violates the function of the mucosal barrier. Via transcytosis, bacteria are taken up by underlying myeloid/dendritic cells. M cells, however, are not antigen-presenting cells but rather act as 'antigen delivery cells' to bona fide dendritic cells for antigen presentation (Dillon and Lo 2019).

The nature of mucosa makes it a selective barrier not only for secretion but also absorption. Compounds of different chemical properties penetrate the epithelium at different rates, by different routes, crossing the cell membrane and entering the cell (transcellular or intracellular route) or passing between cells (intercellular route) (Squier and Kremer 2001). Non-keratinised lining mucosa is relatively more elastic and permeable and thus potentially more suitable for drug or antigen delivery (Kraan et al. 2014). Antigen may not enter directly into the bloodstream but can be trapped by mucosal antigen-presenting DCs. Sublingual or buccal DCs then enter the blood circulation and thence into distant lymphoid organs as *in vivo* sublingual immunisation and antigen-bearing DCs are carried into distant lymph nodes and spleen. Therefore, sublingual and buccal immunisation promotes systemic immunity as well as protecting against pathogens that enter at distant sites such as the respiratory or reproductive tract (Hovav 2018).

The mucosa contains abundant T cells of the conventional type. However, a unique subset exists within the epithelial layer. These T cells express either $\alpha\beta$ or $\gamma\delta$ TCR and mostly express $CD8\alpha\alpha$ homodimers but not $CD8\alpha\beta$ heterodimers. In gastrointestinal (GI) mucosa of mice, the ratio of intraepithelial lymphocyte (IEL) to epithelial cell ranges from 5–10 in small intestine to 40 in colon. IELs in the oral-pharyngeal mucosa are less well studied. Lymphocytes, including IELs and lamina propria (LP) lymphocytes, form a network that ensures the integrity of the mucosal barrier and GI environment (Wu et al. 2014).

2.3 Gingiva

Gingiva is masticatory oral mucosa which attaches to the underlying alveolar bone surrounding the tooth. A thin layer of dense fibrous connective tissue supports the stratified squamous epithelium of the gingiva. Healthy gingiva has a 'salmon' or 'coral pink' appearance, unless it is pigmented due to ethnic origin. Gingiva is divided into three anatomical locations. Figure 2.3 illustrates two of the regions: (i) the free margin of gingiva surrounding the tooth and covering the internal walls of the gingival sulcus; (ii) attached gingiva that is firmly bonded to the underlying periosteum of alveolar bone; and (iii) interdental gingiva (not shown in figure).

The coronal end is several cells thick tapering to a single cell at the apical end. Cells in this layer have wide intercellular spaces which allow two-way movement of fluid and cells (Walmsley et al. 2007). The gingival epithelium may be divided into the oral epithelium covering the external surface of the gingiva, the crevicular epithelium (or oral sulcular epithelium) lining the gingival crevice, and the non-keratinised junctional epithelium (JE) (see Figure 2.3).

The gingival barrier is also subject to constant mechanical damage due to mastication and oral hygiene activities. The connection between the JE and tooth is routinely breached during physiological functions such as chewing and brushing. This becomes vulnerable to transient microbial entry and translocation of oral microbes is reported after chewing and during dental procedures. A remarkable property of JE is the ability to regenerate if damaged or surgically excised in health. A unique immunological system is probably in place for both surveillance and repair. Loss of this balance may lead to destructive inflammation, including development of periodontitis (Moutsopoulos and Konkel 2018).

2.3.1 Gingival Crevicular Fluid

In the healthy sulcus, the amount of gingival crevicular fluid (GCF) is very low. GCF production is mediated by passive diffusion of the extracellular fluid by an osmotic gradient through the basement membrane and then via the JE into the sulcus. In this situation, the GCF is considered as a transudate. GCF increases in inflammatory or infectious states from vasodilation when the permeability of the epithelial barrier and underlying vasculature increases. The resulting GCF is regarded as inflammatory exudate in which the protein concentration is increased in both amount and composition by extent of plasma protein exudation (de Aguiar et al. 2017). GCF contributes to host defence by washing bacterial colonies and their metabolites away from the sulcus (Subbarao et al. 2019).

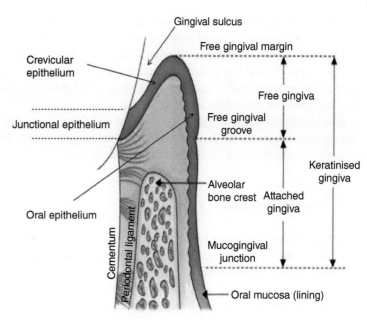

Figure 2.3 Structure of the gingiva. The outermost cells of the junctional epithelium (JE) appear elongated and do not exhibit phenotypic stratification but align with their long axis parallel to the tooth surface. The JE has wide intercellular spaces and thus is highly permeable for water-soluble substances and facilitates the continuous flow of gingival crevicular fluid (GCF). GCF is an exudate found in the sulcus, also known as the periodontal pocket, between the tooth and marginal gingiva. *Source:* Al-Rawee and Abdalfattah 2020/ Peertechz Publications/CC BY 4.0.

Gingival crevicular fluid has diversified composition and carries plasma proteins, cytokines, immunoglobulins and cells. It also serves as the primary pathway for transmigration of polymorphonuclear leucocytes. Even when the gingiva does not appear inflamed clinically, the JE has many polymorphonuclear leucocytes (PMNs) moving through it towards the sulcus. This form an important part of the defence mechanism. The constituents of the immune cells in this local fluid reflect the inflammatory state of the adjacent gingiva (Walmsley et al. 2007).

Bacterial enzymes, bacterial degradation products, host cell degradation products, host mediated enzymes, inflammatory mediators and extracellular matrix proteins, either together or individually, should be detected in higher levels in GCF during the active phase of periodontitis (Subrahmanyam and Sangeetha 2003).

2.3.1.1 Immune Cells in Gingival Crevicular Fluid

Neutrophils constitute 95% of total leucocytes recruited to the gingival crevice in health. Extravasated neutrophils in GCF may mediate microbial surveillance through phagocytosis, degranulation and the secretion of antimicrobial peptides and/ or neutrophil extracellular traps within and outside the tissue (Rijkschroeff et al. 2016).

Like neutrophils, gingival Th17 cells also develop independently of commensal microbe colonisation. This finding is unlike the Th17 cell stimulation situation in the skin and gastrointestinal tract (Park and Lee 2018). *Candida* sp., normal flora in the oral cavity, are quick to become opportunistic in suitable conditions. Neutrophils are a key component of defence against *Candida* and are recruited by interleukin (IL)-17 cells (Yu et al. 2007). IL-17-signalling in epithelial cells also stimulates beta-defensin 3 which has a surveillance role against *C. albicans*.

Tissue neutrophils are critical in oral/periodontal immunity as patients with defective neutrophil production and recruitment present with severe/aggressive periodontal immunopathology. The various gene mutations include ELANE (neutrophil elastase associated severe congenital neutropenia), WAS (Wiskott–Aldrich syndrome), LYST (lysosomal trafficking regulator mutations are responsible for Chediak–Higashi syndrome), CXCR4 (WHIM syndrome) and ITGB2 (integrin b2, involved in leucocyte adhesion deficiency) are neutrophil-related single-gene mutations (Moutsopoulos and Konkel 2018).

Although tissue macrophages are well-known immune cells for mucosal immunity at all other anatomical barriers, their genetic and cellular heterogeneity and differential functionality in the gingiva remain to be clarified (Moutsopoulous and Konkel 2018).

2.4 Lamina Propria

The presence of blood and lymphatic vessels in the lamina propria (LP) suggests gateways for entry and exit of immune cells into the mucosa and epithelium layer. Predendritic cells (pre-DCs) and monocytes enter the LP via the circulation and differentiate there, creating a transitory site for immune cells that subsequently populate the epithelia. Interstitial DCs (iDCs) expressing both CD11c and CD11b represent the major DC subset in the LP of the buccal and gingival mucosae (Hovav 2014). Langerin+ DCs are found in LP (Hovav 2018). Together with the epithelia, LP acts as the effector site or battlefront where activated lymphocytes migrate and relocate to mediate immunity (Wu et al. 2014).

Two special types of macrophages are distinguished in the LP. The melanophage cell ingests melanin granules extruded from melanocytes while the siderophage contains hemosiderin derived from red blood cells (Squier and Brogden 2011).

The blind vessels of lymphatic capillaries that arise in the LP are sites where cells and fluid collect and are carried to lymph nodes. From there, cells are recirculated back into the blood system. DCs capable of entering the blood circulation seed to distant lymph nodes and spleen following sublingual immunisation of mice. This ability is the basis of the 'common mucosal immune system' (Kraan et al. 2014).

In several regions of the oral cavity, there are nodules of lymphoid tissue consisting of crypts formed by invagination of the epithelium into the LP. Leucocytes traffic into these areas from the blood and extensive infiltration of lymphocytes and plasma cells are observed (Squier and Brogden 2011).

2.5 Oral Tolerance

To maintain a healthy stable environment, a balanced immune homeostasis between mucosal immune activation and oral tolerance is in place in the oral cavity. Despite continuous exposure to large amounts of antigens derived from food and microbes, severe inflammatory responses are relatively rare. This character has made it an attractive site for inducing tolerance against allergens. In contrast, this immune regulation has also made it a challenge for mucosal vaccination, resulting in only a few mucosal vaccines being available (Kraan et al. 2014). Other reasons why the oral mucosa does not appear to be easily sensitised include the presence of mucins in saliva, which prevent antigen from reaching the immune cells, antigen dilution and presence of enzymes (Challacombe et al. 2015).

Various immune cells are involved in oral tolerance induction. Oral DCs are of major importance as they constantly monitor changes in oral microbiota, orchestrating the activation and polarisation of naive T cells to decide whether to induce immunity or tolerance. Two major classes are conventional DCs and plasmacytoid DCs (pDCs). Immature conventional DCs patrol tissue microenvironments where an encounter with foreign antigen initiates maturation and migration to the draining lymph nodes (LNs) to present pathogen-derived peptides to CD4$^+$ and CD8$^+$ T cells. In contrast, pDCs are difficult to detect in peripheral tissues; they circulate in the blood and can be found in peripheral lymphoid organs (Hovav 2014).

Oral LCs, on the other hand, regulate by expressing higher levels of Toll-like receptors 2 and 4 (TLR2 and TLR4) compared to epidermal LCs. These cells upregulate co-inhibitory molecules B7-H1 and B7-H3, while decreasing expression of co-stimulatory molecule CD86 (B7-2) in respond to lipopolysaccharide, leading to polarised development of T regulatory (Treg) cells secreting IL-10 and transforming growth factor (TGF) beta (Hovav 2014). Treg cells inhibit the activity and immune response of numerous immune cells, including T cells and macrophages, by producing TGF-beta and IL-10. Studies have demonstrated that TCRαβ1CD8αα1 IELs are associated with intestinal antigen tolerance, immune regulation and antimicrobial function (Wu et al. 2014).

Though gingival resident Foxp3+ regulatory T cells have been described, the low number of these cells and the number of DCs that support Treg generation suggest it may not be the dominant tolerance mechanism at the gingiva (Moutsopoulos and Konkel 2018).

Studying diseased tissue has helped identify potential signalling pathways in tolerance induction. Tolerance to tumour may be relayed through the programmed death ligand 1 (PD-L1) which downregulates T-cell functions and survival. PD-L1 expression has been used in the tumour microenvironment as a tumour-protective mechanism by binding to programmed death receptor 1 (PD-1) expressed on T cells, leading to functional anergy and/or apoptosis of effector T cells (Groeger and Meyle 2019).

Interestingly, this relative ease in induction of oral tolerance has been applied as a therapeutic approach in inflammatory disease where oral exposure to HSP60-derived peptide linked to cholera toxin B subunit ('Behçet's peptide') was able to prevent subsequent development of mucosally induced uveitis (Phipps et al. 2003).

2.6 Submucosa

Supporting the mucosa is the submucosa layer consisting of loose fatty or glandular connective tissue containing major blood vessels, glands and the submucosal plexus (plexus of Meissner). Its composition determines the flexibility of the attachment of oral mucosa to underlying structures. In regions such as gingiva and parts of the hard palate, there is no intervening submucosa and attachment is firm and inelastic (Squier and Brogden 2011). Larger lymphatic vessels are found in the submucosa where lymph ultimately drains into deep cervical lymph nodes. Less frequent are sebaceous glands which may produce antimicrobial properties (Squier and Brogden 2011).

The main APCs in the submucosa are DCs and macrophages. Plasmacytoid DC (pDC) localise in the submucosal tissue in contrast to myeloid (m) DCs in the lamina propria (Hovav 2014). Both CD4 and CD8 T cells are readily found here (Challacombe et al. 2015).

The submucosa may also contain scattered migratory cells, of which mast cells are frequently the predominating type. Mast cells are of myeloid origin derived from the bone marrow. Upon activation, mast cells release a range of preformed mediators, including cytokines, vasoactive amines and enzymes stored in their granules (Walsh 2003). Mast cells have important roles in guarding against invading pathogens. They also play a pathological role and are the cause of hypersensitive allergic diseases. The localisation of mast cells close to surfaces and blood vessels explains the rapid type 1 hypersensitive features associated with the oral cavity.

The submucosa is rich in blood supply brought in through arteries which then branch into the mucosa which, however, do not reach into the epithelial layer. Many minor salivary glands are also located here, producing secretions that reach the mucosal surface via small ducts. Surrounding the ducts is lymphoid tissue (duct-associated lymphoid tissue [DALT] which contributes to the local production of secretory antibodies, particularly IgA [sIgA]). Bacteria may be brought directly into the lymphoid aggregate via ducts of the minor salivary glands (Challacombe et al. 2015).

2.7 Saliva and Salivary Glands

Salivary glands produce watery fluid known as saliva that keeps the oral cavity, teeth and mucosa moist. Secretions of the salivary gland are necessary to make eating, speaking and swallowing comfortable. Saliva is constantly secreted but usually just enough to moisten the mouth and teeth.

Major salivary glands consist of three pairs: (i) the parotid, (ii) submandibular, and (iii) sublingual (Figure 2.4). These glands are located outside the oral cavity and connected with elongated duct systems that conduct the gland secretions into the mouth.

About 600–1000 minor salivary glands reside in the submucosal layer located in different parts of the oral cavity such as the labial, lingual, palatal, buccal, glossopalatine and retromolar areas. They are absent only in the gingiva and the anterior part of the hard palate. These glands connect with short duct channels directly onto the mucosal surface.

A salivary gland is made up of cell clusters (acini) that secrete a watery solution that contains amylase (serous cells) or mucus (mucous cells). As compound glands, collecting ducts from these acini enter the main duct of salivary glands (Figure 2.5). Major salivary glands secrete a unique formulation of saliva depending on this combination of cells. Thus, saliva from parotid glands is watery while submandibular secretions are thick. Secretions from sublingual glands are the thickest and contain the least amount of amylase (Kessler and Bhatt 2018).

2.7.1 Immunity in Salivary Glands

The oral cavity is reported to contain over 700 bacterial species (Challacombe et al. 2015). Saliva is critical in protecting the oral epithelium from multiple harmful substances and regulating the types of oral microbial flora.

The salivary mucus provides a protective physical barrier, producing a 30 μm thick layer over the oral mucosa (Osailan et al. 2012). Furthermore, it contains varieties of factors with antimicrobial properties, namely immunoglobulins (IgA, IgM, IgG), lysozyme, lactoferrin, peroxidases, secretory leucocyte protease inhibitor (SLPI) and antimicrobial peptides such as histatins. Salivary flow also flushes out micro-organisms from oral mucosa and tooth surfaces.

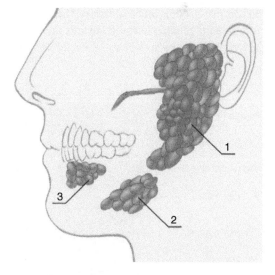

Figure 2.4 Major salivary glands situated external to the oral cavity. 1. Parotid; 2. sublingual; 3. submandibular. *Source:* Goran tek-en/Wikimedia Commons/CC BY-SA 4.

(a)

(b)

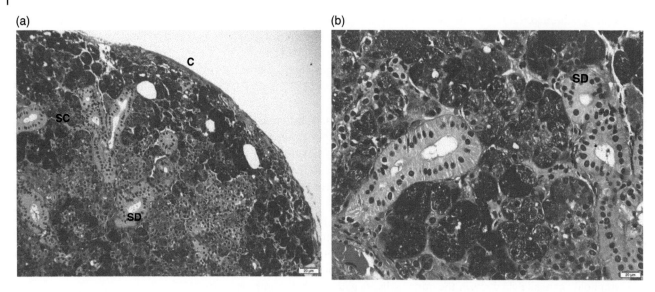

Figure 2.5 (a) Histology of normal salivary gland with outer capsule (C) showing numerous secretory units. (b) Striated ducts (SD) lined by large cuboidal cells surrounded by serous excretory cells (SC) that stain strongly with haematoxylin and eosin (H&E) stain.

Individuals with decreased or no saliva have reduced innate antimicrobial defences that ultimately allow increased oral candidiasis infections. Saliva also helps in balancing the oral pH between 5.5 and 7.0, providing antimicrobial activity (Kraan et al. 2014).

Nevertheless, saliva has been identified as an ideal niche for bacteria as it carries approximately 100 million bacteria/ml (Challacombe et al. 2015).

Duct-associated lymphoid tissue (DALT) that surrounds the ducts of minor salivary glands also contributes to oral-pharyngeal immune compartments and can be the site for induction of the adaptive response and local production of secretory antibodies. Contribution to total salivary IgA is as high as 25%, suggesting a greater contribution than major salivary glands (Nair and Schroeder 1986).

2.8 Mucosa-associated Lymphoid Tissue

In contrast to other mucosal tissues, the oral mucosa in general lacks mucosa-associated lymphoid tissue (MALT) for local immune induction. However, towards the back of the mouth around the oropharyngeal area lies the largest accumulation of lymphoid tissue known as the Waldeyer's ring. This is located just beneath non-keratinised stratified squamous epithelium. These MALTs serve to protect the opening of the pharynx. The Waldeyer's ring consists of the lingual tonsil at the terminal sulcus of the mouth, palatine tonsils at the sides of the oropharynx and adenoids and tubal tonsils at the root of the pharynx (Figure 2.6). The adenoids and tubal palatine are further differentiated ciliated respiratory epithelium. Lingual tonsils are located near other structures, e.g. salivary glands, differentiating them from the palatine tonsils. The tonsils have many deep invaginations of the epithelium into the underlying lymphoid tissue, known as tonsillar crypts.

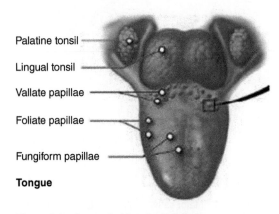

Palatine tonsil

Lingual tonsil

Vallate papillae

Foliate papillae

Fungiform papillae

Tongue

Figure 2.6 Anatomical location of tonsils.
Source: Modified from https://courses.lumenlearning.com/austincc-ap1/chapter/special-senses-taste-gustation/

2.8.1 Tonsil Immunity

Tonsils as MALTs are organised lymphoid follicles (Figure 2.7). They are frequent sites of infection and provide the first line of defence against ingested or inhaled foreign pathogens. Within the lymphoid tissue are channels lined by squamous epithelium that

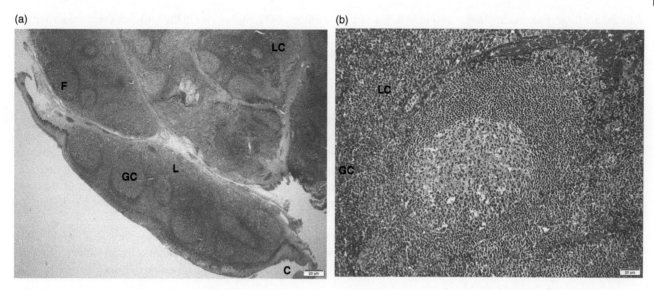

Figure 2.7 Normal histology of tonsil. The luminal surface is lined by stratified squamous epithelium with the underlying lymphoid tissue (L) containing typical lymphoid follicles (F). The lymphoid follicle shows a less intensely stained germinal centre (GC) and the more intensely stained lymphocyte corona (LC) at the periphery. The lymphoid aggregates are penetrated by epithelial crypts (C).

open onto the surface. These are known as crypts which are enriched in microfold or M cells that transport antigens into APCs in lymphoid follicles below. Other APCs residing in mucosa, such as DCs, macrophages and Langerhans cells (LCs), also take up antigens and migrate into MALT (as well as draining lymph nodes) to present to T cells which initiate activation of the adaptive immune responses, including B cells. Other cells in the tonsils that act as APCs include human leucocyte antigen (HLA)-DR-positive endothelial cells and epithelial cells that can potentially process and present antigens to extrafollicular T lymphocytes.

Activation of T cells leads to stimulation of B cells which differentiate into plasma cells to start producing immunoglobulin. The distribution of B cells, T cells and macrophages within adenoids and tonsils is shown in Figure 2.8. Within lymphoid

Figure 2.8 Epithelial and subepithelial distribution of T cells (anti-CD3), B cells (anti-CD20) and macrophages (anti-M13) in sections of human adenoid (a) and tonsils (b). *Source:* Reproduced from Boyaka et al. 2000/ with permission from ELSEVIER.

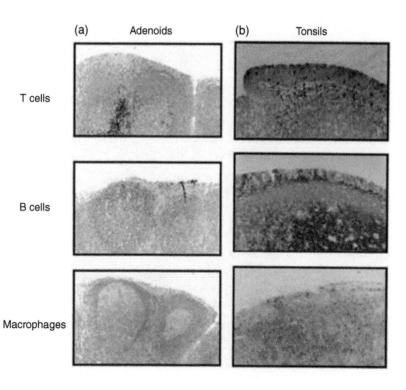

follicles are large, pale macrophages, acting as APCs, scattered among the lymphocytes in the follicles; there are also many mitotic cells within the follicles.

A study by Boyaka et al. (2000) on intraepithelial and subepithelial immune cells in germinal centres of the adenoids and tonsils showed that 25–35% were CD3$^+$ T cells, 60–75% were CD19$^+$ B cells while 5–8% were M13$^+$ macrophages (see Figure 2.8). The lower percentage of T cells is in contrast to higher distribution of these cells in mucosal surfaces of the GI tract.

Naive B cells are able to bind directly to antigens and differentiate to plasma cells producing immunoglobin (Ig) of the IgM type. B cells can act as APCs and may proceed to activate specific T cells. Activated T cells help B cells to switch to plasma cells producing other immunoglobulins such as IgG and IgA. Memory B and T cells are also generated at the same time. More B cells were observed to secrete IgG than IgA in the adenoid and tonsils. Immunoglobulin-secreting B cells also occur in the germinal centres of the lymphoid follicle, the mantle zone, extrafollicular area and reticular sites of the crypt tonsillar epithelium (Boyaka et al. 2000). All these changes are reflected in development of primary follicles into larger and distinct secondary follicles containing germinal centres.

The study by Boyaka et al. (2000) also noted that the majority of T cells in these compartments were CD4$^+$ and TCRαβ and could be induced to produce both Th1 and Th2 cytokines. The features of both T cells and B cells here suggest that the nasopharyngeal-associated lymphoreticular tissues possess both mucosal and systemic properties.

2.9 Lymph Nodes and the Lymphatic System

Lymph nodes are small (few mm to 2 cm), oval-shaped, encapsulated lymphoid organs. Of the 800 lymph nodes present in a human body, 300 are clustered in the head and neck region. The lymph nodes of the head and neck are broadly divided into two groups: (i) a superficial (palpable) ring of lymph nodes and (ii) a vertical group of deep (not easily palpable) lymph nodes.

Superficial lymph nodes are arranged in a 'ring' shape, extending from underneath the chin to the posterior aspect of the head and neck (Figure 2.9). These lymph nodes receive lymph from the scalp, face and neck and ultimately drain into the deep lymph nodes. Deep lymph nodes are organised into a vertical chain, located close to the internal jugular vein within the carotid sheath. The efferent vessels from the deep cervical lymph nodes converge to form the jugular lymphatic trunks (Watkinson 2006).

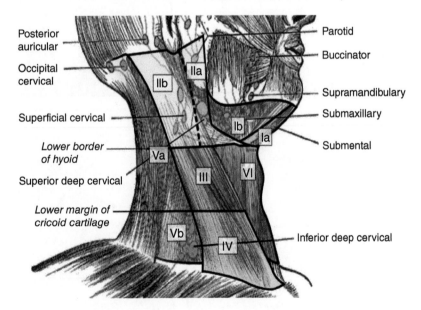

Figure 2.9 Superficial cervical lymph nodes and lymph node levels. *Source:* Mikael Häggström/Wikimedia Commons/CC0 1.0.

All lymphatic vessels that arise in the lamina propria of the oral mucosa ultimately drain into the deep cervical lymph nodes (Squier and Brogden 2011), either directly or indirectly via nodes in outlying groups. Immunogenic cells and fluid carrying antigens from nearby tissue enter lymph nodes through open-ended lymphatic capillaries. The first lymph node that the surrounding tissue drains into is known as the sentinel lymph node.

Lymphatic capillaries and arteries converge to form larger lymphatic collecting vessels and lymphatic trunks and finally become the thoracic duct which joins the blood system at the subclavian veins. This connectivity allows the lymphatic fluid from nearby tissue to be relocated into the blood circulation. Unlike MALTs, lymph nodes have no direct interactions with environmental antigens.

2.9.1 Lymph Node Immunity

Immunologically speaking, a sentinel lymph node is the target destination of the antigen-bearing LCs and DCs that are initially located in the mucosal epithelia and lamina propria. Once migrated to a lymph node, draining the sublingual and buccal area, antigen-bearing DCs are able to activate CD8 T cells. Upon activation, T and B cells that leave the site of the initial antigen presentation enter the circulation and disperse to selected mucosal sites, where they differentiate into memory or effector cells. The activation of CD4 T lymphocytes leads to the induction of antigen-specific helper cells.

T (Th cells) and/or regulatory T cells (Tregs) mediate immune responses, whereas CD8 T cells facilitate the induction of cytotoxic T lymphocyte (CTL) responses. The tissue destination of these cells appears to be largely determined by site-specific integrins.

At the lymph node, LCs and DCs present the antigens they carry to T cells located in primary follicles. Upon activation of the T cells, the primary follicles develop into secondary follicles with germinal centres where memory cells are generated similar to lymphoid follicles in MALTs (Figure 2.10). Here, B cells are differentiated into plasma cells to start producing antibodies. Increased proliferation of effector cells and production of antibodies also cause lymph nodes to swell and become palpable during an infection.

Interestingly, keratinocytes and DCs of the oral mucosa do not elicit an immune response against commensal microbial flora. Using molecular pattern recognition receptors, these cells are able to differentiate between commensal and pathogenic micro-organisms. Conversely, commensal microbes induce immune tolerance rather than immune elimination protocols which results in either lack of T-cell activation in response to immunogenic presentation of antigens or suppression of activity of effector T cells by regulatory T cells (Feller et al. 2013).

(a)　　　　　　　　　　　　　　　　　(b)

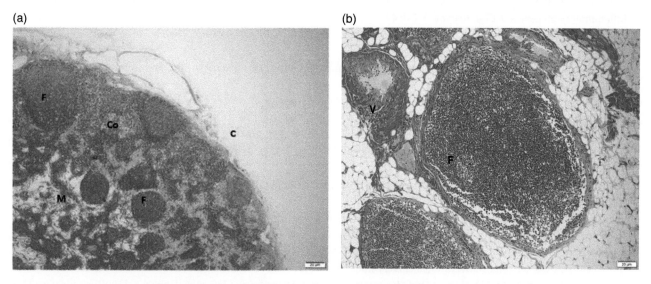

Figure 2.10 (a) Histology of the lymph node surrounded by a capsule (C) which comprises an outer cortex (Co) and an inner medulla (M). (b) The cortex contains lymphoid follicles (F) which develop into the germinal centre.

2.10 Conclusion

The immune system of the oral cavity has many defence mechanisms that prevent entry and conduct removal of harmful microbes. This is essential as the mouth forms the gateway where food and air-borne micro-organisms are daily challenges to the oral environment. In addition, the oral cavity is also involved in mastication and oral hygiene. Nevertheless, the immune system is able to balance its antimicrobial response and tolerance to harmless food and aeroantigens which extends to the oral microbiome that also has important beneficial roles. It is interesting to note that the immunity generated is not limited to mucosal but extends to systemic responses. Understanding the oral immune system is also important for development of vaccines as well as therapies to suppress proinflammatory diseases.

References

Abreu, M.T., Fukata, M. and Arditi, M. (2005). TLR signaling in the gut in health and disease. *J. Immunol.* 174: 4453–4460.

Al-Rawee, R.Y. and Abdalfattah, M.M. (2020). Anatomy respect in implant dentistry. assortment, location, clinical importance. *J. Dent. Probl. Solut.* 7 (2): 068–078.

Boyaka, P.N., Wright, P.F., Marinaro, M. et al. (2000). Human nasopharyngeal-associated lymphoreticular tissues. Functional analysis of subepithelial and intraepithelial B and T cells from adenoids and tonsils. *Am. J. Pathol.* 157 (6): 2023–2035.

Challacombe, S.J., Shirlaw, P.J. and Thornhill, M.H. (2015). Immunology of diseases of the oral cavity. In: *Mucosal Immunology*, 4e (eds J. Mestecky, W. Strober, M. Russell et al.). Cambridge, MA: Academic Press.

Cook, S.L., Bull, S.P., Methven, L., Parker, J.K. and Khutoryanskiy, V.V. (2017). Mucoadhesion: a food perspective. *Food Hyrocolloids* 72: 281–296.

de Aguiar, M.C.S., Perinetti, G. and Capelli Jr, J. (2017). The gingival crevicular fluid as a source of biomarkers to enhance efficiency of orthodontic and functional treatment of growing patients. *BioMed Res. Int.* 2017: 3257235.

Dillon, A. and Lo, D.D. (2019). M cells: intelligent engineering of mucosal immune surveillance. *Front. Immunol.* 10: 1499.

Feller, L., Altini, M., Khammissa, R.A.G., Chandran, R., Bouckaert, B. and Lemmer, J. (2013). Oral mucosal immunity. *Oral Surg. Oral Med. Oral Patho.l Oral Radiol.* 116(5): 576–583.

Groeger, S. and Meyle, J. (2019). Oral mucosal epithelial cells. *Front. Immunol.* 10: 208.

Hovav, A.H. (2014). Dendritic cells of the oral mucosa. *Mucosal Immunol.* 7 (1): 27–37.

Hovav, A.H. (2018). Mucosal and skin Langerhans cells – nurture calls. *Trends Immunol.* 39 (10): 788–800.

Kagnoff, M.F. and Eckmann, L. (1997). Epithelial cells as sensors for microbial infection. *J. Clin. Invest.* 100: 6–10.

Kessler, A.T. and Bhatt, A.A. (2018). Review of the major and minor salivary glands, part 1: anatomy, infectious, and inflammatory processes. *J. Clin. Imaging Sci.* 8: 47.

Kraan, H., Vrieling, H., Czerkinsky, C., Jiskoot, W., Kersten, G. and Amorij, J.P. (2014). Buccal and sublingual vaccine delivery. *J. Control. Release* 190: 580–592.

Matsopoulos, N.M. and Konkel, J.E. (2018). Tissue-specific immunity at the oral mucosal barrier. *Trends Immunol.* 39 (4): 276–287.

Nair, P.N.R. and Schroeder, H.E. (1986). Duct-associated lymphoid tissue (DALT) of minor salivary glands and mucosal immunity. *Immunology* 57: 171–175.

Osailan, S.M., Pramanik, R., Shirlaw, P., Proctor, G.B. and Challacombe, S.J. (2012). Clinical assessment of oral dryness: development of a scoring system related to salivary flow and mucosal wetness. *Oral Surg. Oral Med. Oral Pathol. Oral Radiol.* 114: 597–603.

Park, Y.J. and Lee, J.K. (2018). The role of skin and orogenital microbiota in protective immunity and chronic immune-mediated inflammatory disease. *Front. Immunol.* 8: 1955.

Phipps, P.A., Stanford, M.R., Sun, J.B. et al. (2003). Prevention of mucosally induced uveitis with a HSP60-derived peptide linked to cholera toxin B subunit. *Eur. J. Immunol.* 33: 224–232.

Rijkschroeff, P., Jansen, I., van der Weijden, F. et al. (2016). Oral polymorphonuclear neutrophil characteristics in relation to oral health: a cross-sectional, observational clinical study. *Int. J. Oral Sci.* 8: 191–198.

Squier, C. and Brogden, K. (2011). *Human Oral Mucosa: Development, Structure and Function.* Hoboken, NJ: Wiley-Blackwell.

Squier, C. and Kremer, M.J. (2001). Biology of oral mucosa and esophagus. *J. Natl Cancer Inst. Monogr.* 29: 7–15.

Subbarao, K.C., Nattuthurai, G.S., Sundararajan, S.K., Sujith, I., Joseph, J. and Syedshah, Y.P. (2019). Gingival crevicular fluid: an overview. *J. Pharm. Bioallied Sci.* 11 (Suppl 2): S135–S139.

Subrahmanyam, M.V. and Sangeetha, M. (2003). Gingival crevicular fluid: a marker of the periodontal disease activity. *Indian J. Clin. Biochem.* 18 (1): 5–7.

Walmsley, A.D., Walsh, T.F., Lumley, P.J. et al. (2007). The healthy mouth. In: *Restorative Dentistry*, 2e. Philadelphia, PA: Elsevier.

Walsh, L.J. (2003). Mast cells and oral inflammation. *Crit. Rev. Oral Biol. Med.* 14(3): 188–198.

Watkinson, J.C. (2006). Management of cervical lymph nodes in differentiated thyroid cancer. In: *Practical Management of Thyroid Cancer: A Multidisciplinary Approach* (eds E.L. Mazzaferri, C. Harmer, U. Mallick and P. Kendall-Taylor). London: Springer, London.

Wu, R.Q., Zhang, D.F., Tu, E. and Chen, Q.M. (2014). The mucosal immune system in the oral cavity – an orchestra of T cell diversity. *Int. J. Oral Sci.* 6: 125–132.

Yu, J.J., Ruddy, M.J., Wong, G.C. et al. (2007). An essential role for IL-17 in preventing pathogen-initiated bone destruction: recruitment of neutrophils to inflamed bone requires IL-17 receptor-dependent signals. *Blood* 109: 3794–3802.

3

Mechanisms of Immune Responses

Mohammad Tariqur Rahman

University of Malaya, Kuala Lumpur, Malaysia

3.1 Introduction

The human body is responsive to any physiological insult, be it internal or external. To maintain a healthy condition, the body needs both arms and armour to fight against those insults. From a molecule or cell, to an organ level, the human body is equipped with those weapons, which we call the immune system of the body. Fuller details of those components are given in Chapter 1.

The healthy state of a human body refers to a natural state of balance, i.e. homeostasis of all its physiological systems. This homeostasis can be disrupted by many forms of harmful events and agents such as trauma, micro-organisms and unwanted cells such as cancerous or apoptotic cells. The immune system responds to these disruptions and restores homeostasis to maintain a state of health.

This chapter will describe the fundamental mechanisms of how immune responses work against harmful agents. Biologically speaking, the immune response is how the body prevents, recognises and defends against a harmful agent, be it foreign or indigenous.

The core functions of the immune response include the following aspects.

- Prevention of the entry of harmful agents. In the case where the agents are of indigenous origin, the immune system prevents their further spread.
- In the case where the harmful agents manage to enter the body, the immune surveillant troopers use their tools to recognise those agents.
- Once recognised, activated immune responses destroy the harmful agents and restore balance.

Although these core functions appear as independent mechanisms of the immune system, they are integrated and work in concert to maintain homeostasis. Furthermore, preventing the entry of a harmful agent such as a pathogen, and its subsequent recognition and defence against it can act non-specifically against any pathogen or against a particular type of pathogen.

While non-specific immune responses, also called *innate* immune responses, are mostly pre-existing forms of defence mechanism, specific forms of immune response, also called *adaptive* or *acquired* immune responses, develop as the pathogen is recognised. In the following sections of this chapter, the mechanisms of both innate and adaptive immune responses will be discussed (Figures 3.1 and 3.2).

3.2 Innate Immune Mechanisms

Soon after birth, a human body encounters many potentially harmful agents including infectious micro-organisms from which protection is necessary to maintain homeostasis. While certain forms of innate immune mechanisms involve triggers resulting from disruptions to homeostasis caused by non-infectious or infectious means, the other forms are always ready to do their job.

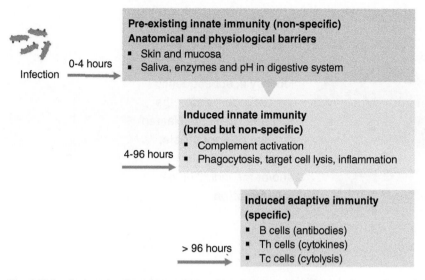

Figure 3.1   Progression from innate immunity to adaptive immunity

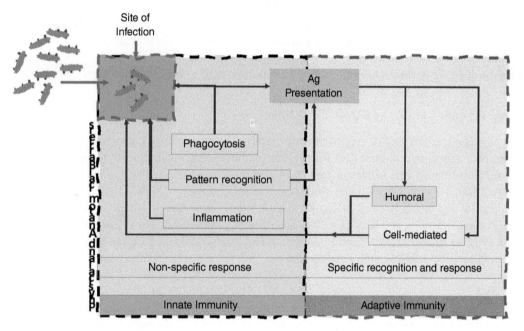

Figure 3.2   Interplay between innate and adaptive immunity.

A number of common pre-existing anatomical and physiological barriers in the form of physical, biochemical and cellular components provide protection by preventing the entry, invasion or spread of unwanted micro-organisms and particles. Therefore, the innate immune system includes all aspects of the host's immune defence mechanisms that are encoded in their mature functional forms by the germline genes of the host. Those components prevent their entry, invasion and spread, irrespective of the specific nature, type and mode of causing harm by the agents to the body; hence the name non-specific or innate immunity (Figure 3.3).

3.2.1   Preventing Entry Using Anatomical and Physiological Barriers

A number of anatomical and physiological barriers in the form of physical, biochemical and cellular components provide protection by preventing the entry, invasion or spread of harmful agents and events.

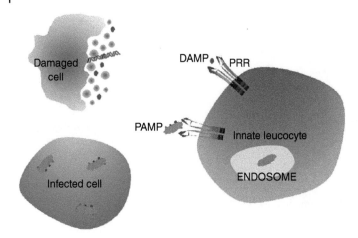

Binding of PAMPs or DAMPs to the PRRs activates an innate leucocyte, subsequently the pathogen and/or the damaged cells are cleared through **phagocytosis, targeted cell lysis** and/or the induction of **inflammation**

Figure 3.3 Activation of the innate immune response.

The anatomical and physiological barriers which form the first line of defence in the immune response include epithelial cell layers that express tight cell-to-cell contacts (tight junctions, cadherin-mediated cell interactions and others); the secreted mucus layer that overlays the epithelium in the respiratory, gastrointestinal and genitourinary tracts; the epithelial cilia that sweep away this mucus layer, permitting it to be constantly refreshed after it has been contaminated with inhaled or ingested particles; hydrolytic enzymes in body secretions such as saliva, tears and skin oils; mucus which traps bacteria and small particles; skin; and low pH of stomach acids.

With respect to the discipline of dentistry, salivary secretions play an important role in protection of the oral environment.

3.2.2 Non-specific Recognition and Defence against Harmful Agents

When the anatomical and physiological barriers fail to prevent entry of harmful agents such as pathogens, other forms of innate immunity come into play. These involve the components of the immune system which work non-specifically to recognise pathogens and subsequently activate cellular events to protect the host. These innate immune mechanisms require the release of certain triggers resulting from trauma, injury, cell infection or death. Mostly, these forms of innate immunity include soluble proteins and bioactive small molecules that are either constitutively present in biological fluids (such as the complement proteins, defensins and ficolins 1–3) or are released from cells as they are activated, including cytokines that regulate the function of other cells, chemokines that attract inflammatory leucocytes, lipid mediators of inflammation, reactive free radical species and bioactive amines and enzymes that also contribute to tissue inflammation. Innate immune response mechanisms also involve cell surface proteins or secreted proteins, such as the pattern recognition proteins.

All these elements of the innate or non-specific immune mechanism mediate the innate response against a broad range of pathogens. This is different from what happens in the adaptive immune response where the participating cells recognise unique molecular structures on pathogens, commonly known as antigens (Ag), using their unique Ag receptors.

3.2.3 Pattern Recognition

When a cell is damaged or dying, with or without any infectious agents, specific host macromolecules called damage-associated molecular patterns (DAMPs) are released and appear on the surface of the damaged cell. If the damage involves a foreign body such as a pathogen, it furnishes common molecular structures on its own surface or on the surface of the cell it has infected. These structures are called pathogen-associated molecular patterns (PAMPs). Therefore, cell damage or death in the absence of a pathogen gives rise to DAMPs only, but both DAMPs and PAMPs will be present when a pathogen invades. Innate leucocytes initiate innate responses by the recognition of such DAMPs and PAMPs.

Innate leucocytes use their pattern recognition molecules (PRMs) to recognise DAMPs and PAMPs. Some PRMs are membrane bound and others are soluble. PRMs that are expressed on the surface of innate leucocytes are called pattern recognition receptors (PRRs). Common examples of PRRs are Toll-like receptors (TLRs) and sugar chain-recognising molecules called lectins.

Once recognised by PRMs or PRRs, based on the DAMP or PAMP, subsequent clearance of the pathogens or unwanted cells involves complement-mediated cell lysis, inflammation and/or phagocytosis.

3.2.4 Complement Activation

The complement system comprises a complex system of enzymes that circulate in the blood in an inactive state. Once activated, the complement system starts interacting with the invading pathogen and eventually destroys it.

3.2.5 Inflammation

Inflammation is a type of innate immune response that occurs when tissues are injured by bacteria, trauma, toxins, heat or other harmful insult.

Inflammation begins upon binding of a ligand, generally a part of a pathogen, with the innate leucocyte PRRs. The binding results in intracellular signal transduction leading to the transcription and synthesis of various 'proinflammatory' cytokines. Eventually the damaged cells release histamine, bradykinin and prostaglandins, causing blood vessels to leak fluid at the damaged site. These cytokines in turn drive events responsible for the influx of first innate and later (if necessary) adaptive leucocytes into the site of injury or infection. The redness and swelling we commonly associate with inflammation are its outward physical signs. The same cytokines can also cause damage to healthy tissue and impair immune function, if left to operate unchecked.

If properly regulated, inflammation promotes a localised gathering of the cells and molecules necessary to repair tissue damage and clear pathogens and is beneficial for restoration of tissue homeostasis. Once the restoration is completed with the elimination of the damaging agents, inflammation is expected to resolve naturally. However, if the inflammation fails to resolve and becomes chronic, excessive or prolonged, it will undermine homeostasis and may become pathological. Thus, properly controlled inflammation is part of a healthy innate response and essential for homeostasis.

3.2.6 Phagocytosis

Phagocytosis ('eating of cells') is an important innate immune mechanism by which a number of cells of the immune system recognise, engulf and destroy foreign cells as well as damaged or dead cells and extracellular matrix.

The cells involved in phagocytosis are commonly called phagocytes and include neutrophils, macrophages and dendritic cells (DCs). Neutrophils mainly engulf and destroy pathogens, while macrophages and DCs engulf not only pathogens but also dead host cells, cellular debris and host macromolecules. All these phagocytes use their surface-bound PRR to carry out phagocytosis. The most potent types of antigen-presenting cells (APC) are the broad class of DC present in most tissues of the body and concentrated in the secondary lymphoid tissues. A second type of DC, designated as plasmacytoid DC, produces type I interferon which plays roles in antiviral host defence and autoimmunity. Both myeloid stem cells and common lymphoid progenitors can be differentiated to conventional and plasmacytoid DC.

The phagocytes originate from two distinct lineages of haematopoietic cells: (i) the myeloid cells, i.e. granulocytes such as polymorphonuclear neutrophils (PMNs) and eosinophils, and (ii) the mononuclear-phagocytic cells, i.e. monocytes (immature cells circulating in the bloodstream) and macrophages.

Neutrophils produce reactive oxygen species (ROS) to kill bacterial pathogens. They also produce enzymes that are useful for tissue remodelling and repair following injury. Thus, neutrophils are involved not only in clearance of microbial pathogens but also in repair of tissue injury. Neutrophils are also known to produce tumour necrosis factor (TNF) and interleukin (IL)-12 which carry out other immunoregulatory roles.

Monocytes and macrophages phagocytose microbes that are bound to either immunoglobulin (Ig) or complement components. They use nitric oxide to kill microbial pathogens. Monocytes and macrophages produce IL-12 and IFN-gamma to exert their regulatory role in adaptive immune responses. Thus, these cells are also key players in the adaptive immune response. Activated macrophages also produce IL-6, TNF, IL-10, IL-1 receptor antagonist and transforming growth factor (TGF) beta.

Eosinophils are the most prominent cells in most allergic responses. Basophils and mast cells are key initiators of immediate hypersensitivity responses, which is attributed to their cell surface receptors for IgE named FcεRI. Mast cells and, more prominently, basophils can release substantial amounts of IL-4 which is known to induce allergic immune responses.

Once they have engulfed and internalised the harmful foreign agents, macrophages and DCs present one or more unique parts of these agents, better known as processed Ag, on their cell surfaces. This processed Ag on the surface of the phagocytes is used by adaptive leucocytes to initiate the production of antibodies (Ab) against the foreign agent. These cells are then activated and mediate antigen-specific protection, an important component of adaptive immunity.

The process of phagocytosis involves several phases. A brief description of events during those phases is given in reference to engulfing a bacterium.

3.2.6.1 Chemotaxis

Tissue damage due to bacterial infection can cause the release of chemical products at the site of infection such as formyl peptides of microbes, complement activation products, cytokines and chemokines, leukotrienes and products of coagulation and fibrinolysis. These products direct the movement of innate leucocytes toward the site of infection, hence the name chemotaxis.

3.2.6.2 Opsonisation

Soon after invasion, a bacterial cell is coated by a number of cellular macromolecules called *opsonins*, such as complement fragments C3b, iC3b and C4b, immunoglobulins IgG and IgM, mannose-binding lectin, C-reactive protein and others. The process of bacterial coating by the opsonin is called opsonisation. This coating neutralises the negative charge on the surface of bacteria and enables their firm adhesion to the surface of phagocytic cells.

3.2.6.3 Engulfment

Following the binding of a bacterium through opsonins, the phagocyte starts to form pseudopods to enclose it. Thus, the bacterium is internalised or engulfed, resulting in the formation of the *phagosome*. The phagosome subsequently fuses with granules (lysosomes) containing antimicrobial enzymes, forming the *phagolysosome*.

3.2.6.4 Degradation

Within the phagolysosme, various antimicrobial substances help to digest the foreign material, destroy bacteria or inhibit their growth. These microbicidal mechanisms include the production of lysozyme, acidic hydrolases, neutral proteases, lactoferrin, bacterial permeability-increasing protein, cathelicidins, defensins and reactive oxygen and nitrogen species.

3.2.7 Target Cell Lysis

Unwanted cells such as cancer cells and cells infected with intracellular pathogens express certain DAMPs and/or PAMPs on their cell surfaces. The expression of these surface markers makes them 'target cells' for destruction by cells of the innate system. Innate leucocytes use their PRRs to recognise the target cells and initiate a complex process resulting in lysis of the unwanted cells. These types of innate responses are carried out primarily by neutrophils, macrophages and another type of innate leucocyte called a natural killer (NK) cell.

3.3 Adaptive Immune Mechanisms

The adaptive immune mechanism depends on long-lived cells that persist in an apparently dormant state but can exert effector functions rapidly after second and subsequent encounter(s) with a specific pathogen. With respect to the order of events, adaptive immune mechanisms are activated after the innate host defence response. Unlike innate immunity, the adaptive response is characterised by specificity, division of labour, memory, diversity and tolerance, permitting it to contribute in a more specific manner to act prominently and effectively against specific pathogens or toxins when they are encountered subsequently. Two major groups of blood cells, namely B lymphocytes (B cells) and T lymphocytes (T cells), are the key players of the adaptive system.

3.3.1 Specificity

One of the key features of adaptive immunity is recognition of a specific pathogen. In contrast to the 'broad' recognition mediated by PRMs in innate immunity, the 'specific' recognition of a pathogen, more particularly an antigen of the target pathogen, is aided by the specific antigen receptors on the surfaces of T and B lymphocytes, namely T-cell receptors (TCRs) and B-cell receptors (BCRs) respectively. Each lymphocyte expresses thousands of copies of a unique receptor. Interaction of these antigen receptors with the target antigen triggers activation of the lymphocyte. Some of these proteins interact directly and specifically with antigen, while others convey the intracellular signals triggered by antigen binding into the cytoplasm and nucleus of the lymphocyte, resulting in the activation and subsequent proliferation of the lymphocyte to generate short-lived daughter effector cells. These effector cells carry out the function of eliminating the specific target pathogen.

3.3.2 Division of Labour

Different subsets of lymphocytes such as B cells, cytotoxic T cells (Tc), and helper T cells (Th) play different yet concerted roles to eliminate the target pathogen. The role of B cells in recognising an antigen is fundamentally different from that used by Tc and Th lymphocytes.

3.3.2.1 B Cells Recognise Intact Ag

The BCR binds an intact antigen, which may be either a soluble molecule or a molecule present on the surface of a pathogen. This results in the production of daughter effector cells called *plasma cells*, all of which synthesise and secrete a specific antibody (Ab) against the target Ag, thus establishing a *humoral response*. However, Abs are unable to penetrate cell membranes or to attack an intracellular pathogen.

3.3.2.2 T Cells Recognise Processed Ag Presented with MHC Molecule

Unlike the BCR, the TCR does not recognise an intact and native Ag. A TCR binds a short peptide derived from a protein Ag which is processed and presented at the surface of a host cell such as a DC, with the aid of a MHC molecule. A TCR recognises this 'MHC–processed Ag' complex on the surface of the host cell. Peptides from the processed Ag can be bound to either MHC class I or MHC class II molecules (Figure 3.4).

A subset of T cells, namely Tc cells, recognise the 'MHC I–processed Ag' complex. The activated Tc cell proliferates and differentiates into identical daughter effector cells called cytotoxic T lymphocytes (CTL). Almost all body cells have MHC class I molecules, which is a double-edged sword. Having MHC I molecules on the surface makes a cell a potential target for CTL. However, CTL cannot attack them as it needs a 'MHC I–processed Ag' complex. Since most host cells do not have the ability to phagocytose a pathogen, it is only after infection with an intracellular pathogen that a host cell displays a 'MHC I–processed Ag' complex and subsequently is recognised by the TCR of CTLs. This is the beneficial aspect of having MHC I molecules on the surface of all host cells which helps in the clearance of infected host cells.

The second subset of T cells, Th cells, recognise antigenic peptides that a DC presents with MHC class II molecules. MHC class II molecules are expressed only by certain cell types that can act as specialised APCs, including DCs, macrophages

Figure 3.4 Cellular interactions needed for immune response.

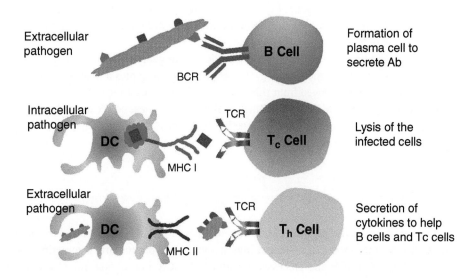

and activated B cells. When the TCR of a Th effector cell recognises this 'MHC II–processed Ag', the cell is stimulated to produce cytokines that assist B cells and Tc cells to become fully activated. Thus, Th cells contribute to both humoral and cell-mediated adaptive responses. In addition, cytokines secreted by Th cells stimulate innate leucocytes, thereby reinforcing innate immunity.

3.3.3 Immunological Memory

Cells of the adaptive immune system can 'remember' the encounter with an antigen. Upon subsequent exposures to a given pathogen, the effector functions are fast and effective. A constant supply of resting B and T cells is maintained throughout the body, with each lymphocyte expressing its complement of unique receptor proteins, thus continuing to maintain the immunological memory.

Once activated through an antigen-specific BCR or TCR, the respective daughter cells give rise to the short-lived effector cells required to eliminate the pathogen, as well as long-lived memory cells that persist in the tissues essentially in a resting state until a subsequent exposure to the same pathogen. The attack on the pathogen by this first round of effector cells is called the *primary immune response*. The second (or subsequent) exposure to the same pathogen is countered by clonally selected effector cells, which is collectively called the *secondary immune response*. New populations of memory cells are also produced during the secondary response, ensuring that the host maintains long-term or even lifelong immunity to that pathogen.

3.3.4 Diversity

While the innate immune responses are based on the genetically fixed anatomical and physiological mechanisms, the weapons of the adaptive immune system are genetically diverse and forever evolving through encounters with new pathogens or antigens. That offers a limitless number of options, at least theoretically, for us to fight against any pathogens using the adaptive immune mechanism. This enormous diversity arises from the combined actions of several genetic rearrangement mechanisms that are available for the genes encoding the TCRs, BCRs and Abs. For example, the BCR and TCR genes are translated from a large collection of pre-existing gene segments by a mechanism called *somatic recombination*. A specific combination of gene segments used to synthesise a TCR or BCR makes a lymphocyte and its daughter cells unique from any other subsets of lymphocytes. The ability to produce vast numbers of B and T cells clones guarantees that there will be at least one clone expressing a unique receptor sequence for every Ag encountered during the host's life span.

3.3.5 Tolerance

On one hand, the cells of the adaptive immune system such as B, Tc (CTL) and Th cells have enormous potential to produce their clones by rearranging genes to synthesise BCR, TCR or Ab to target virtually any Ag. At the same time, these cells also avoid attacking their own cells and tissues, unless they are infected or become abnormal for some reason such as malignancy. This avoidance is called tolerance.

The random somatic recombination or genetic rearrangements of each antigen give rise to the ability to encode receptors that recognise self-molecules (self Ag). If this possibility becomes a reality, the self-targeting lymphocytes must be identified and then either removed from the body entirely or at least inactivated, to ensure that the individual has an effective lymphocyte repertoire that does not attack healthy tissue. These cells can be eliminated at the early lymphocyte stage called *central tolerance*. If some of the self-targeting lymphocytes escape central tolerance, they will be eliminated during the second stage of tolerance, called *peripheral tolerance*.

3.4 Key Molecules and Interactions in Adaptive Immune Mechanisms

A number of molecules participate in different types of interactions involved in adaptive immune mechanisms. Central to these interactions are receptor–ligand interactions, more particularly interactions between Ag and Ab, PRR and DAMP/PAPM, MHC molecules and processed Ag, and TCR/BCR and Ag presented by MHC molecules.

3.4.1 Antigen

Biochemically, antigens are mostly proteins (polypeptide chains) and polysaccharides. Lipids (fats) and nucleic acids (DNA or RNA) can act as antigens if they are complexed with polypeptide chains. The abbreviation 'Ag' stands for its involvement as an antibody generator. According to that abbreviation, an Ag is a molecule that can activate the adaptive immune response mechanism for the production of Ab, which then can bind the Ag and aids its clearance. However, practically, an Ag can also bind to both TCR or BCR (B cell-bound Ab).

As far as the binding is concerned, Ab binds to a specific site of an antigenic molecule that is called an *epitope*. Therefore, it is possible that an antigenic agent such as a pathogen can have multiple Ab binding sites (epitopes) (Figure 3.5a).

It is not only the harmful pathogens that carry antigenic properties, i.e. have the potential to activate immune mechanisms to produce Ab. A protein molecule from a healthy individual can be antigenic to another healthy individual, as is obvious in cases of blood transfusion. At the same time, self-molecules can also act as Ag. To eliminate any possibility to react against self-Ag, immune cells are trained to distinguish between 'self' and 'non-self' so that they do not provoke any immune reaction. This training is called the negative selection of T cells and takes place in the thymus.

A continuous sequence of amino acids of a polypeptide chain can act as a *continuous epitope*. However, an epitope may not necessarily consist of sequential amino acids. Different amino acids from different parts of the polypeptide chain often come in close contact because of conformational or structural folding. Thus, an epitope may consist of amino acids which belong to different sequences in the primary structure of a polypeptide chain, which is called a *discontinuous or conformational epitope* (Figure 3.5b).

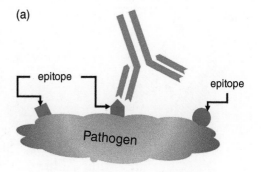

(a)

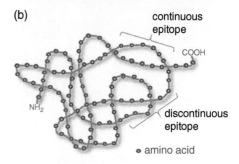

(b)

Figure 3.5 (a) The epitope. (b) Continuous and discontinuous epitopes.

3.4.2 Antibody

Biochemically, antibodies are globular-shaped glycoproteins which are also called immunoglobulins (Ig), referring to their globular structure and role in the immune system. Antibodies are secreted by B cells, mostly by differentiated B cells also called plasma cells. Antibodies are present either in the secreted form, i.e. circulating freely in the circulation, or membrane bound on the surface of a B cell as the B-cell receptor (BCR).

In its three-dimensional structure, an antibody molecule consists of four polypeptide chains: two identical heavy chains and two identical light chains. The two heavy chains are connected with each other by disulfide bonds (-S-S-). At the same time, one light chain and one heavy chain are connected also using disulfide bonds (-S-S-) (Figure 3.6).

Each heavy chain consists of three constant domains (C_H 1–3) and one variable domain (V_H). Each light chain consists of one constant domain (C_L) and one variable domain (V_L). Note that domain refers to a part of a polypeptide chain that has unique structural and functional features. The variable domains of both heavy and light chains carry the antigen binding site, known as the antigen binding fragment (F_{ab}). The constant domains of the heavy chains are called the fragment crystallisation (F_c).

Based on the variation in the amino acid sequences of the F_c region, Ig molecules are divided into five major isotypes or classes as follows.

- *Ig A*: mostly found in different secretions in mucosal areas, such as the gut, respiratory tract and urogenital tract; prevents colonisation by pathogens. Also found in saliva, tears and breast milk. IgA often exists as a dimer in different secretions, where two monomers are bound with a secretory molecule (υ).
- *Ig D*: found on the surface of B cells where it acts as an antigen receptor. It has been shown to activate basophils and mast cells to produce antimicrobial factors.
- *Ig E*: mostly involved in inflammatory responses where IgE binds to allergens and triggers histamine release from mast cells and basophils. Known to protect from parasitic worms.

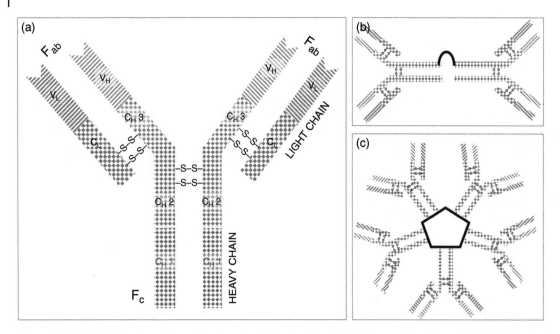

Figure 3.6 General structure of an antibody molecule having two light chains and two heavy chains (a). Dimer of secretory IgA (b) and pentamer of IgM (c).

- *Ig G*: the most common form of Ig in the circulation, fighting against many invading pathogens. IgG crosses the placenta and gives passive immunity to the fetus.
- *Ig M*: mostly expressed on the surface of B cells as a monomer or secreted as a pentamer. IgM is known to eliminate pathogens in the early stages of adaptive (humoral) immunity until there is sufficient IgG. Immature B cells, which have never been exposed to an antigen, express only the IgM isotype in a cell surface-bound form.

3.4.3 Major Histocompatibility Complex Molecules

Major histocompatibility complex (MHC) refers to a group of genes while the MHC molecules refer to its translated products. The presence of MHC molecules enables T cells to distinguish self- and non-self-Ag, thus avoiding any possible immune response against self-Ag, i.e. autoimmune reaction. T cells recognise the antigenic peptides through TCR. In fact, a specific TCR has no affinity for the target antigenic peptide alone. At the same time, the same TCR has very low affinity for any other antigenic peptides even if it forms a complex with an MHC molecule. Thus, T cells can only recognise the target antigenic peptide when it is presented in association with a specific MHC molecule, a phenomenon called *MHC restriction*.

The MHC molecules (also called the human leucocyte-associated [HLA] antigens) are a class of cell surface glycoproteins that present peptide fragments of antigenic proteins, which need to be cleared. The MHC I molecules present peptides that are synthesised within the cell, while the MHC II molecules present peptides that are proteolytically processed after ingesting the antigenic agent by the cell.

3.4.3.1 HLA I or MHC I

There are three major HLA I molecules, HLA-A, -B and -C, each encoded by a distinct gene. The HLA I molecules are heterodimers consisting of a transmembrane alpha-chain, also known as the class I heavy chain having three domains (alpha-1, alpha-2, alpha-3), associated with beta-2-microglobulin (beta-2m) protein. The extracellular alpha-1 and alpha-2 domains form a groove in which antigenic peptides can bind, thus presenting the target Ag to the TCR. The alpha-3 domain interacts with the CD8 molecule on cytotoxic T cells (Tc). This restricts recognition of antigenic peptides that are presented in class I HLA molecules to CD8$^+$ Tc cells.

Under certain circumstances, exogenous Ags which are not internally processed by APC can also be internalised by endocytosis and presented through HLA class I molecules. This uptake of exogenous antigens and display to T cells in HLA class I proteins is known as *cross-presentation*. Cross-presentation is particularly important in inducing an immune response against those viruses which escape Ag processing through the endogenous pathway.

3.4.3.2 HLA II or MHC II

The class II HLA molecules consist of two transmembrane polypeptide chains, namely alpha and beta chains (Figure 3.7). There are three major class II proteins designated HLA-DR, HLA-DQ, and HLA-DP. Both alpha and beta chains contain a short cytoplasmic domain, a transmembrane domain and two extracellular domains (alpha-1 and alpha-2, or beta-1 and beta-2). In its 3D structure, the alpha and beta chains form a pair where the alpha-1 and beta-1 form a peptide-binding groove. The alpha-2 and beta-2 domains bind the antigenic peptide and the beta-2 domain interacts with the CD4 molecule of the helper T cells (Th).

Class II proteins are expressed constitutively on monocytes, macrophages, B cells and DCs, all of which present antigens to CD4$^+$ Th cells. The target antigenic peptides are loaded into the class II peptide-binding groove via the 'exogenous' pathway that starts with endocytosis or phagocytosis of extracellular pathogens such as most bacteria, parasites and virus particles that have been released from infected cells as well as pollens, venoms and alloantigens. The ingested antigens are processed to linear peptide fragments by proteolysis after fusion of lysosomes with the phagocytic vacuoles or endosomes to form an acidic compartment.

3.4.3.3 Antigen Presentation by CD 1 (Not HLA)

The transmembrane protein CD1 molecules are structurally similar to class I HLA, having three extracellular domains and associating with beta-2-microglobulin. The alpha-1 and alpha-2 domains of CD1 molecules also associate similar to class I MHC molecules to form a binding groove to bind glycolipid components of microbial pathogens. The CD1–glycolipid complex is recognised by T cells that use the gamma/delta TCR. Glycosphingolipids, a class of carbohydrate-containing lipids found in both eukaryotic and prokaryotic cells, can also be presented by the CD1 molecule to NK cells.

3.4.4 T-cell Receptor

The T-cell receptor (TCR) is a heterodimer composed of two different protein chains. About 95% of all human TCRs consists of an alpha chain and a beta chain, while the rest consist of a gamma chain and a delta chain. This ratio changes during ontogeny and in diseased states such as leukaemia.

The T-cell receptor (TCR) is expressed on the surface of T cells and binds processed peptide Ags presented by MHC molecules. Different TCRs can recognise the same Ag, while different Ags can be bound by the same TCR. Binding of TCR with antigenic peptide and MHC activates T lymphocytes to initiate a series of biochemical events resulting in subsequent immune responses such as helping B cells to produce Ab.

Figure 3.7 Basic structure of MHC molecules.

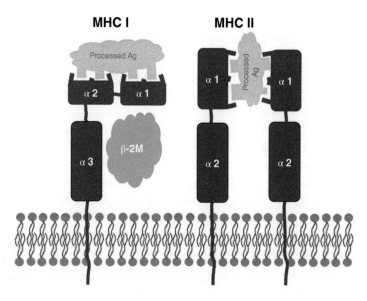

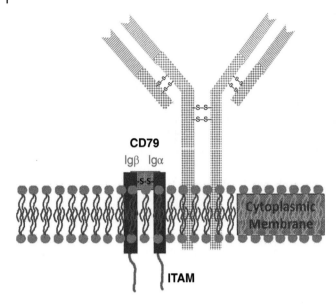

Figure 3.8 The BCR complex consists of an Ig molecule for Ag binding, also known as the membrane immunoglobulin (mIg). The mIg is similar to a monomeric structure of IgG, having two light chains and two heavy chains. In addition to the mIg molecule, the BCR complex also contains a heterodimer subunit, containing Ig-alpha and Ig-beta chains bound together by disulfide bridges, also known as the signal transduction moiety. Each member of the dimer spans the plasma membrane and has a cytoplasmic tail bearing an immunoreceptor tyrosine-based activation motif (ITAM).

3.4.5 B-cell Receptor

The B-cell receptors (BCR) are basically Ig molecules that form a type 1 transmembrane receptor protein usually located on the outer surface of B cells. The BCR is composed of two parts: (i) a membrane-bound Ig molecule of IgD, IgM, IgA, IgG or IgE which are mostly identical to a monomeric version of their secreted forms; and (ii) a signal transduction moiety also known as CD79 which is a heterodimer of Ig-alpha/Ig-beta (Figure 3.8). Disulfide bridges connect the Ig isotype and the signal transduction region. Pre-B cells that do not generate any Ig molecule normally carry both Ig-alpha and Ig-beta to the cell surface.

The major functions of BCRs are (i) initiating the signal transduction, involving changes in receptor oligomerisation, and (ii) mediating internalisation for subsequent processing of the Ag and presentation of peptides to helper T cells.

When a B cell is activated by its first encounter with an Ag that binds to its receptor (also called the *cognate Ag*), the cell proliferates and differentiates to generate a population of antibody-secreting plasma B cells and memory B cells.

3.5 Comparison Between Innate and Adaptive Immune Mechanisms

Innate Immune Mechanism	Adaptive Immune Mechanism
Depends on pre-existing barriers and mechanisms which do not require genetic rearrangements.	Depends on somatic gene rearrangements to enable cells to act against specific pathogens.
Cells of the innate immune mechanisms called 'innate leucocytes' express PRMs of limited diversity that collectively and quickly recognise a wide range of pathogens non-specifically.	Cells of the adaptive immune mechanisms called 'adaptive leucocytes' express an almost infinite number of extremely diverse receptors which are specific to the pathogen.
Response is triggered by binding between PRM and damage-associated molecular patterns (DAMPs) or pathogen-associated molecular patterns (PAMPs).	Response is triggered by antigen receptor binding to a unique antigen derived from a specific pathogen, which often involves MHC molecules.
The number of innate leucocytes remains largely unchanged as they do not proliferate upon recognising and responding to any pathogen.	Adaptive leucocytes proliferate to produce large numbers of unique effector daughter cells.
Responding cells are short-lived and do not have any memory of earlier encounters.	Responding cells are long-lived and a part of the daughter cell carries the memory.
Degree of defence is similar upon repeated exposure to the same pathogen, but often is very fast.	Degree of defence is stronger and faster with repeated exposure to the same pathogen.

3.6 Immune Deficiencies

Deficiencies of phagocytic mechanism result in pyogenic or granulomatous bacterial infections of the respiratory tract, lymph nodes, skin, mucosa and visceral organs caused by several bacterial spp. namely *Staphylococcus aureus*, *Serratia marcescens*, *Klebsiella* sp., *Salmonella* sp., *Escherichia coli* and *Pseudomonas aeruginosa*, and fungal spp. such as *Candida* sp. and *Aspergillus* sp.

Primary immunodeficiencies due to abnormal numbers of phagocytes result in severe congenital neutropenia and cyclic neutropenia. Impaired ability to migrate, engulf or destroy foreign pathogens linked to leucocyte adhesion deficiencies may lead to chronic granulomatous disease, specific granule deficiency, myeloperoxidase deficiency and other conditions.

Further Reading

A. Agrawal, P.P. Singh, B. Bottazzi, C. Garlanda, A. Mantovani. Pattern recognition by pentraxins. *Adv Exp Med Biol*, 653 (2009), pp. 98–116.

A. Balato, D. Unutmaz, A.A. Gaspari. Natural killer T cells: an unconventional T-cell subset with diverse effector and regulatory functions. *J Invest Dermatol*, 129 (2009), pp. 1628–1642.

A. Strasser, P.J. Jost, S. Nagata. The many roles of FAS receptor signaling in the immune system. *Immunity*, 30 (2009), pp. 180–192.

A.D. Kennedy, F.R. DeLeo. Neutrophil apoptosis and the resolution of infection. *Immunol Res*, 43 (2009), pp. 25–61.

A.P. Sjoberg, L.A. Trouw, A.M. Blom. Complement activation and inhibition: a delicate balance. *Trends Immunol*, 30 (2009), pp. 83–90.

C.D. Allen, T. Okada, J.G. Cyster. Germinal-center organization and cellular dynamics. *Immunity*, 27 (2007), pp. 190–202.

C.J. Melief. Mini-review: regulation of cytotoxic T lymphocyte responses by dendritic cells: peaceful coexistence of cross-priming and direct priming? *Eur J Immunol*, 33 (2003), pp. 2645–2654.

C.L. Abram, C.A. Lowell. The ins and outs of leukocyte integrin signaling. *Annu Rev Immunol*, 27 (2009), pp. 339–362.

D.I. Godfrey, H.R. MacDonald, M. Kronenberg, M.J. Smyth, L. Van Kaer. NKT cells: what's in a name? *Nat Rev Immunol*, 4 (2004), pp. 231–237.

D.P. Huston. The biology of the immune system. *JAMA*, 278 (1997), pp. 1804–1814.

F. Sallusto, A. Lanzavecchia. Heterogeneity of CD4+ memory T cells: functional modules for tailored immunity. *Eur J Immunol*, 39 (2009), pp. 2076–2082.

F.A. Bonilla, H.C. Oettgen. Adaptive immunity. *J Allergy Clin Immunol*, 125 (2010), pp. S33–S40.

G. Sonderstrup, H.O. McDevitt. DR, DQ, and you: MHC alleles and autoimmunity. *J Clin Invest*, 107 (2001), pp. 795–796.

H. Schmidlin, S.A. Diehl, B. Blom. New insights into the regulation of human B-cell differentiation. *Trends Immunol*, 30 (2009), pp. 277–285.

H. von Boehmer, P. Kisielow, H. Kishi, B. Scott, P. Borgulya, H.S. The expression of CD4 and CD8 accessory molecules on mature T cells is not random but correlates with the specificity of the alpha beta receptor for antigen. *Immunol Rev*, 109 (1989), pp. 143–151.

H.W. Schroeder, L. Cavacini. Structure and function of immunoglobulins. *J Allergy Clin Immunol*, 125 (2010), pp. S41–S52.

J. Wu, V. Groh, T. Spies. T cell antigen receptor engagement and specificity in the recognition of stress-inducible MHC class I-related chains by human epithelial gamma delta T cells. *J Immunol*, 169 (2002), pp. 1236–1240.

J.F. Miller. The discovery of thymus function and of thymus-derived lymphocytes. *Immunol Rev*, 185 (2002), pp. 7–14.

L. Van Kaer. Accessory proteins that control the assembly of MHC molecules with peptides. *Immunol Res*, 23 (2001), pp. 205–214.

L.D. Notarangelo Primary immunodeficiencies. *J Allergy Clin Immunol*, 125 (2010), pp. S182–S194.

L.R. Thomas, R.M. Cobb, E.M. Oltz. Dynamic regulation of antigen receptor gene assembly. *Adv Exp Med Biol*, 650 (2009), pp. 103–115.

M. Benoit, B. Desnues, J.L. Mege. Macrophage polarization in bacterial infections. *J Immunol*, 181 (2008), pp. 3733–3739.

M. Colonna, B. Pulendran, A. Iwasaki. Dendritic cells at the host-pathogen interface. *Nat Immunol*, 7 (2006), pp. 117–120.

M. Harboe, T.E. Mollnes. The alternative complement pathway revisited. *J Cell Mol Med*, 12 (2008), pp. 1074–1084.

M. Jankovic, R. Casellas, N. Yannoutsos, H. Wardemann, M.C. Nussenzweig. RAGs and regulation of autoantibodies. *Annu Rev Immunol*, 22 (2004), pp. 485–501.

M.C. Carroll. Complement and humoral immunity. *Vaccine*, 26 (suppl 8) (2008), pp. I28–I33.

M.C. Carroll. The complement system in regulation of adaptive immunity. *Nat Immunol*, 5 (2004), pp. 981–986.

M.P. Longhi, C.L. Harris, B.P. Morgan, A. Gallimore. Holding T cells in check—a new role for complement regulators? *Trends Immunol*, 27 (2006), pp. 102–108.

N. Garbi, S. Tanaka, F. Momburg, G.J. Hammerling. Impaired assembly of the major histocompatibility complex class I peptide-loading complex in mice deficient in the oxidoreductase ERp57. *Nat Immunol*, 7 (2006), pp. 93–102.

N.S. Joshi, S.M. Kaech. Effector CD8 T cell development: a balancing act between memory cell potential and terminal differentiation. *J Immunol*, 180 (2008), pp. 1309–1315.

Natural killer cell tolerance licensing and other mechanisms. *Adv Immunol*, 101 (2009), pp. 27–79.

P.J. Bjorkman. MHC restriction in three dimensions: a view of T cell receptor/ligand interactions. *Cell*, 89 (1997), pp. 167–170.

R. Konig, S. Fleury, R.N. Germain. The structural basis of CD4-MHC class II interactions: coreceptor contributions to T cell receptor antigen recognition and oligomerization-dependent signal transduction. *Curr Top Microbiol Immunol*, 205 (1996), pp. 19–46.

R. Medzhitov. Recognition of microorganisms and activation of the immune response. *Nature*, 449 (2007), pp. 819–826.

R.M. Zinkernagel, P.C. Doherty. The discovery of MHC restriction. *Immunol Today*, 18 (1997), pp. 14–17.

S. Caillat-Zucman. Molecular mechanisms of HLA association with autoimmune diseases. *Tissue Antigens*, 73 (2009), pp. 1–8.

S. Gordon. Alternative activation of macrophages. *Nat Rev Immunol*, 3 (2003), pp. 23–35.

S.G. Tangye, D.M. Tarlinton. Memory B cells: effectors of long-lived immune responses. *Eur J Immunol*, 39 (2009), pp. 2065–2075.

S.J. Ono. Molecular genetics of allergic diseases. *Annu Rev Immunol*, 18 (2000), pp. 347–366.

S.J. Turley, K. Inaba, W.S. Garrett, M. Ebersold, J. Unternaehrer, R.M. Steinman, et al. Transport of peptide-MHC class II complexes in developing dendritic cells. *Science*, 288 (2000), pp. 522–527.

S.P. Commins, L. Borish, J.W. Steinke. Immunologic messenger molecules: Cytokines, interferons, and chemokines. *J Allergy Clin Immunol*, 125 (2010), pp. S53–S72.

S.R. Schwab, J.G. Cyster Finding a way out: lymphocyte egress from lymphoid organs. *Nat Immunol*, 8 (2007), pp. 1295–1301.

T. Kurosaki, M. Hikida. Tyrosine kinases and their substrates in B lymphocytes. *Immunol Rev*, 228 (2009), pp. 132–148.

T. Nitta, S. Murata, T. Ueno, K. Tanaka, Y. Takahama Thymic microenvironments for T-cell repertoire formation. *Adv Immunol*, 99 (2008), pp. 59–94.

U. Holmskov, S. Thiel, J.C. Jensenius. Collectins and ficolins: humoral lectins of the innate immune defense. *Annu Rev Immunol*, 21 (2003), 547–578.

W.J. Burlingham. A lesson in tolerance—maternal instruction to fetal cells. *N Engl J Med*, 360 (2009), pp. 1355–1357.

Y. Minai-Fleminger, F. Levi-Schaffer. Mast cells and eosinophils: the two key effector cells in allergic inflammation *Inflamm Res*, 58 (2009), pp. 631–638.

Y.X. Fu, D.D. Chaplin. Development and maturation of secondary lymphoid tissues. *Annu Rev Immunol*, 17 (1999), pp. 399–433.

4

Immune Responses in Wound Healing of Oral Tissues

Firdaus Hariri[1] and Reezal Ishak[2]

[1] *University of Malaya, Kuala Lumpur, Malaysia*
[2] *Universiti Kuala Lumpur Institute of Medical Science Technology, Kuala Lumpur, Malaysia*

4.1 Introduction

The oral cavity is a vital component in the human body as it is part of a complex system which contributes to important functions such as mastication, digestion and speech. It is surrounded by the upper and lower lips at the outer aspect and is in continuity with the labial mucosa in the inner aspect of the cavity. The inner part comprises various major anatomical soft and hard tissue structures which include the labial mucosa, gingiva, teeth and tongue.

As the oral cavity is essential in human daily activities, the area is often subjected to different types of persistent physical contact and irritation. It may be mild and non-traumatising such as teeth brushing and food chewing, but may lead to different types of injury when the area is exposed to traumatising impact such as in laceration wounds or burns.

4.2 Types of Oral Tissues

The upper and lower lips are two flexible muscular folds extending from the corners of the mouth to the nasal columella base and the mentolabial sulcus. The outer skin of the lips outside the vermillion border is similar to other facial skin and contains adnexal structures such as hair follicles, sebaceous glands and eccrine sweat glands. Thin stratum corneum forms part of the vermillion and this area contains dermal blood vessels and occasionally ectopic sebaceous glands (Figure 4.1).

Internally, the lips are in continuity with the labial mucosa which meets the alveolar mucosa. The buccal mucosa is located at the inner part of the cheek and forms the lateral wall of the oral cavity. There are many minor salivary glands in both labial and buccal mucosa. The oral mucosa is lined by the protective stratified squamous epithelium which is partially keratinised on the gingiva and hard palate. Underneath the buccal mucosa is the buccinator muscle and buccal fat pad which contribute to the cheek contour. Sensory innervation to these structures is supplied by branches of the maxillary and mandibular nerves whereas motor innervation is provided by the facial nerve.

The other major components are the teeth and tongue. The teeth are firmly supported by the alveolar bone with periodontal ligaments. There are 20 deciduous teeth in children which will be gradually replaced by a set of 32 permanent teeth, in the normal population. The tongue is a muscular structure and is a primary component in mastication and deglutition. It is also well vascularised and the dorsal surface of the tongue is keratinised with the presence of papillae.

4.3 Categories of Oral Tissue Injury

As the oral cavity is often exposed to various types of physical and mechanical contacts, soft tissue trauma is considered as the most common tissue injury. Conditions such as linea alba, buccal mucosa and lip biting, inflammatory papillary hyperplasia and traumatic ulcers are examples. Also, denture stomatitis is an example of prosthesis-associated oral tissue injury.

Immunology for Dentistry, First Edition. Edited by Mohammad Tariqur Rahman, Wim Teughels and Richard J. Lamont.
© 2023 John Wiley & Sons Ltd. Published 2023 by John Wiley & Sons Ltd.

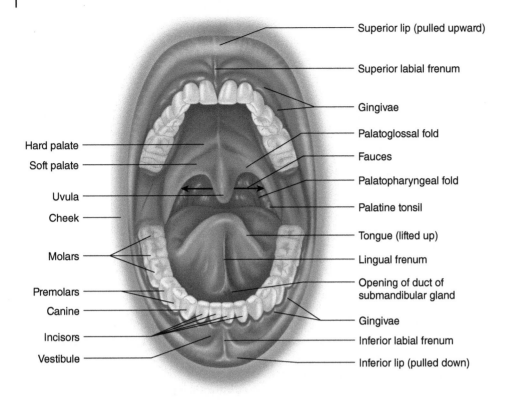

Superior lip (pulled upward)

Superior labial frenum

Gingivae

Palatoglossal fold

Fauces

Palatopharyngeal fold

Palatine tonsil

Tongue (lifted up)

Lingual frenum

Opening of duct of
submandibular gland

Gingivae

Inferior labial frenum

Inferior lip (pulled down)

Hard palate

Soft palate

Uvula

Cheek

Molars

Premolars

Canine

Incisors

Vestibule

Figure 4.1 Oral tissue structures.

Severe injury from major accidents such as falls, sports-related injuries and motor vehicle accidents may cause oral tissue lacerations (Figure 4.2). Iatrogenic injury to oral tissues includes laceration wounds secondary to intraoral procedures. The degree of laceration is dependent on the nature of injury and location of impact. Oral tissue laceration can be superficial or deep and in a severe cases may extend through multiple layers.

Chemical injuries may include chemical burns and allergic stomatitis. Intervention-associated oral tissue injuries such as oral mucositis and actinic cheilitis may occur in patients receiving radiation therapy. Less common oral tissue injuries include secondary injury from electrical and thermal burns such as from hot water or from contact heat of a dental handpiece.

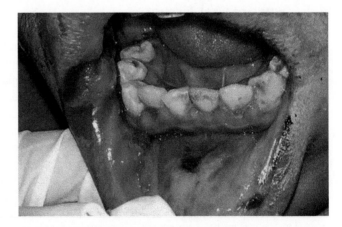

Figure 4.2 Lacerations of the lips and labial mucosa following a motor vehicle accident.

4.4 Stages of Wound Healing

Wound healing is a complex systemic process that follows a series of physiological interactions that affect healing development. The different phases of the healing process involve haemostasis, inflammation, proliferation and tissue remodelling.

4.4.1 Haemostasis Phase

The haemostasis phase happens immediately after injury. It includes interactions within the extracellular matrix which plug the injury site with blood clot and formation of a wound matrix, which is complete in a few hours. Various resident cells, infiltrating leucocytes and soluble mediators are recruited to the wound site. Different clotting factors are initiated from the injured tissues and a cascade of events follows through vasoconstriction in order to reduce blood loss. This response is triggered by platelets and leads to a blood clot filling up the wound site with growth factors and cytokines. Exposed collagen activates thrombocytes and this causes aggregation in order to remove any invading micro-organisms.

The blood clot containing fibrin molecules forms the provisional matrix that traps aggregated platelets and becomes the main part of the fibrin web. The fibrin web is also composed of fibronectin, vitronectin and thrombospondins which form the basis of a scaffold structure for the migration of leucocytes, fibroblasts and endothelial cells.

Inactive clotting enzyme proteases are bound to the surface of the provisional matrix and become activated. This subsequently expedites the cascade of clotting processes. In addition, chemotactic factors released by platelets attract leucocytes to the wound site. The presence of growth factors and cytokines released by both platelets and leucocytes will activate the inflammation process (Figure 4.3). These growth factors include platelet-derived growth factor (PDGF), transforming growth factor (TGF)-alpha, TGF-beta, vascular endothelial growth factor (VEGF) and basic fibroblast growth factor (bFGF). The presence of PDGF and TGF-beta subsequently attracts neutrophils and monocytes to the site and initiates the inflammatory response. Chemoattractants generated by the complement system in the form of C5a or from bacterial waste products such as f-Met-Leu-Phe provide additional signals for the recruitment of neutrophils. This event sets up the next phase of the healing process.

4.4.2 Inflammation Phase

The inflammation phase is the hallmark of the healing process and is often represented by the classic signs of inflammation based on rubor (redness), calor (heat), tumor (swelling) and dolor (pain) at the wound site. Phagocytes such as neutrophils, monocytes and macrophages are the key cells in the inflammation phase and migrate into the blood clot. These cells begin to remove cell debris and the blood clot which in turn releases soluble mediators including proinflammatory cytokines in the form of interleukin (IL)-1, IL-6, IL-8 and tumour necrosis factor (TNF)-alpha and growth factors (PDGF, TGF-alpha, TGF-beta, VEGF and bFGF).

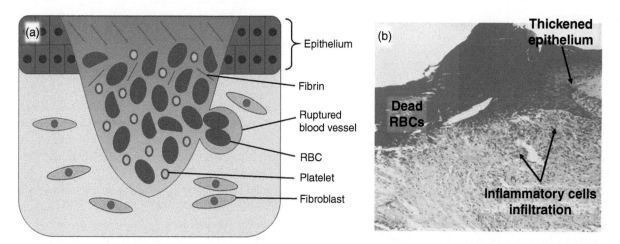

Figure 4.3 Haemostasis phase. (a) The body's physiological response prevents blood loss from ruptured blood vessels upon injury by forming a fibrin clot which consists of trapped red blood cells. Platelets subsequently release growth factors and initiate the repair process. (b) Breached epithelial cell lining due to an inflicted wound. Accumulation of dead red blood cells has plugged the bleeding wound and this is followed by the infiltration of inflammatory cells at the site. The epithelium appears thickened as the cells prepare for the next phase of the healing process.

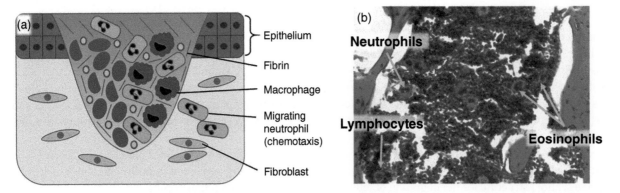

Figure 4.4 Inflammation phase. (a) Immediately after injury, the inflammation phase is initiated. Activated neutrophils begin to attach onto the endothelial cell walls of the blood vessels surrounding the wound, change shape and migrate through the cells' tight junctions to the wound site (chemotaxis). Monocytes/macrophages arrive at the wound site either by leaving the blood circulation or through migration and proliferation of resident macrophages. (b) The hallmark of the inflammatory response is the presence of leucocytes at the wound site. Neutrophils are among the first cells of cellular defence that arrive at the location and are followed by other white blood cells such as eosinophils, lymphocytes and macrophages (not pictured).

The soluble mediators activate and recruit fibroblasts together with epithelial cells for the next phase of the healing process. The fibroblasts secrete collagen fibres and help bind the wound together. In addition, chemoattractive cytokines, collectively known as chemokines, activate and recruit neutrophils, macrophages, eosinophils and basophils to the site. Chemokines also act as the regulatory mechanism for leucocytes during development and normal health conditions.

Neutrophils are the first line of defence in the inflammation phase and the first to respond to the soluble mediators released. Neutrophils remove any foreign materials and kill invading micro-organisms through phagocytosis. Usually, the number of neutrophils at the wound site starts to diminish after a few days due to apoptotic cell death and they are gradually replaced by tissue macrophages (Figure 4.4). In addition to resident macrophages, the majority of macrophages are recruited from the blood as circulating monocytes. Once recruited, the circulating monocytes become activated macrophages. Similar to neutrophils, the role of activated macrophages is to kill invading bacteria and remove cellular debris during the healing process. Depletion of the amount of activated macrophages and the absence of neutrophils in the wound marks the conclusion of the inflammation phase and the beginning of the proliferation phase.

4.4.3 Proliferation Phase

4.4.3.1 Re-epithelialisation Process

During the proliferation phase, the main focus is to cover the wound surface in a process known as re-epithelialisation. The epithelial cells proliferate across the wound surface and through the blood clot. The epidermis will grow upward and bond together until the full thickness of the skin is restored. The most prominent step at this stage is the migration of keratinocytes over the wound. Keratinocytes are the major cell type of the epidermis and the outermost layer. Unlike in the skin, keratinocyte migration and re-epithelialisation happens rather rapidly in the oral mucosa.

The hypoxic condition of the wound promotes the migration of epithelial cells. Thus, the function of keratinocytes is crucial for an effective re-epithelialisation process. Clinically, re-epithelialisation is the sign of healing, but this is not the final process. It is followed by granulation of tissues and reformation of the vascular network.

Fibroblasts are the key cells in the proliferation phase. Migration of fibroblasts into the extracellular matrix depends on interaction with and recognition by the matrix component. The synthesis of collagen and fibronectin which makes up the new extracellular matrix needed by fibroblasts is regulated by cytokines, PDGF and TGF-beta.

The new extracellular matrix will close the tissue gaps and re-establish mechanical strength at the wound site. Fibroblasts change their morphology during migration and accumulation within the extracellular matrix as the healing process takes place. The concentration gradient of cytokines, PDGF and TGF-beta dictates the direction of fibroblast migration within the extracellular matrix, whereas proteolytic enzymes in the form of matrix metalloproteinases (MMPs) are secreted in order to clear the path for movement into the wound site.

Once fibroblasts have migrated into the extracellular matrix and integrate, the proliferation process begins. Fibroblasts interact with the fibrin matrix and initiate the synthesis of components for granulation tissues which include collagen, proteoglycans and elastin. There are at least 20 individual types of collagen that have been recognised but collagen type III is predominantly synthesised during this process. Subsequently, the production of collagen starts to increase while the amount of fibroblasts reduces gradually in the tissues.

4.4.3.2 Angiogenesis Process

For tissues to maintain viability, the damaged vascular networks must be regenerated in a process known as angiogenesis. This process is initiated by growth factors including bFGF, PDGF and VEGF. The formation of new vascular networks starts with binding of growth factors to the receptors on the endothelial cells of remaining blood vessels, which consequently activates the cascade of intracellular signals. Activated endothelial cells then secrete proteolytic enzymes that dissolve the basement membranes of the extracellular matrix. As a result, the endothelial cells are able to migrate into the wound site and begin to proliferate by forming buds or sprouts.

The presence of superficial adhesion molecules such as integrins influences the action of endothelial cells. In addition, MMPs help endothelial proliferation by lysing the surrounding tissue matrix. When sprouts extending from the endothelial cells encounter another sprout, they becomes a small tubular vessel which progressively forms a new vascular loop. The new vascular loop later differentiates and matures into arteries and venules. The process continues until the vascular network is sufficiently repaired. This newly developed vascular network gives the granular appearance to the granulation tissue and the angiogenesis process is complete after primary blood flow at the wound site has been restored.

4.4.3.3 Granulation Tissue Formation

Granulation tissue formation consists of new capillary buds, fibroblasts, phagocytes and randomly organised collagen bundles. This is a transitional replacement phase for dermis which progressively matures and is replaced by fibrous scar tissue. At this stage, the angiogenesis process is not entirely complete and the tissue is highly vascularised. The wound site appears red and the tissue may be traumatised easily. It is during this transitional phase that the fibrin matrix is gradually replaced. Fibroblasts still play a significant role and contribute to the production of collagen and substances for the extracellular matrix which include fibronectin, proteoglycans, glycosaminoglycans and hyaluronic acid. The extracellular matrix eventually becomes the scaffolding for cellular adhesion and organises the movement, growth and differentiation of cells within it.

The granulation tissue has an increased metabolic rate compared to normal dermis. This facilitates the cellular activities required for migration and differentiation, and protein synthesis. At the end of this phase, fibroblasts are degraded, and the extracellular matrix is reorganised and remodelled. The number of fibroblasts is reduced by myofibroblast differentiation and terminated through apoptosis. The proliferation phase and re-epithelialisation process are illustrated in Figure 4.5a and 4.5b, respectively.

4.4.4 Tissue Remodelling

The last phase of wound healing is remodelling. Rearrangement of collagen fibres steadily increases the tensile strength of the wound and the granulation tissue starts to mature into scar tissue. The production of collagen type III in the proliferative phase is now replaced by stronger collagen type I which is organised in small parallel bundles. The presence of myofibroblasts at the site triggers wound contractions through numerous attachments to the collagen. The tissue of a healed wound will never be as strong as normal healthy tissue that has never been wounded. However, the tensile strength of epithelial cells is enhanced mainly by collagen fibre reorganisation during granulation and improved covalent cross-linking of collagen molecules by the enzyme lysyl oxidase. This enzyme is secreted by fibroblasts into the extracellular matrix. The tensile strength of the repaired tissue will continue to improve slowly for several months until it reaches about 80% of normal tissue strength.

Several different classes of proteolytic enzymes are involved in this remodelling phase and these are produced by the cells within the wound site at different times throughout the healing process. MMPs and serine proteases are the two

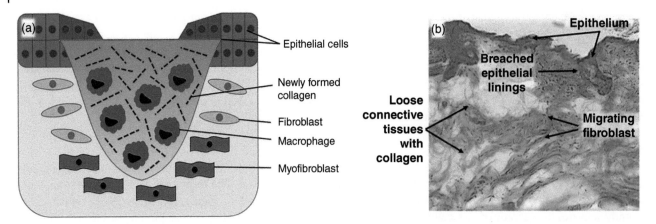

Figure 4.5 Proliferation phase. (a) Activated macrophages from the circulation and resident macrophages move into the injury site. The cells destroy foreign materials and at the same time release proteases that remove denatured extracellular matrix. Macrophages also secrete growth factors that stimulate epithelial cells and fibroblasts to proliferate. Myofibroblasts contribute to the healing process of connective tissues and restoration of tissue integrity. (b) Cellular restructuring and progressive re-epithelialisation process of the breached epithelial linings at the wound location. The granulation tissue formation is characterised by the migration of fibroblasts and the presence of loose connective tissue with newly formed collagen.

most important families of enzymes involved in the remodelling phase. The specific MMPs involved during the healing process include collagenases, gelatinases and stromelysins. Collagenases act by degrading intact molecules of fibrillar collagen, while gelatinases degrade damaged fibrillar collagen. In addition, stromelysins effectively break down proteoglycans.

One of the most important serine proteases in this process is neutrophil elastase that has broad substrate specificity and can cause damage to many protein molecules. In normal physiological conditions, these proteolytic enzymes are highly regulated by specific enzyme inhibitors produced by cells within the wound site. The enzyme inhibitors for MMPs are known as tissue inhibitors of matrix metalloproteinases (TIMPs), and for serine protease are named alpha-1-protease inhibitor and alpha-2 macroglobulin. The completion of this remodelling phase is a result of balanced and tightly regulated activity of the proteases (Figure 4.6).

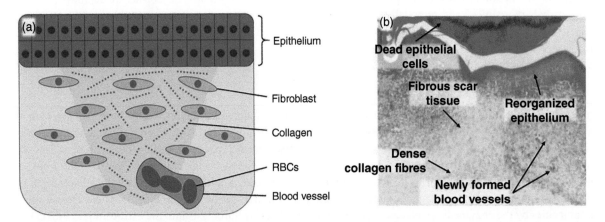

Figure 4.6 Tissue remodelling phase. (a) The initial disorganised repaired tissue is gradually replaced by extracellular matrix that closely resembles the normal uninjured tissue. Oral mucosa wounds normally show very little to almost no visible scar formation and the final structure is visually more similar to the original tissues. (b) The final step of the wound healing process is the tissue remodelling phase. The epithelium is reorganised to resemble the previous normal structure with dead epithelial cells sloughing off the surface. Collagen fibres became denser and fibrous scar tissue is noticeable underneath the epithelium. Newly formed blood vessels can also be identified at the end of this remodelling phase.

4.5 Role of Leucocytes in Wound Healing

Leucocytes, also known as white blood cells, are part of the body's immune system. These cells help to fight off invading micro-organisms, harmful foreign materials and other forms of damage. Leucocytes consist of different types of cells, namely granulocytes, which include neutrophils, eosinophils and basophils; monocytes and lymphocytes (T cells and B cells). These cells are actively involved in inflammatory responses immediately after the onset of tissue injury. Injuries to the tissue lead to the recruitment of inflammatory cells from the circulation in response to soluble mediators released by the wound. Among these cells, neutrophils and macrophages are the most significant leucocytes during the inflammatory response and onset of the healing process.

4.5.1 Neutrophils

Neutrophils are recruited to the wound site in response to the activated complement pathway, platelet degranulation and bacterial by-products. Neutrophils are the first inflammatory cells to arrive at the site after the release of soluble mediators. These cells are the first line of defence against any invading foreign micro-organisms and decline in numbers if infection is absent. Neutrophils leave the blood circulation through a process called extravasation and reside at the site for about 2–5 days after the injury.

The extravasation process involves important interactions between adhesion molecules, such as cellular adhesion molecules (CAMs), selectins and cadherins, and receptors, particularly integrins which are associated with the plasma membranes of neutrophils and endothelial cells. In the beginning, circulating neutrophils loosely adhere onto the endothelial cells of blood vessels via selectin molecules which cause them to roll on the surface of the endothelial cells. As neutrophils roll, they become activated by the presence of chemoattractants in the form of growth factors, cytokines or bacterial by-products, which leads to firm adhesion on the endothelial cells. This action is a result of integrin receptors binding with ligands such as intracellular adhesion molecules (ICAM) and vascular cell adhesion molecules (VCAM) that are expressed on the endothelial cells. Consequently, neutrophils change their spherical form into a flattened shape which allows the cells to squeeze through the tight junction between the endothelial cells of the blood vessels.

Neutrophils migrate to the wound site in a directed motion known as chemotaxis towards an increasing concentration gradient of chemotactic stimuli and into the extracellular matrix. Neutrophils also produce and release mediators such as TNF-alpha and IL-1 which amplify the inflammatory response by recruiting fibroblasts and epithelial cells. Furthermore, neutrophils start the debridement process at the wound site by releasing high levels of proteases (neutrophil elastase and neutrophil collagenase), and generate reactive oxygen species in order to kill microbes during the phagocytosis process.

The chronicity of inflammation is associated with the continuing presence of microbes in the wound and prolonged recruitment of neutrophils. In normal circumstances, the number of neutrophils at the wound site starts to deplete after about 2–3 days through apoptosis and they are gradually replaced by tissue monocytes.

4.5.2 Macrophages

Macrophages originating as circulating monocytes arrive at the wound site approximately 2–3 days after injury. Activated tissue macrophages play an important role in regulating the healing process, particularly for the proliferative phase of healing. Monocytes migrate to the wound site through an extravasation process similar to neutrophils and differentiate into activated tissue macrophages after stimulation by growth factors, chemokines, cytokines and fragments of degraded extracellular matrix. The many functions of these macrophages include host defence, resolution of inflammatory processes, tissue restoration and supporting cell proliferation.

In addition, macrophages remove necrotic tissues through the actions of secreted MMPs and elastase. Macrophages are unique because they are known to have the most effective means of removing neutrophils. By responding to neutrophils and their products, macrophages can identify and actively ingest apoptotic neutrophils. Macrophages also play an essential role in the proliferative phase of wound healing through the synthesis of numerous growth factors and cytokines which include TGF-alpha, TGF-beta, PDGF, VEGF, bFGF, IL-1 and IL-6. These growth factors are responsible for recruiting and activating fibroblasts, and subsequently organise the formation of new tissue matrix, while the cytokines promote angiogenesis. The role of macrophages is integral to resolving inflammatory reactions and for optimal wound healing. The presence of activated macrophages at the wound site results in enhanced tissue repair.

4.6 Spectrum of Wound Healing in the Oral Cavity

Due to the nature of its function, the oral surface is regularly exposed to harmful substances and pathogenic organisms. The warm, moist environment of the oral mucosa is particularly ideal for bacterial growth, but it rarely becomes infected or forms scar tissue. In fact, wounds in the oral mucosa heal rather rapidly compared to the skin. Tissue healing in the oral mucosa follows similar phases of wound healing as the skin, but obvious differences exist. The differences between oral and skin wound healing range from macroscopic representation of wound closure to the cellular progression of inflammation and re-epithelialisation.

Environmental factors are one of the most obvious differences in the healing process of oral mucosa. The presence of saliva provides a moist, warm environment in the oral cavity. In addition to cytokines and protease inhibitors, saliva contains an abundance of important growth factors such as TGF-alpha, VEGF and TGF-beta. Although not exclusively, this distinctive environmental characteristic is linked to the improved healing process in the oral mucosa. The different properties of cells within the oral mucosa and skin structure such as fibroblasts and keratinocytes also contribute to the healing process. Additionally, different states of immunity could be one of the contributing factors that expedite wound healing in the oral mucosa.

Having extensive blood microcirculation in the oral mucosa gives better access for inflammatory cells to reach the wound site and is considered to be beneficial for wound healing. The interactions between the fundamental properties of the cells within the oral mucosa together with surrounding tissue environment and immune system in some measure may explain the improved wound healing progress. The epithelium of the oral mucosa is intrinsically prepared to be repaired through different mechanisms largely because it is subjected to pathogen exposure and extreme mechanical load regulated by extrinsic factors in the microenvironment. It has been reported that the presence of commensal micro-organisms in the oral biofilm has a beneficial influence by increasing the proliferation of keratinocytes and expression of host defence proteins in the oral mucosa barrier.

The scarless outcome of wound healing in the oral cavity also suggests that some phases of the healing process have been altered. Reduced inflammatory reaction of wounds in the oral mucosa is quite similar to the fetal wound healing model which heals without a scar. During the angiogenesis process of healing, new blood vessels are formed in both skin and oral mucosa. Experimental evidence has shown that wounds in the oral mucosa have very little or no obvious scar formation due to reduced capillary growth and less inflammation. Wounds in the oral mucosa appear to have reduced inflammatory cellular infiltration and exhibit low levels of inflammatory cytokines. Consequently, this response contributes towards lower fibroblast activity and modified collagen deposition.

The intensified re-epithelialisation in the oral mucosa indicates that a proliferative stem cell population is working progressively. A multipotent stem cell population exists within the lamina propria of the connective tissue layer in the oral mucosa, named human oral mesenchymal stem cells (hOMSCs). The hOMSCs are a self-renewing group of cells that can differentiate into osteoblasts, chondroplasts, adipocytes and neuronal cell lineages, which is very important for oral mucosa wound healing. Recent technological advances have revealed that the oral mucosa is a rich source of stem cells which could be utilised for the treatment of wounds and wound healing research.

The unique oral mucosa environment gives an advantage during wound healing compared to the skin. Wound healing in the oral mucosa progresses rapidly with minimal scar tissue and is marked by decreased inflammatory reactions and reduced angiogenesis. This exceptional healing mechanism is the outcome of both intrinsic and extrinsic factors that work together during the wound healing process in the oral cavity.

Recommended Reading Lists

DiPietro, L.A., Schrementi, M. (2018). Oral Mucosal Healing. Wound Healing: Stem Cells Repair and Restorations, Basic and Clinical Aspects, 125–132. John Wiley & Sons, Inc. https://doi.org/10.1002/9781119282518.ch10

Gibbs, S., Roffel, S., Meyer, M., Gasser, A. (2019). Biology of Soft Tissue Repair: Gingival Epithelium in Wound Healing and Attachment to the Tooth and Abutment Surface. *European Cells & Materials*, Volume 38, 63–78. https://doi.org/10.22203/eCM.v038a06

Gourdie, R.G., Myers, T.A. (2013). Wound Regeneration and Repair: Methods and Protocols. New York, Humana Press. https://doi.org/10.1007/978-1-62703-505-7

MacLeod, A.S., Kwock, J.T. (2018). Inflammation in Wound Repair: Role and Function of Inflammation in Wound Repair. Wound Healing: Stem Cells Repair and Restorations, Basic and Clinical Aspects, 177–194. John Wiley & Sons, Inc. https://doi.org/10.1002/9781119282518.ch14

Reinke, J.M., Sorg, H. (2012). Wound Repair and Regeneration. *European Surgical Research, Volume* 49(1), 35–43. https://doi.org/10.1159/000339613

Schultz, G.S., Chin, G.A., Moldawer, L., Diegelmann, R.F. (2011). Principles of Wound Healing. In R. Fitridge (Eds.) et. al., Mechanisms of Vascular Disease: A Reference Book for Vascular Specialists, 423–450. University of Adelaide Press. https://doi:10.1017/UPO9781922064004.024

Smith, P.C., Martínez, C. (2018). Wound Healing in the Oral Mucosa. In: Bergmeier, L. (Eds) Oral Mucosa in Health and Disease, 77–90. Springer, Cham. https://doi.org/10.1007/978-3-319-56065-6_6

5

Stem Cell Immunology
Sabri Musa and Ngui Romano

University of Malaya, Kuala Lumpur, Malaysia

5.1 Introduction

Stem cells are generally defined as cells with the ability to self-renew by dividing over an indefinite period throughout the life of an individual and which, under appropriate conditions and specific signals, can develop into various cell lineages with different characteristics and specialised functions (i.e. differentiation) (Slack 2008; Telles et al. 2011; Zomer et al. 2015). Thus, they are unique human cells that can develop into many different cell types and, in some cases, fix damaged tissues. In other words, stem cells are undifferentiated cells distinguished by their capacity for autoregeneration and asymmetric division, indicating daughter stem cells with a stronger commitment to proliferation and cell differentiation. Stem cells are present in almost all tissues in the body, including neural (Gage 2000), gastrointestinal (Potten 1998) and adipose tissue (Cawthorn et al. 2012), and in hepatic (Forbes et al. 2002), haematopoietic (Weissman 2000), epidermal (Watt 1998) and mesenchymal stem cells (Pittenger et al. 1999) (Figure 5.1).

5.2 General Characteristics of Stem Cells

The classic definition of a stem cell requires that it possesses the two characteristics of self-renewal and differentiation (i.e. potency). Self-renewal is also known as cell proliferation and involves the ability of the cell to go through numerous cycles of growth and division while maintaining its undifferentiated state (Slack 2008; Telles et al. 2011; Zomer et al. 2015). The two mechanisms that ensure the maintenance of stem cell populations are asymmetric cell division and stochastic differentiation. In the former, a stem cell divides into a mother cell, which is identical to the original stem cell, and a differentiated daughter cell. When a stem cell self-renews, it divides and does not disrupt the undifferentiated state. In stochastic differentiation, a stem cell grows and divides into two different daughter cells, while another stem cell undergoes mitosis and produces two stem cells identical to the original (Shenghui et al. 2009).

Another stem cell characteristic is its capacity to differentiate into specialised cell types, also known as potency (Figure 5.2). Based on their differentiation potential, stem cells are classified as totipotent, pluripotent, multipotent, oligopotent and unipotent (Malaver-Ortega et al. 2012). Totipotent and pluripotent stem cells relate to embryonic stem cells (ESC) with the former found in the zygote in the early stages of development, of up to 32 cell embryos. Pluripotent cells are found in the blastocyst's inner cell mass, usually between 32 and 64 cells (Mitalipov and Wolf 2009). Totipotent cells can generate all forms of cell types, including embryonic and extraembryonic tissues. Pluripotent stem cells are also known as the most primitive stem cells and can produce all the cell types in an organism. Pluripotent stem cells (PSCs) can produce three germ layers, namely the endoderm, mesoderm and ectoderm (Brevini et al. 2007). Multipotent stem cells are present in various adult organs and differentiate into many cell types (Beyer Nardi and da Silva 2006). Oligopotent cells cannot differentiate while unipotent stem cells can only generate one mature cell type. Thus, oligopotent and unipotent stem cells are called progenitor cells (Mitalipov and Wolf 2009).

Figure 5.1 Characteristics of mesenchymal stem cells (MSCs). Multipotent stem cells can (i) proliferate, (ii) self-renew, (iii) undergo uncommitted differentiation and (iv) experience committed differentiation to form (a) haematopoietic, (b) muscular, (c) epithelial, (d) neuronal and (e) fat (adipose) cells.

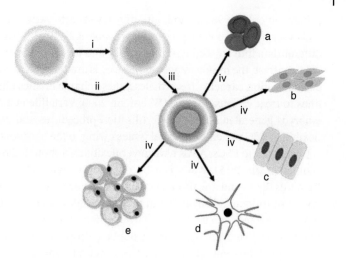

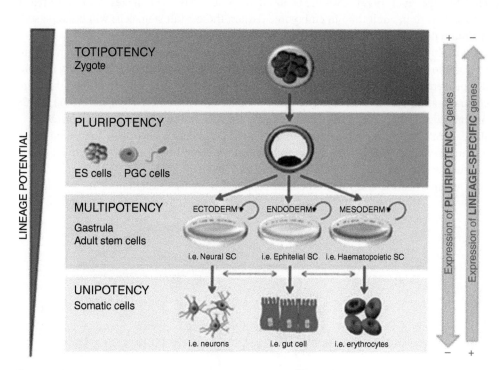

Figure 5.2 Lineage of human development potency. *Source:* Adapted from Berdasco and Esteller (2011).

The traditional developmental dogma follows the differentiation of totipotent stem cells to PSCs, PSCs to multipotent stem cells, multipotent stem cells to unipotent stem cells, and finally, mature cells. Both their self-renewal capacity and differential potential are reduced during their journey from totipotent to mature cell state.

5.3 Types of Stem Cells

Stem cells are primarily classified as ESCs and adult stem cells (ASCs) (Rimondini and Mele 2009). This classification is based on their residency (Guleria et al. 2014). The ESC lines were first established in mice in 1981 (Evans and Kaufman 1981), and the first characterisation of an ESC line in humans was in 1988 (Thomson et al. 1998). ESCs are derived from the inner cell mass of the blastocyst during early embryonic (morula stage) development. They are pluripotent, meaning that they can spontaneously turn into more than one type of cell or multicellular structures in vitro, known as embryonic bodies

(Thomson et al. 1998). In addition, they give rise to various types of specialised cells, including cardiomyocytes, neurons and other haematopoietic progenitors (Evans et al. 1990; Verfaillie et al. 2002). Two advantages of ESCs are the capacity to differentiate into any cell type in the body and to self-replicate for numerous generations.

In contrast, the disadvantages of these cells are the ethical issues involved and their virtually unlimited proliferation and differentiation capacity. Nevertheless, these characteristics allow in vitro manipulation to produce specific precursor cell lines to treat various diseases (Weissman 2000; Verfaillie et al. 2002). ESCs used in research today originate from unused embryos generated by in vitro fertilisation procedures and donated to science for research purposes. Despite their high flexibility, ESC use entails ethical issues owing to the blastocyst destruction required for isolating them.

In contrast to ESCs, ASCs have lower flexibility although they are notable for their abundance, easy access and high yield (Zomer et al. 2015). ASCs can be defined as stem cells found in any developed tissues in organisms (Bongso and Richards 2004) and are also known as somatic or postnatal stem cells (Egusa et al. 2012). They are undifferentiated multipotent or unipotent cells found in most adult tissues and organs, and can only differentiate into a limited number of cell types. These cells can be harvested from different tissues in the body, such as bone marrow, umbilical cord, amniotic fluid, brain tissue, liver, pancreas, cornea, dental pulp and adipose tissue (Guleria et al. 2014) (Figure 5.3). Types of ASCs include haematopoietic stem cells (HSCs), MSCs, neural stem cells (NSCs), ESCs and skin stem cells (SKCs). The most recognised ASCs are mesenchymal stem cells (Pittenger et al. 1999). ASCs are believed to reside in 'stem cell niches', a specific area of each tissue. Although fewer cells are present in adult than in embryonic tissues, these adult stem cells will undergo self-renewal and differentiation to maintain healthy tissues and repair injured ones (Egusa et al. 2012).

Mesenchymal stem cells are adult multipotent stem cells and can be isolated from various adult or fetal tissues and membranes (Bianchi et al. 2001; Filioli Uranio et al. 2011). MSCs have two unique properties. The first is their capacity for self-renewal beyond Hayflick's limit, a property shared by embryonic stem cells. The second is their ability to differentiate into mesenchymal and non-mesenchymal mature cell lines such as fat, bone, cartilage and neural cells (Caplan, 1991). MSCs can be harvested from various adult tissues such as bone marrow, adipose tissue, skin and tissues of the orofacial area.

Extensive studies have been done on MSCs from various sources. In dentistry, several MSCs have been discovered in the last few decades, such as bone marrow stem cells (BMSCs) from orofacial bones, dental tissue-derived stem cells, oral mucosa-derived stem cells, periosteum-derived stem cells and salivary gland-derived stem cells (SGSCs) (Egusa et al. 2012). MSCs are involved in the growth, wound healing and replacement of cells lost daily by exfoliation or in pathological

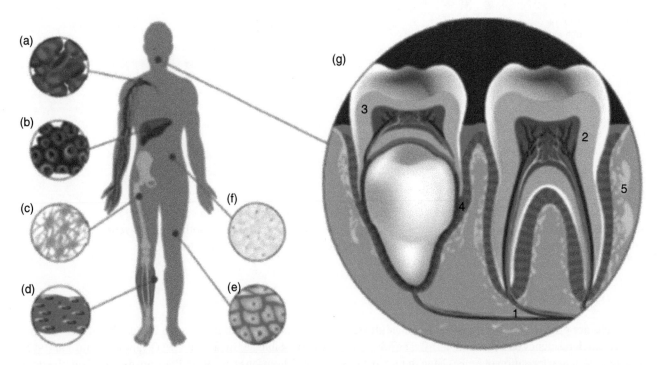

Figure 5.3 Sources of stem cells in humans. The diagram shows some tissue sources of adult stem cells: (a) peripheral blood, (b) liver, (c) bone marrow, (d) muscles, (e) skin, (f) adipose tissue and (g) dental tissues (1 apical dental papilla, 2 adult pulp, 3 pulp of deciduous teeth, 4 periodontal ligament, and 5 alveolar). *Source:* Adapted from Hernández-Monjaraz et al. (2018).

conditions. Studies have shown that they induce repair in neural, hepatic and skeletal muscle after infusion in preclinical and clinical models (Su et al. 2014; Kim and Park 2017). These characteristics make them potential candidates for tissue engineering and repair (Rohban and Pieber 2017).

The discovery of MSCs and their multipotency attributes has opened an entirely new field in medical research. This is due to the range of cells that multipotent stem cells can differentiate into (Pittenger et al. 1999). This allows the cells to be used in regenerative medicine as they can support tissue repair and differentiate, form and replace permanently lost tissue (Bussolati 2011). To be defined as MSCs, the cells must have the ability to form osteoblasts, chondroblasts and adipocytes (Dominici et al. 2006). They can be derived from bone marrow, placenta, umbilical cord blood, adipose tissue, adult muscle, corneal stroma and dental sources (Prockop 1997).

While several MSCs exist, their source tissue provides subtle differences in character and differentiation potential. For example, umbilical cord stem cells have a lower ability to form adipocytes but greater osteogenic capacity (Kern et al. 2006; Han et al. 2017). Recent advances in regenerative medicine have brought dental-derived MSCs to the fore as suitable candidates for regenerative medicine. This is also due to the fewer controversial ethical issues involving their use and their easier availability. The first MSCs isolated from dental origin were derived from the third molar dental pulp (Gronthos et al. 2000) and deciduous and periodontal ligaments (Miura et al. 2003; Seo et al. 2004).

The primary outcomes of MSCs of dental origin have been minimal. However, they have led to the cultivation and scaling up of MSCs using human platelet lysates in providing autologous settings for cell-based regenerative medicine (Govindasamy et al. 2011). Long-term cultivation has been considered for obtaining sufficient cells which retain their plasticity for therapeutic use. In addition, investigations have revealed the ability of human periodontal ligament stem cells (PDLSCs) to differentiate into hepatic cells and insulin-producing cells, indicating their propensity to differentiate into endodermal lineage (Kawanabe et al. 2010; Lee et al. 2014). On this point, MSCs of dental origin need not be limited to tooth regeneration purposes but can go beyond that. Nevertheless, many unanswered questions regarding this relatively untapped resource remain in terms of isolation, expansion, parameters for monitoring clinical efficacy and the proper biological source of dental MSCs in enough numbers for therapeutic purposes.

Another type of ASC is induced pluripotent stem cells (iPSCs). These ASCs have been changed in a lab using nuclear reprogramming methods to more resemble embryonic stem cells. Takahashi and Yamanaka (2006) were the first scientists to report that human stem cells could be changed in this way, in 2006. They successfully converted fibroblasts into pluripotent stem cells by modifying the expression of only four genes. This achievement represents the origin of iPSCs. Human iPSCs are similar to ESCs in morphology, proliferation, surface antigens, gene expression, epigenetic status of pluripotent cell-specific genes and telomerase activity. In addition, they are pluripotent and able to differentiate into all cell types from three germ layers in vitro, and capable of forming teratomas. iPSCs are somatic cells that have been reprogrammed to a pluripotent state by introducing a group of transcription factors including OCT4, SOX2, KLF4 and C-MYC into the genomes of mice (Takahashi and Yamanaka 2006) and human somatic cells (Takahashi et al. 2007). The discovery of such technology is based on the hypothesis that nuclear reprogramming is a process driven by factors that play a critical role in maintaining the pluripotency of ESCs (Takahashi and Yamanaka 2006).

The research field of induced pluripotency has grown exponentially in recent years. Efficiency, reliability and security are essential to ensure the success of these reprogramming processes. Conventional reprogramming techniques depend on the stable integration of transgenes but they can introduce the risk of insertional mutagenesis. Hence, several non-integrative reprogramming techniques have been successfully established to improve the quality of the generated MSCs (Diecke et al. 2014).

The advantage of iPS technology is that it can generate specific stem cells. A classic example was demonstrated in a study by Freund et al. (2010) who successfully generated cardiomyocytes from the skin fibroblast in a patient with hereditary haemorrhagic telangiectasia. Nevertheless, there have been a few other breakthroughs in this field. Ieda et al. (2010) used a combination of cardiac transcription factors to directly reprogram cardiac fibroblast into cardiomyocytes. Yoshida and Yamanaka (2011) proposed iPSCs as a potential source for cardiac regeneration if reprogramming efficiency can be improved and safety issues are addressed before progressing to clinical application.

5.4 Immunology of Stem Cells

In basic terms, the immune system is a collection of cells and proteins that function as protection against foreign antigens. Generally, it has two lines of defence: innate immunity and adaptive immunity. Innate immunity is the first immunological, non-specific (antigen-independent) mechanism for fighting an intruding pathogen. It is a rapid immune response, occurring within minutes or hours after aggression, and has no immunological memory. Therefore, it cannot recognise or 'memorise' the same pathogen should the body be exposed to it in the future.

On the other hand, adaptive immunity is antigen dependent and antigen specific with memory capacity. This enables the host to mount a more rapid and efficient immune response upon subsequent exposure to a similar antigen. Thus, there is much synergy between the adaptive immune system and its natural counterpart. However, they are not mutually exclusive mechanisms of host defence. Instead, they are complementary, with defects in either system resulting in host vulnerability that can provoke illness or disease (Turvey and Broide 2010; Bonilla and Oettgen 2010; Murphy et al. 2007).

The primary function of innate immunity is the recruitment of immune cells to sites of infection and inflammation through the production of cytokines which are small proteins involved in cell-to-cell communication. Cytokine production leads to the release of antibodies and other proteins and glycoproteins that activate the complement system. The complement system is a biochemical cascade that identifies and opsonises foreign antigens, rendering them susceptible to phagocytosis, a process whereby cells engulf microbes and remove cell debris. Innate immune responses also promote clearance of dead cells or antibody complexes and remove foreign substances present in the body. They can also activate adaptive immune responses through a process known as antigen presentation. Numerous cells are involved in innate immune responses, including phagocytes (macrophages and neutrophils), dendritic cells, mast cells, basophils, eosinophils, natural killer (NK) cells and lymphocytes (T cells) (Turvey and Broide 2010).

On the other hand, adaptive immunity, also referred to as acquired or specific immunity, is activated after the infection is established. The adaptive immune response is specific to the pathogen, meaning that it recognises a specific 'non-self' antigen in the presence of 'self' antigens. It then generates pathogen-specific immunological effector pathways that eliminate specific pathogens or pathogen-infected cells. Acquired immunity also develops an immunological memory after an initial response to a specific pathogen that can rapidly eliminate such a pathogen should subsequent infections occur. This process of acquired immunity is the basic principle in vaccinations as it also provides long-lasting protection. For example, persons who recover from measles are protected against it during their lifetime. Like the innate system, the acquired system includes both humoral and cell-mediated immunity components. The adaptive immune system includes T cells, which are activated through antigen-presenting cells (APCs), and B cells (Bonilla and Oettgen 2010).

An intrinsic property of multipotent stem cells is their ability to differentiate in vitro into tissue-specific cells under appropriate cellular signalling conditions. Because of this characteristic, the genetic reprogramming of somatic cells or MSCs to produce pluripotent-derived stem cells from embryonic tissues has been studied widely in clinical settings, especially in regenerative medicine (Tena and Sachs 2014). However, several limitations influence its application in a clinical setting, including delivery, cell culture differentiation and immunological rejection. Thus, understanding the properties of stem cells and the in vitro and in vivo immune responses they elicit is important for designing successful protocols to overcome these immunological limitations.

5.4.1 Immunogenicity and Immunomodulatory Effects of Stem Cells

One of the most intriguing features of MSCs, more correctly known as multipotent stem cells, is that they can facilitate tissue regeneration by differentiating into several cell types, escaping immune recognition and inhibiting immune responses. In other words, they can be used as an immune-privileged 'Band-aid' without elicitation of inflammation and immune responses (Bradley et al. 2002). Therefore, MSCs may serve as immunosuppressive agents in inflammatory and other autoimmune diseases (Rasmusson 2006). The immunomodulatory effects of MSCs seem to be achieved by multiple mechanisms inhibiting proinflammatory cells and simultaneously activating other immune cells that shift the balance toward regeneration.

Additionally, there is a possibility for their use in transplantation due to their immune-suppressive property. The immunomodulatory and anti-inflammatory effects of MSCs help deal with graft rejection and autoimmune diseases. Allogeneic MSC transplantations are possible, but the xenogeneic model results in transplant rejection (Grinnemo et al. 2004). For example, transplantation of allogeneic undifferentiated murine ESCs in the heart causes cardiac teratomas, which are immunologically rejected after several weeks. The increased inflammation and upregulation of the class I and II major histocompatibility complex (MHC) has been associated with such rejection (Nussbaum et al. 2007). Another in vivo study using differentiated ESCs transplanted into ischaemic myocardium showed an accelerated immune response compared with undifferentiated ESCs, indicating that ESC immunogenicity increases upon differentiation (Swijnenburg et al. 2005). In addition, in vitro results of studies on the expression of human leucocyte antigens (HLA) and the immunological properties of differentiated and undifferentiated MSCs show that both have immunosuppressive effects and may thus be able to be used in transplantations with minimal risk of rejection (Le Blanc et al. 2003). MSCs do not cause allogeneic or xenogeneic lymphocyte proliferation, and they interfere with B cell and dendritic cell development (Marti et al. 2011).

Mesenchymal stem cells can influence both innate and adaptive immune responses and are proven to control various immune cells such as T cells, B cells, NK cells, dendritic cells and neutrophils while stimulating T-regulatory cells (Wada et al. 2013). The effect of MSCs on innate and adaptive immunity involves the suppression of inflammatory markers such as interleukin (IL)-1-beta, tumour necrosis factor alpha and IL-6, together with an increase in protective cytokines such as IL-10, prostaglandin E2 and indoleamine 2,3 dioxygenases (IDO) (Moreira et al. 2017). These properties contribute to the low immunogenicity characteristics of MSCs. Recent findings suggest that MSCs have different immunomodulatory effects on the same types of immune cells and are influenced by the microenvironment or the state of disease. These findings show that MSCs can change their effects to protect the body in dealing with diseases under different conditions (Gao et al. 2016).

5.4.2 Mesenchymal Stem Cells and Dendritic Cells/Monocytes/Macrophages

Studies show that MSCs could promote the polarisation of monocytes/macrophages toward an anti-inflammatory/immune-regulatory (type 2) phenotype (Deng et al. 2016). Furthermore, they have been demonstrated to directly inhibit differentiation into type 1 phenotype and dendritic cells (DCs) (Jiang et al. 2005). In other words, it is generally accepted that cells produced from DC progenitors lack the proper DC phenotype and have impaired functions in the presence of MSCs, but not in control DCs (Spaggiari and Moretta 2013). Jiang et al. (2005) studied the effects of MSCs on monocyte-derived DCs, noting that mature DCs have reduced CD83 expression when treated with MSCs, thus suggesting their immature status. This was accompanied by reduced expression of presentation molecules, co-stimulatory molecules and IL-12 secretion. It was concluded that the MSCs act to suppress the differentiation of monocytes into DCs.

The polarisation of macrophages toward the type 2 phenotype can be promoted by the MSCs-secreted IL-1 receptor antagonist (IL-1-RA) (Luz-Crawford et al. 2016). The anti-inflammatory monocytes secrete a high level of IL-10. The increased production of IL-10 mediated by MSCs has been demonstrated in a sepsis model in mice. In their study, Németh et al. (2009) demonstrated that IL-10 neutralisation could reverse the beneficial effects of bone marrow-derived MSCs on overall survival in mice. In contrast, levels of IL-12p70, tumour necrosis factor (TNF)-alpha and IL-17 expression are decreased. This process is mediated by the MSC-produced IL-6 and hepatocyte growth factor (HGF) (Deng et al. 2016; Melief et al. 2013).

Besides IL-10, high levels of MHC class II, CD45R and CD11b are also expressed by MSC-primed monocytes which are capable of suppressing T-cell activity regardless of FoxP3$^+$ regulatory T cells (Tregs) (Ko et al. 2016). The formation of FoxP3$^+$ Tregs from naive CD4$^+$ T cells produces supernatants of type 2 macrophages, highlighting the role of soluble factors in MSC-mediated immunomodulation (Schmidt et al. 2016). Monocyte-induced Treg formation is mediated by monocyte-produced chemokine (C-C motif) ligand 18 (CCL-18) and monocyte-released transforming growth factor (TGF)-beta-1 (Melief et al. 2013; Schmidt et al. 2016).

During their differentiation into type 2 macrophages, they bind and re-release TGF-beta-1 macrophages, thus contributing to the Tregs' MSC-induced formation (Melief et al. 2013; Schmidt et al. 2016). MSC-induced Treg formation is significantly reduced by the neutralisation of CCL-18 (Melief et al. 2013). CCL-18 can turn memory CD4$^+$ T cells into CD4$^+$CD25$^+$Foxp3$^+$ Tregs with increased IL-10 and TGF-beta-1 production. Also, CCL-18-pretreated Tregs inhibit CD4$^+$CD25$^-$ effector T-cell proliferation via the activation of G-protein-coupled receptors (Chang et al. 2010). In addition, DCs can be differentiated into tolerogenic DCs by macrophage type 2-derived CCL-18, and are thus capable of priming Treg formation (Melief et al. 2013; de Witte et al. 2018) (Figure 5.4a).

The migration and maturation of DCs are also suppressed by MSCs (Ge et al. 2010). In the presence of MSCs, the capability of DCs to support antigen-specific CD4$^+$ T-cell proliferation and display an MHC class II–peptide complex is reduced (English et al. 2008). TNF-alpha secretion by mature type 1 DCs is also significantly reduced if co-cultured with MSCs, while anti-inflammatory mature type 2 DCs show increased secretion of IL-10 (Aggarwal and Pittenger 2005).

Braza et al. (2016) successfully demonstrated a cytokine-independent pathway for the MSC-induced polarisation of monocytes/macrophages through phagocytosis in a mouse model (Figure 5.4b). The lung macrophages phagocytosed MSCs, resulting in the monocytes transforming into a type 2 immunosuppressive phenotype (Braza et al. 2016). The depletion of phagocytic cells demonstrates their crucial role in MSC-mediated immunomodulation as the absence of monocytes, macrophages and DCs negates the ability of MSCs to suppress T-cell proliferation (Eggenhofer et al. 2011).

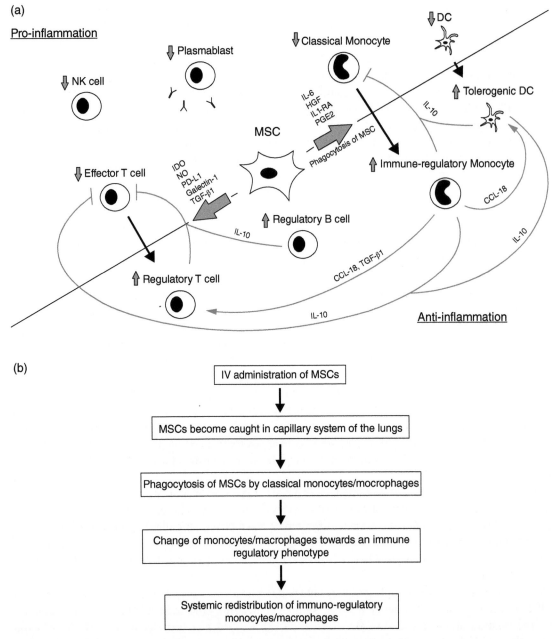

Figure 5.4 (a) Proposed interaction of MSCs with host immune cells. (b) Proposed pathway of MSC-mediated anti-inflammation via phagocytosis of MSCs by de Witte et al. (2018) and Braza et al. (2016). *Source:* Adapted from Weiss and Dahlke (2019).

5.4.3 Mesenchymal Stem Cells and T Cells

T cells have the most crucial role in the immune system. The inhibition of T-cell proliferation and cytokine production is related to the anti-inflammatory and immunosuppressive properties of MSCs (Wada et al. 2013). MSCs have been reported to block the response of naive and memory T cells towards their associated antigens. It has been suggested that MSCs physically inhibit T cell and APC contact in non-cognate interactions (Krampera et al. 2003). In other words, MSCs suppress T-cell proliferation. Several studies show that MSCs could suppress the proliferation of CD4$^+$ and CD8$^+$ T-cell subsets (Duffy et al. 2011). When interacting with DCs, MSCs can change from proinflammatory Th1 to anti-inflammatory Th2 cells, including inducing a change in the cytokine profile toward anti-inflammation (Wang et al. 2008; Ge et al. 2010). In addition, Gieseke et al. (2010) have shown that MSCs can directly inhibit the proliferation of CD4$^+$ and CD8$^+$ T cells without the presence of other immune cells, and that this process is partially mediated by MSC-derived galectin-1.

Thus, MSCs can suppress T-cell activation. At the same time, MSCs can induce an irreversible T-cell hyporesponsiveness and apoptosis via the secretion of PD-L1 (Davies et al. 2017) (Figure 5.4a).

Moreover, MSCs can control immune responses by promoting the apoptosis of activated T cells through cell-to-cell contact in the FAS ligand (FASL)/FAS-mediated death pathway. This increases the production of Tregs, leading to immune tolerance (Wang et al. 2012). The role of MSCs in facilitating the in vitro and in vivo formation of Tregs has been revealed in several studies (Aggarwal and Pittenger 2005; Ge et al. 2010). Tregs are essential for immune homeostasis as they prevent autoimmunity (Marson et al. 2007). Ge et al. (2010) demonstrated that MSCs can induce Tregs as well as playing an essential role in tolerance induction in a kidney allograft transplantation model.

The upregulation of Tregs induced by MSCs is not the result of an expansion of pre-existing natural Tregs. Instead, it is due to the induction of Tregs from conventional T cells (Engela et al. 2013; Khosravi et al. 2017). In a neutralisation study, Melief et al. (2013) showed that the generation of Tregs is TGF-beta-1 mediated and that MSCs constitutively secrete TGF-beta-1. However, the presence of monocytes was proven to be essential for the formation of Tregs as TGF-beta-1 alone seems not to be sufficient (Melief et al. 2013).

5.4.4 Mesenchymal Stem Cells and Natural Killer Cells

Natural killer cells function in the innate immune system. It has been found that MSCs can change the phenotype and arrest the growth, cytokine production and cytotoxicity of HLA class I-expressing targets through cell-to-cell contact or soluble factors (Sotiropoulou et al. 2006). In addition, human MSCs are known to reduce the secretion of interferon (IFN)-gamma from NK cells (Aggarwal and Pittenger 2005); that is, they are potent inhibitors of the proliferation of NK cells. In addition, MSCs also constrain important NK cell effector functions such as cytolytic activity and cytokine production, and this combined effect would inhibit the activities of NK cells. Several studies have shown impaired cytotoxic activity and cytokine production by NK cells after co-culture with MSCs involving MSC-secreted prostaglandin E2 (PGE2), IDO, TGF-beta-1, IL-6 and nitric oxide (NO) (Sato et al. 2007; Spaggiari et al. 2008; Deng et al. 2016) (Figure 5.4a).

5.4.5 Mesenchymal Stem Cells and B cells

B cells play a significant role in facilitating humoral immunity in the adaptive immune system, where their primary function is to secrete antibodies in response to antigens. By blocking IFN-gamma production in T cells, MSCs block the growth of B cells and the formation of plasma cells. In other words, MSCs directly interact with B cells to reduce plasmablast formation and promote the induction of regulatory B cells (Bregs) (Franquesa et al. 2015). This is augmented by the reduced production of B cell activating factor (BAFF) by DCs (Fan et al. 2016). In addition, Bregs have immunosuppressive properties through which they provide immunological tolerance (Rosser and Mauri 2015).

Carter et al. (2011) reveal that IL-10-producing Bregs could transform effector CD4[+] T cells into Foxp3[+] Tregs. Breg formation and IL-10 production stimulated by MSCs seem to depend on direct cell-to-cell contact or at least on the proximity of the corresponding cells, rather than being mediated via soluble factors (Luk et al. 2017). Nevertheless, this shows that active cell metabolism is needed to stimulate MSCs to form the Bregs and their suppressive effects on T-cell proliferation (Luk et al. 2016, 2017).

Another study demonstrated that MSC-secreted IL-1-RA could also inhibit B-cell differentiation via a cytokine-triggered mechanism (Luz-Crawford et al. 2016). Moreover, MSCs also inhibit the proliferation of B cells in the presence of T cells (Luk et al. 2017). It is postulated that this could be due to T cell-secreted IFN-gamma, as IFN-gamma pretreated MSCs can inhibit B-cell proliferation (Luk et al. 2017).

Meanwhile, Corcione et al. (2006) showed the in vitro inhibition of human MSC B-cell proliferation, differentiation and chemotaxis. B-cell proliferation was inhibited through arresting the G0/G1 phase of the cell cycle. At the same time, inhibition of B-cell differentiation was seen in the impaired production of IgM, IgG and IgA. Chemotactic properties were affected as evidenced by the CXCR4, CXCR5 and CCR7 B-cell expression, and CXCL12, the CXCR4 ligand, and CXCL13, the CXCR5 ligand, chemotaxis (Corcione et al. 2006).

5.5 Mesenchymal Stem Cell Growth Factors

Growth factors are essential for development, influencing stem cell differentiation, modulating the growth of tissues and organs during embryogenesis, and in physiological tissue repair. They can also induce differentiation for specific lineage and control tissue engineering processes for therapeutics (Casagrande et al. 2011). Unfortunately, tissue regeneration is not achievable with the number of MSCs obtainable from donors, and this is compounded by the issue of MSC survival after transplantation. However, factors that are acknowledged to control cell growth, motility, viability and morphogenesis might help deal with these issues, aside from other trophic factors. Thus, the ex vivo expansion of MSCs incorporates the use of growth factors. Aside from influencing cell proliferative and pro-survival ability, growth factors can also affect differentiation. However, they should not stimulate differentiation at an early stage as this results in low numbers of early-differentiating progenitors (Rodrigues et al. 2010).

The various functions of MSCs are attributed to the different factors secreted, including TGF-beta, HGF, primary fibroblast growth factor (FGF) and vascular endothelial growth factor (VEGF), which promote cell proliferation and angiogenesis, especially of fibroblasts and epithelial or endothelial cells. In addition, insulin growth factor (IGF) 1, IL-6 and stanniocalcin-1 play an apoptotic role in fibroblasts. At the same time, VEGF, HGF and TGF-beta-1 can protect endothelial cells from apoptosis (Pers et al. 2015). Furthermore, MSCs appear to express cytokines such as TGF-beta, VEGF, epidermal growth factor (EGF) and various other molecules that can induce tissue repair (Freitag et al. 2016).

Rodrigues et al. (2010) gave three essential criteria for choosing growth factors for MSC proliferation and expansion. The first is the need for the growth factor to lengthen proliferation for several population doublings to produce a significant number of MSCs before undergoing differentiation. The second is the ability of the growth factor to be a substitute for an animal serum for proliferation to remove the use of xenographic substances and decrease the chances of variability. The third is the requirement of modes for localised and controlled delivery to maintain the mitogenic and protective signals for preventing the uncontrolled proliferation of MSCs.

Expression of various growth factors such as the platelet-derived growth factor (PDGF), essential fibroblast growth factor and VEGF in the normal state or as a response to toxic stimuli such as injury or hypoxia is related to paracrine-mediated angiogenesis of dental pulp stem cells (DPSCs) (Marei and Backly 2018). Osathanon et al. (2014) compared the effects of chemical and growth factor induction protocols on the neurogenic differentiation of DPSCs. The chemical induction protocol failed to enhance the expression of neuronal mRNA. However, the growth factor induction protocol incorporating FGF resulted in an increase in neurogenic markers for mRNA and protein, with increases in gamma-aminobutyric acid receptor expression indicating the neuronal-like function of the cells. Thus, the study concluded that the growth factor protocol is preferable to chemical induction for studying the neuronal differentiation of DPSCs.

5.6 Conclusion

Innate immunity is the first immunological mechanism activated to fight against infectious agents. It is a rapid immune response and occurs minutes or hours after aggression by pathogens. This is followed by adaptive immunity to eliminate pathogens. A unique feature of adaptive immunity is its ability to develop immunological memory to 'record' its experiences with various pathogens. This leads to effective and rapid immune responses upon subsequent exposure to similar pathogens. There is a significant synergy between the adaptive immune system and its innate counterpart, and defects in either can lead to immunopathological disorders.

Although stem cell application as an alternative treatment in clinical settings remains in its infancy, there has been substantial progress in research-related stem cells over the past decade. Factors such as delivery methods, cell culture differentiation and immunological rejection need to be fully understood and explored to provide insights for the successful utilisation of multipotent stem cells in clinical settings.

References

Aggarwal, S. and Pittenger, M.F. (2005). Human mesenchymal stem cells modulate allogeneic immune cell responses. *Blood* 105 (4): 1815–1822.

Berdasco, M. and Esteller, M. (2011). DNA methylation in stem cell renewal and multipotency. *Stem Cell Res. Ther.* 2 (5): 42.

Beyer Nardi, N. and da Silva Meirelles, L. (2006). Mesenchymal stem cells: isolation, in vitro expansion and characterization. *Hand. Exp. Pharmacol.* 174: 249–282.

Bianchi, G., Muraglia, A., Daga, A., Corte, G., Cancedda, R. and Quarto, R. (2001). Microenvironment and stem properties of bone marrow-derived mesenchymal cells. *Wound Repair Regen.* 9 (6): 460–466.

Bongso, A. and Richards, M. (2004). History and perspective of stem cell research. *Best Pract. Res. Clin. Obstet. Gynaecol.* 18 (6): 827–842.

Bonilla, F.A. and Oettgen, H.C. (2010). Adaptive immunity. *J. Allergy Clin. Immunol.* 125 (2): S33–40.

Bradley, J.A., Bolton, E.M. and Pedersen, R.A. (2002). Stem cell medicine encounters the immune system. *Nat. Rev. Immunol.* 2 (11): 859–871.

Braza, F., Dirou, S., Forest, V. et al. (2016). Mesenchymal stem cells induce suppressive macrophages through phagocytosis in a mouse model of asthma. *Stem Cells* 34 (7): 1836–1845.

Brevini, T.A., Tosetti, V., Crestan, M., Antonini, S. and Gandolfi, F. (2007). Derivation and characterization of pluripotent cell lines from pig embryos of different origins. *Theriogenology* 67 (1): 54–63.

Bussolati, B. (2011). Stem cells for organ repair. *Organogenesis* 7 (2): 95–95.

Caplan, A.I. (1991). Mesenchymal stem cells. *J. Orthopaed. Res.* 9 (5): 641–650.

Carter, N.A., Vasconcellos, R., Rosser, E.C. et al. (2011). Mice lacking endogenous IL-10-producing regulatory B cells develop exacerbated disease and present with an increased frequency of Th1/Th17 but a decrease in regulatory T cells. *J. Immunol.* 186 (10): 5569–5579.

Casagrande, L., Cordeiro, M.M., Nör, S.A. and Nör, J.E. (2011). Dental pulp stem cells in regenerative dentistry. *Odontology* 99 (1): 1–7.

Cawthorn, W.P., Scheller, E.L. and MacDougald, O.A. (2012). Adipose tissue stem cells: the great WAT hope. *Trends Endocrinol Metab* 23 (6): 270–277.

Chang, Y., de Nadai, P., Azzaoui, I. et al. (2010). The chemokine CCL18 generates adaptive regulatory T cells from memory CD4+ T cells of healthy but not allergic subjects. *FASEB J.* 24 (12): 5063–5072.

Corcione, A., Benvenuto, F., Ferretti, E. et al. (2006). Human mesenchymal stem cells modulate B-cell functions. *Blood* 107: 367–372.

Davies, L.C., Heldring, N., Kadri, N. and Le Blanc, K. (2017). Mesenchymal stromal cell secretion of programmed death-1 ligands regulates T cell mediated immunosuppression. *Stem Cells* 35 (3): 766–776.

Deng, Y., Zhang, Y., Ye, L. et al. (2016). Umbilical cord-derived mesenchymal stem cells instruct monocytes towards an IL10- producing phenotype by secreting IL6 and HGF. *Sci. Rep.* 6: 37566.

deWitte, S.F.H., Luk, F., Sierra Parraga, J.M. et al. (2018). Immunomodulation by therapeutic mesenchymal stromal cells (MSC) is triggered through phagocytosis of MSC by monocytic cells. *Stem Cells* 36 (4): 602–615.

Diecke, S., Jung, S.M., Lee, J. and Ju, J.H. (2014). Recent technological updates and clinical applications of induced pluripotent stem cells. *Korean J. Intern. Med.* 29 (5): 547–557.

Dominici, M., Le Blanc, K., Mueller, I. et al. (2006). Minimal criteria for defining multipotent mesenchymal stromal cells. The International Society for Cellular Therapy position statement. *Cytotherapy* 8 (4): 315–317.

Duffy, M.M., Ritter, T., Ceredig, R. and Griffin, M.D. (2011). Mesenchymal stem cell effects on T-cell effector pathways. *Stem Cell Res. Ther.* 2 (4): 34.

Eggenhofer, E., Steinmann, J.F., Renner, P. et al. (2011). Mesenchymal stem cells together with mycophenolate mofetil inhibit antigen presenting cell and T cell infiltration into allogeneic heart grafts. *Transplant Immunol.* 24 (3): 157–163.

Egusa, H., Sonoyama, W., Nishimura, M., Atsuta, I. and Akiyama, K. (2012). Stem cells in dentistry – Part I: Stem cell sources. *J. Prosthodont. Res.* 56 (3): 151–165.

Engela, A.U., Hoogduijn, M.J., Boer, K. et al. (2013). Human adipose tissue derived mesenchymal stem cells induce functional de-novo regulatory T cells with methylated FOXP3 gene DNA. *Clin. Exp. Immunol.* 173 (2): 343–354.

English, K., Barry, F.P. and Mahon, B.P. (2008). Murine mesenchymal stem cells suppress dendritic cell migration, maturation, and antigen presentation. *Immunol. Lett.* 115 (1): 50–58.

Evans, M.J. and Kaufman, M.H. (1981). Establishment in culture of pluripotential cells from mouse embryos. *Nature* 292 (5819): 154–156.

Evans, M.J., Notarianni, E., Laurie, S. and Moor, R.M. (1990). Derivation and preliminary characterization of pluripotent cell lines from porcine and bovine blastocysts. *Theriogenology* 33 (1): 125–128.

Fan, L.X., Hu, C.X., Chen, J.J., Cen, P.P., Wang, J. and Li, L.J. (2016). Interaction between mesenchymal stem cells and B-cells. *Int. J. Molec. Sci.* 17 (5): 650.

Filioli Uranio, M., Valentini, L., Lange-Consiglio, A. et al. (2011). Isolation, proliferation, cytogenetic, and molecular characterization and in vitro differentiation potency of canine stem cells from foetal adnexa: a comparative study of amniotic fluid, amnion, and umbilical cord matrix. *Molec. Reprod. Dev.* 78 (5): 361–373.

Forbes, S., Vig, P., Poulsom, R., Thomas, H. and Alison, M. (2002). Hepatic stem cells. *J. Pathol.* 197 (4): 510–518.

Franquesa, M., Mensah, F.K., Huizinga, R. et al. (2015). Human adipose tissue-derived mesenchymal stem cells abrogate plasma blast formation and induce regulatory B cells independently of T helper cells. *Stem Cells* 33 (3): 880–891.

Freitag, J., Bates, D., Boyd, R. et al. (2016). Mesenchymal stem cell therapy in the treatment of osteoarthritis: reparative pathways, safety and efficacy – a review. *BMC Musculoskel. Disord.* 17: 230.

Freund, C., Davis, R. P., Gkatzis, K., Ward-van Oostwaard, D. and Mummery, C. L. (2010). The first reported generation of human induced pluripotent stem cells (iPS cells) and iPS cell-derived cardiomyocytes in the Netherlands. *Netherlands Heart J.* 18 (1): 51–54.

Gage F.H. (2000). Mammalian neural stem cells. *Science* 287 (5457): 1433–1438.

Gao, F., Chiu, S.M., Motan, D.A. et al. (2016). Mesenchymal stem cells and immunomodulation: current status and future prospects. *Cell Death Dis.* 7 (1): e2062.

Ge, W., Jiang, J., Arp, J., Liu, W., Garcia, B. and Wang, H. (2010). Regulatory T-cell generation and kidney allograft tolerance induced by mesenchymal stem cells associated with indoleamine 2,3-dioxygenase expression. *Transplantation* 90 (12): 1312–1320.

Gieseke, F., Böhringer, J., Bussolari, R., Dominici, M., Handgretinger, R. and Müller, I. (2010). Human multipotent mesenchymal stromal cells use galectin-1 to inhibit immune effector cells. *Blood* 116 (19): 3770–3779.

Govindasamy, V., Ronald, V.S., Abdullah, A.N. et al. (2011). Differentiation of dental pulp stem cells into islet-like aggregates. *J. Dent. Res.* 90 (5): 646–652.

Grinnemo, K. H., Månsson, A., Dellgren, G. et al. (2004). Xenoreactivity and engraftment of human mesenchymal stem cells transplanted into infarcted rat myocardium. *J. Thorac. Cardiovasc. Surg.* 127 (5): 1293–1300.

Gronthos, S., Mankani, M., Brahim, J., Robey, P.G. and Shi, S. (2000). Postnatal human dental pulp stem cells (DPSCs) in vitro and in vivo. *Proc. Natl Acad. Sci. USA* 97 (25): 13625–13630.

Guleria, M., Dua, H., Rohila, S. and Sharma, A.K. (2014). Stem cells in dentistry. *Indian J. Dent. Sci.* 6 (4): 107–111.

Han, I., Kwon, B.S., Park, H.K. and Kim, K.S. (2017). Differentiation potential of mesenchymal stem cells is related to their intrinsic mechanical properties. *Int. Neurourol. J.* 21 (Suppl 1): S24–S31.

Hernández-Monjaraz, B., Santiago-Osorio, E., Monroy-García, A., Ledesma-Martínez, E. and Mendoza-Núñez, V.M. (2018). Mesenchymal stem cells of dental origin for inducing tissue regeneration in periodontitis: a mini-review. *Int. J. Molec. Sci.* 19 (4): 944.

Ieda, M., Fu, J. D., Delgado-Olguin, P. et al. (2010). Direct reprogramming of fibroblasts into functional cardiomyocytes by defined factors. *Cell* 142 (3): 375–386.

Jiang, X.X., Zhang, Y., Liu, B. et al. (2005). Human mesenchymal stem cells inhibit differentiation and function of monocyte-derived dendritic cells. *Blood* 105 (10): 4120–4126.

Kawanabe, N., Murata, S., Murakami, K. et al. (2010). Isolation of multipotent stem cells in human periodontal ligament using stage-specific embryonic antigen-4. *Differentiation* 79 (2): 74–83.

Kern, S., Eichler, H., Stoeve, J., Klüter, H. and Bieback, K. (2006). Comparative analysis of mesenchymal stem cells from bone marrow, umbilical cord blood, or adipose tissue. *Stem Cells* 24 (5): 1294–1301.

Khosravi, M., Karimi, M.H., Hossein Aghdaie, M., Kalani, M., Naserian, S. and Bidmeshkipour, A. (2017). Mesenchymal stem cells can induce regulatory T cells via modulating miR-126a but not miR-10a. *Gene* 627: 327–336.

Kim, H.J. and Park, J.S. (2017). Usage of human mesenchymal stem cells in cell-based therapy: advantages and disadvantages. *Dev. Reprod.* 21 (1): 1–10.

Ko, J.H., Lee, H.J., Jeong, H.J. et al. (2016). Mesenchymal stem/stromal cells precondition lung monocytes/macrophages to produce tolerance against allo- and autoimmunity in the eye. *Proc. Natl Acad. Sci. USA* 113 (1): 158–163.

Krampera, M., Glennie, S., Dyson, J. et al. (2003). Bone marrow mesenchymal stem cells inhibit the response of naive and memory antigen-specific T cells to their cognate peptide. *Blood* 101 (9): 3722–3729.

Le Blanc, K. (2003). Immunomodulatory effects of fetal and adult mesenchymal stem cells. *Cytotherapy* 5 (6): 485–489.

Lee, J.S., An, S.Y., Kwon, I.K. and Heo, J.S. (2014). Trans differentiation of human periodontal ligament stem cells into pancreatic cell lineage. *Cell Biochem. Function* 32: 605–611.

Luk, F., de Witte, S.F., Korevaar, S.S. et al. (2016). Inactivated mesenchymal stem cells maintain immunomodulatory capacity. *Stem Cells Dev.* 25 (18): 1342–1354.

Luk, F., Carreras-Planella, L., Korevaar, S.S. et al. (2017). Inflammatory conditions dictate the effect of mesenchymal stem or stromal cells on B cell function. *Front. Immunol.* 8: 1042.

Luz-Crawford, P., Djouad, F., Toupet, K. et al. (2016). Mesenchymal stem cell-derived interleukin 1 receptor antagonist promotes macrophage polarization and inhibits B cell differentiation. *Stem Cells* 34 (2): 483–492.

Malaver-Ortega, L.F., Sumer, H., Liu, J. and Verma, P.J. (2012). The state of the art for pluripotent stem cells derivation in domestic ungulates. *Theriogenology* 78 (8): 1749–1762.

Marei, M.K. and Backly, R.M.E. (2018). Dental mesenchymal stem cell-based translational regenerative dentistry: from artificial to biological replacement. *Front. Bioeng. Biotechnol.* 6: 49.

Marson, A., Kretschmer, K., Frampton, G.M. et al. (2007). Foxp3 occupancy and regulation of key target genes during T-cell stimulation. *Nature* 445 (7130): 931–935.

Marti, L.C., Ribeiro, A.A.F. and Hamerschlak, N. (2011). Immunomodulatory effect of mesenchymal stem cells. *Einstein J. Biol. Med.* 9 (2 Pt.1): 224–228.

Melief, S.M., Geutskens, S.B., Fibbe, W.E. and Roelofs, H. (2013). Multipotent stromal cells skew monocytes towards an anti-inflammatory interleukin-10-producing phenotype by production of interleukin-6. *Haematologica* 98 (6): 888–895.

Mitalipov, S. and Wolf, D. (2009). Totipotency, pluripotency and nuclear reprogramming. *Adv. Biochem Eng. Biotechnol.* 114: 185–199.

Miura, M., Gronthos, S., Zhao, M. et al. (2003). SHED: Stem cells from human exfoliated deciduous teeth. *Proc. Natl Acad. Sci. USA* 100 (10): 5807–5812.

Moreira, A., Kahlenberg, S. and Hornsby, P. (2017). Therapeutic potential of mesenchymal stem cells for diabetes. *J. Molec. Endocrinol.* 59 (3): R109–R120.

Murphy, K.M., Travers, P. and Walport, M. (2007). *Janeway's Immunobiology*, 7e. New York: Garland Science.

Németh, K., Leelahavanichkul, A., Yuen, P.S. et al. (2009). Bone marrow stromal cells attenuate sepsis via prostaglandin E (2)-dependent reprogramming of host macrophages to increase their interleukin-10 production. *Nat. Med.* 15 (1): 42–49.

Nussbaum, J., Minami, E., Laflamme, M.A. et al. (2007). Transplantation of undifferentiated murine embryonic stem cells in the heart: teratoma formation and immune response. *FASEB J.* 21 (7): 1345–1357.

Osathanon, T., Sawangmake, C., Nowwarote, N. and Pavasant, P. (2014). Neurogenic differentiation of human dental pulp stem cells using different induction protocols. *Oral Dis.* 20 (4): 352–358.

Pers, Y.M., Ruiz, M., Noel, D. and Jorgensen, C. (2015). Mesenchymal stem cells for the management of inflammation in osteoarthritis: state of the art and perspectives. *Osteoarthritis Cartilage* 23 (11): 2027–2035.

Pittenger, M.F., Mackay, A.M., Beck, S.C. et al. (1999). Multilineage potential of adult human mesenchymal stem cells. *Science* 284 (5411): 143–147.

Potten, C.S. (1998). Stem cells in gastrointestinal epithelium: numbers, characteristics, and death. *Phil. Trans. Roy. Soc. London B Biol. Sci.* 353 (1370): 821–830.

Prockop, D.J. (1997). Marrow stromal cells as stem cells for nonhematopoietic tissues. *Science* 276 (5309): 71–74.

Rasmusson, I. (2006). Immune modulation by mesenchymal stem cells. *Exp. Cell Res.* 312 (12): 2169–2179.

Rimondini, L. and Mele, S. (2009). Stem cell technologies for tissue regeneration in dentistry. *Minerva Stomatol.* 58 (10): 483–500.

Rodrigues, M., Griffith, L.G. and Wells, A. (2010). Growth factor regulation of proliferation and survival of multipotential stromal cells. *Stem Cell Res. Ther.* 1 (4): 32.

Rohban, R. and Pieber, T.R. (2017). Mesenchymal stem and progenitor cells in regeneration: tissue specificity and regenerative potential. *Stem Cells Int.* 2017: 5173732.

Rosser, E.C. and Mauri, C. (2015). Regulatory B cells: origin, phenotype, and function. *Immunity* 42 (4): 607–612.

Sato, K., Ozaki, K., Oh, I. et al. (2007). Nitric oxide plays a critical role in suppression of T-cell proliferation by mesenchymal stem cells. *Blood* 109 (1): 228–234.

Schmidt, A., Zhang, X.M., Joshi, R.N. et al. (2016). Human macrophages induce CD4(+) Foxp3(+) regulatory T cells via binding and re-release of TGF-β. *Immunol. Cell Biol.* 94 (8): 747–762.

Seo, B.M., Miura, M., Gronthos, S. et al. (2004). Investigation of multipotent postnatal stem cells from human periodontal ligament. *Lancet* 364 (9429): 149–155.

Shenghui, H.E., Nakada, D. and Morrison, S.J. (2009). Mechanisms of stem cell self-renewal. *Annu. Rev. Cell Dev. Biol.* 25: 377–406.

Slack, J.M. (2008). Origin of stem cells in organogenesis. *Science* 322 (5907): 1498–1501.

Sotiropoulou, P.A., Perez, S.A., Gritzapis, A.D., Baxevanis, C.N. and Papamichail, M. (2006). Interactions between human mesenchymal stem cells and natural killer cells. *Stem Cells* 24 (1): 74–85.

Spaggiari, G.M. and Moretta, M. (2013). Cellular and molecular interactions of mesenchymal stem cells in innate immunity. *Immunol. Cell Biol.* 91 (1): 27–31.

Spaggiari, G.M., Capobianco, A., Abdelrazik, H., Becchetti, F., Mingari, M.C. and Moretta, L. (2008). Mesenchymal stem cells inhibit natural killer cell proliferation, cytotoxicity, and cytokine production: role of indoleamine 2, 3-dioxygenase and prostaglandin E2. *Blood* 111(3): 1327–1333.

Su, X.W., Broach, J.R., Connor, J.R., Gerhard, G.S. and Simmons, Z. (2014). Genetic heterogeneity of amyotrophic lateral sclerosis: implications for clinical practice and research. *Muscle Nerve* 49 (6): 786–803.

Swijnenburg, R.J., Tanaka, M., Vogel, H. et al. (2005). Embryonic stem cell immunogenicity increases upon differentiation after transplantation into ischemic myocardium. *Circulation* 112 (9 Suppl): I166–I172.

Takahashi, K. and Yamanaka, S. (2006). Induction of pluripotent stem cells from mouse embryonic and adult fibroblast cultures by defined factors. *Cell* 126 (6): 663–676.

Takahashi, K., Tanabe, K., Ohnuki, M. et al. (2007). Induction of pluripotent stem cells from adult human fibroblasts by defined factors. *Cell* 131 (5): 861–872.

Telles, P.D., Machado, M.A., Sakai, V.T. and Nör, J.E. (2011). Pulp tissue from primary teeth: new source of stem cells. *J. Appl. Oral Sci.* 19 (3): 189–194.

Tena, A. and Sachs, D.H. (2014). Stem cells: immunology and immunomodulation. *Dev. Ophthalmol.* 53: 122–132.

Thomson, J.A., Itskovitz-Eldor, J., Shapiro, S.S. et al. (1998). Embryonic stem cell lines derived from human blastocysts. *Science* 282 (5391): 1145–1147.

Turvey, S.E. and Broide, D.H. (2010). Innate immunity. *J. Allergy Clin. Immunol.* 125 (2 Suppl 2): S24–S32.

Verfaillie, C.M., Pera, M.F. and Lansdorp, P.M. (2002). Stem cells: hype and reality. *Hematology Am. Soc. Hematol. Educ. Program*, 369–391.

Wada, N., Gronthos, S. and Bartold, P.M. (2013). Immunomodulatory effects of stem cells. *Periodontology* 2000 (63): 198–216.

Wang, L., Zhao, Y. and Shi, S. (2012). Interplay between mesenchymal stem cells and lymphocytes: implications for immunotherapy and tissue regeneration. *J. Dent. Res.* 91 (11): 1003–1010.

Wang, Q., Sun, B., Wang, D. et al. (2008). Murine bone marrow mesenchymal stem cells cause mature dendritic cells to promote T-cell tolerance. *Scand. J. Immunol.* 68 (6): 607–615.

Watt, F.M. (1998). Epidermal stem cells: markers, patterning and the control of stem cell fate. *Phil. Trans. Roy. Soc. London B Biol. Sci.* 353 (1370): 831–837.

Weiss, A. and Dahlke, M.H. (2019). Immunomodulation by mesenchymal stem cells (MSCs): Mechanisms of action of living, apoptotic, and dead MSCs. *Front. Immunol.* 10: 1191.

Weissman, I.L. (2000). Translating stem and progenitor cell biology to the clinic: barriers and opportunities. *Science* 287 (5457): 1442–1446.

Yoshida, Y. and Yamanaka, S. (2011). iPS cells: a source of cardiac regeneration. *J. Molec. Cell. Cardiol.* 50 (2): 327–332.

Zomer, H.D., Vidane, A.S., Gonçalves, N.N. and Ambrósio, C.E. (2015). Mesenchymal and induced pluripotent stem cells: general insights and clinical perspectives. *Stem Cells Clon. Adv. Appl.* 8: 125–134.

6

Trace Elements in Oral Immunology

Wan Izlina Wan-Ibrahim, Zamri Radzi and Noor Azlin Yahya

Universiti Malaya, Kuala Lumpur, Malaysia

6.1 Minerals and Trace Elements

A mineral is a naturally occurring element of an inorganic solid or chemical compound that is normally crystalline and formed as a result of a geological process (Nickel 1995). Besides being water soluble, a mineral has a definite chemical composition and an ordered internal structure. Certain minerals such as calcium, sodium, potassium, chlorine, magnesium and phosphorus are required by the body in larger amounts (more than 100 mg/day), and are hence known as macronutrients. On the other hand, the term 'trace element' is used based on the prevailing concentration in the body, where the minerals are required in smaller amounts (below 100 mg/day for adults). These consist of transition elements, namely vanadium, chromium, manganese, iron, cobalt, copper, zinc and molybdenum, and non-metal elements, namely selenium, fluorine and iodine (Mehmet Sinan 2018).

Based on nutritional significance, the World Health Organization (WHO) classified the trace elements into three categories: (i) essential trace elements (iodine, zinc, selenium, copper, molybdenum, chromium); (ii) trace elements that are probably essential (manganese, silicon, nickel, boron, vanadium); and (iii) potentially toxic elements, some possibly with essential functions (fluoride, lead, cadmium, mercury, arsenic, aluminium, lithium, stannum) (WHO 1996). However, according to Frieden's classification, elements are divided into three groups, based on the amount found in tissues (Frieden 1985). Earlier, Frieden's categorical classification of elements divided 29 elements that are present in the human body into five major groups (Frieden 1974).

Human serum seems to harbor at least 14 elements, namely copper, zinc, selenium, iron, strontium, molybdenum, manganese, lead, arsenic, chromium, cobalt, vanadium, cadmium and rubidium (Liu et al. 2017). However, the human salivary composition of elements varies from that of serum in terms of types and amount. Saliva mostly contains chromium, copper, iron, manganese, rubidium and zinc, along with other elements such as calcium, potassium, magnesium, sodium, nickel, plumbum, phosphate and sulfur (Ruiz Roca et al. 2019). These micronutrients are imperative to maintain a healthy status by aiding various biological functions and metabolic processes, including forming the body's defence system. However, deficiency or excess of trace elements may cause detrimental effects on human health.

The difference between the toxic level and optimal intake of trace elements varies from one to another. Trace elements can be acquired by the human body via various routes, such as food, drinking water, inhalation of air and dermal contact. Table 6.1 lists the recommended daily intake (RDI), recommended dietary allowance (RDA), tolerable upper intake level and dietary sources of some essential trace elements.

The bioavailability and utilisation of trace elements depend on intrinsic or physiological variables attributed to their absorptive process and metabolic interactions, as well as extrinsic or dietary variables related to the solubility and mobility of the trace elements within the food and the mucosal uptake in the gut lumen (WHO 1996). Understanding the relationship between bioavailability and utilisation of trace elements is important to identify and regulate the risk of deficiency or excess.

Immunology for Dentistry, First Edition. Edited by Mohammad Tariqur Rahman, Wim Teughels and Richard J. Lamont.

Table 6.1 Daily requirement of trace elements.

Trace element	Recommended daily intake (RDI)	Recommended dietary allowance (RDA)	Tolerable upper intake level	Dietary sources
Selenium	70 µg	Children 1 to 3 years old: 20 µg/day; 4 to 8 years old: 30 µg/day; 9 to 13 years old: 40 µg/day Adults and children 14 years old and above: 55 µg /day Pregnancy: 60 µg /day Lactation: 70 µg /day	The safe upper limit for selenium is 400 µg a day in adults	Liver, kidney, seafood, muscle meat, cereal, cereal products, dairy products, fruits and vegetables
Iron	18 mg	Children 1 to 3 years old: 7 mg/day; 4 to 8 years old: 10 mg/day; 9 to 13 years old: 8 mg/day Boys 14 to 18 years old: 11 mg/day Girls 14 to 18 years old: 15 mg/day Adults: 8 mg/day for men aged 19 and older and women aged 51 and older Women 19 to 50 years old: 18 mg/day Pregnancy: 27 mg/day Lactation: 10 mg/day	Infants and children from birth to the age of 13: 40 mg/day Children aged 14 and adults (including pregnancy and lactation): 45 mg/day	Haem iron: liver, meat, poultry, fish Non-haem iron: cereals, green leafy vegetables, legumes, nuts, oilseeds, jaggery, dried fruits
Copper	2 mg	Children 1 to 3 years old: 340 µg /day; 4 to 8 years old: 440 µg/day; 9 to 13 years old: 700 µg/day; 14 to 18 years old: 890 µg/day Men and women aged 19 years and older: 900 µg/day Pregnancy: 1000 µg/day Lactation: 1300 µg/day	Children 1 to 3 years old: 1 mg/day; 4 to 8 years old: 3 mg/day; 9 to 13 years old: 5 mg/day; 14 to 18 years old: 8 mg/day Adults 19 years old and above (including lactation): 10 mg/day Pregnancy: 8 mg/day	Oysters, other shellfish, whole grains, beans, nuts, potatoes, organ meats (kidney, liver), dark leafy greens, dried fruits, yeast
Zinc	15 mg	Infants and children 7 months old to 3 years old: 3 mg/day; 4 to 8 years old: 5 mg/day; 9 to 13 years old: 8 mg/day Girls 14 to 18 years old: 9 mg/day Boys and men aged 14 and older: 11 mg/day Women 19 years old and above: 8 mg/day Pregnant women: 11 mg/day Lactating women: 12 mg/day	Infants: 4-5 mg/day Children 1 to 3 years old: 7 mg/day; 4 to 8 years old: 12 mg/day; 9 to 13 years old: 23 mg/day; 14 to 18 years old: 34 mg/day Adults 19 years old and above (including pregnancy and lactation): 40 mg/day	Animal food: meat, milk, fish The bioavailability of zinc in vegetable food is low
Cobalt	6 µg	Infants: 0.5 µg Children 1–3 years old: 0.9 µg; 4–8 years old: 1.2 µg; 9–13 years old: 1.8 µg Older children and adults: 2.4 µg Pregnancy: 2.6 µg Lactation: 2.8 µg	Not known	Fish, nuts, green leafy vegetables (broccoli, spinach), cereals, oats

Element	Amount	Age-based requirements	Toxicity / Upper levels	Best sources
Chromium	120 µg	Children 1 to 3 years old: 11 µg; 4 to 8 years old: 15 µg; Boys 9 to 13 years old: 25 µg; Men 14 to 50 years old: 35 µg; Men 51 years old and above: 30 µg; Girls 9 to 13 years old: 21 µg; 14 to 18 years old: 24 µg; Women 19 to 50 years old: 25 µg; 51 years old and above: 20 µg; Pregnancy: 30 µg; Lactation: 45 µg	Doses larger than 200 µg are toxic	Best sources: processed meats, whole grains, spices
Molybdenum	75 µg	Children 1 to 3 years old: 17 µg/day; 4 to 8 years old: 22 µg/day; 9 to 13 years old: 34 µg/day; 14 to 18 years old: 43 µg/day; Men and women aged 19 years and above: 45 µg/day; Pregnancy and lactation: 50 µg/day	Children: 300–600 µg /day; Adults (including pregnancy and lactation): 1100–2000 µg /day	Animal food: liver; vegetables: lentils, dried peas, kidney beans, soybeans, oats, barley
Fluorine	In drinking water: 0.5 to 0.8 mg	Children 1 to 3 years old: 0.7mg; 4 to 8 years old: 1 mg; 9 to 13 years old: 2 mg; 14 to 18 years old: 3 mg; Men 19 years old and above: 4 mg; Women 14 years old and above (including pregnancy or lactation): 3 mg	0.7–9 mg for infants; 1.3 mg for children 1 to 3 years of age; 2.2 mg for children 4 to 8 years old; 10 mg for children above 8 years old, adults, and pregnancy and lactation	Drinking water, foods (sea fish and cheese), tea

Source: Adapted from Bhattacharya et al. (2016).

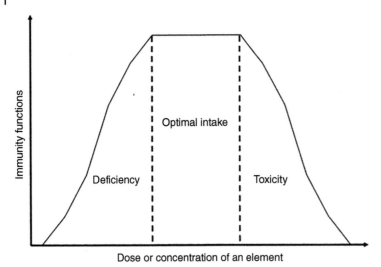

Figure 6.1 Typical dose–response curve for essential trace elements.

6.2 Homeostasis of Trace Elements and Immunity

The human body keeps a delicate balance of redox modulations by homeostatic regulation of the amount of trace elements and minerals. Imbalance, caused by either deficiency or overload disorders, could lead to oxidative stress and deleterious effects on the ability to maintain a healthy immune system (Laur et al. 2020). Disturbances in the homeostatic regulation of trace elements may lead to the development of various pathological states and diseases (Mehri 2020). It is of paramount importance to regulate the immune response to prevent excessive reactions that could lead to autoimmunity and chronic inflammation (Huang et al. 2012). The window of optimal performance or effects of trace elements is often depicted as a dose–response curve as in Figure 6.1.

In general, the homeostasis of trace elements depends on four principal mechanisms: absorption, distribution, biotransformation and excretion of the elements (Grochowski et al. 2019; Zheng and Monnot 2012). The homeostasis of certain trace elements is also dependent on the bioavailability of other minerals and other dietary factors. For example, zinc and copper have mutual antagonistic effects, where an increase in zinc will decrease the level of copper, and vice versa. In zinc-deficient rats, significant changes were observed in the excretion, reabsorption and redistribution of not only copper but the other 11 minerals and trace elements, including iron, selenium and zinc itself (Yu et al. 2019).

6.3 Effects of Minerals and Trace Elements on Immune Response

Micronutrients and other associated co-factors have been found to significantly modulate the immune response. This synergistic relationship works by enhancing the body's resistance to diseases. Deficiency and excess of micronutrients impact the function of the immune system by affecting the innate immune system and adaptive antibody responses (Alpert 2017; Maggini et al. 2007). Dysregulation of the immune response increases the susceptibility of the host to infections, where an increase in morbidity and mortality is evident (Maggini et al. 2007).

Trace elements play various biological roles (Table 6.2) but their most predominant function in the human body is as co-factors and/or catalysts in the enzyme system. Trace elements work synergistically with vitamins too, contributing to the body's natural defence system by supporting physical barriers (maintenance of skin and mucosa layer), cellular immunity and antibody production (Maggini et al. 2007). It has been shown that deficiency in certain vitamins, minerals and trace elements such as vitamins A, C, D, E, B6, B12, iron, selenium, copper and zinc in humans and animals could alter the body's immunocompetence (Alpert 2017; Beck 1999; Wintergerst et al. 2007).

6.3.1 Selenium (Se)

Selenium has active roles in many crucial cellular processes involving both the innate and acquired immune response. Dietary Se, where the predominant ingested form exists as selenomethionine, can be contributed by the consumption of grains, vegetables, fruits, seafood, dairy products, muscle meat, liver and kidney (Bhattacharya et al. 2016). Depending on

Table 6.2 Major biological functions of trace elements.

Trace element	Major biological functions
Selenium	Regulation of redox reactions
	Cellular functions and maintenance
	Oxidant defence enzymes
	Immunity
Magnesium	Enzyme co-factor
	Physiological calcium antagonist
	Involved in vitamin metabolism
	Synthesis of hormones, proteins, nucleic acids
Iron	Oxygen transport
	Respiration
	Amino acid and lipid metabolism
	Redox reactions
	Immune cell proliferation and maturation
Manganese	Enzyme co-factor
	Bone metabolism
	Protein, lipid and carbohydrate metabolism
	Immunity
Copper	Enzyme co-factor
	Energy production
	Iron metabolism
	Connective tissue maturation
	Neurotransmission
	Cell activation
	Immunity
Zinc	Protein, lipid and carbohydrate metabolism
	Bone metabolism
	Regulation of cell cycle and cell division
	Immunity

the average Se status of the population and the biological state of the individual, the RDI of Se ranges from 55 to 75 µg. A lactating mother, however, generally requires a higher amount of Se (Avery and Hoffmann 2018). In 2019, dos Santos et al. carried out a systematic review to identify and map the global status of urinary Se in healthy children. It was concluded that urinary Se is pertinent to one's health, and it ranges from 7.7 to 145 µg/l (dos Santos et al. 2019). However, the cut-off value in the child population is yet to be confirmed (Campos et al. 2021).

The incorporation of Se into selenoproteins reflects its role in the regulation of redox reactions, oxidative stress, antioxidant functions and inflammation. Furthermore, Se is also involved in several physiological systems including the central nervous system, male reproductive system, endocrine system, muscle function and cardiovascular system (Avery and Hoffmann 2018; Hoffmann and Berry 2008; Huang et al. 2012; Kamwesiga et al. 2015).

Selenoproteins have one or more residues of the non-standard amino acid selenocysteine, designed as the twenty-first amino acid. The incorporation of selenocysteine occurs co-translationally by the ribosome during protein synthesis (Böck 2013; Huang et al. 2012). To date, 25 selenoproteins have been identified in humans (Avery and Hoffmann, 2018). These include glutathione peroxidases, thioredoxin reductases, iodothyronine deiodinase, methionine-R-sulfoxide reductase and selenophosphate synthetase 2. Se and selenoproteins promote cell signalling events during the activation, differentiation and proliferation of immune cells that trigger the innate and adaptive immune response. Dietary Se may have an impact on various leucocytic effector functions by increasing the expression of selenoproteins and this affects their capability to adhere, migrate, undergo phagocytosis and induce cytokine secretion during the episode of immune response (Huang et al. 2012).

Increased intake of Se enhances both humoral and cell-mediated immune responses and these have been demonstrated in many studies (Alpert 2017; Avery and Hoffmann 2018; Hoffmann and Berry 2008; Kamwesiga et al. 2015; Spallholz et al. 1990; Spallholz and Stewart 1989). Enhanced humoral immunity towards various antigens has been observed in animal studies upon dietary supplementation of Se, where immunoglobulin titres were found to be elevated (Spallholz and Stewart 1989). The opposite happened when the animals either had a Se deficiency or were fed with a toxic amount of Se.

In vitro studies have confirmed that the immunomodulatory actions of Se include increasing the production of interleukin (IL)-2 by activated $CD4^+$ cells and its receptor expression leading to the generation of cytotoxic T lymphocytes and natural killer cells (Stone et al. 2010). Se supplementation has been shown to significantly reduce the rate of $CD4^+$ cell count in antiretroviral therapy in naive HIV patients (Kamwesiga et al. 2015). In humans, microarray data demonstrated that Se supplementation affects the pathways involving ribosomal protein and translation factor gene expression in peripheral lymphocytes (Pagmantidis et al. 2008). It was hypothesised that the upregulation of these genes is related to the selenoproteins' biosynthesis machinery and higher lymphocyte activity. Se supplementation in adults with marginal Se status increased the production of interferon (IFN)-gamma, IL-10, $CD4^+$ cells and an earlier peak of T-cell proliferation, while humoral immune response remained unaffected (Broome et al. 2004).

Se deficiency may increase the case fatality rate in serious illnesses (Karacabey and Ozdemir 2012). At the same time, Se deficiency was found to cause a decrease in IgM and IgG titres, impaired neutrophil chemotaxis and antibody production by the lymphocytes, increased $CD4^+$ T cells, and decreased $CD8^+$ and $CD4^-/CD8^-$ thymocytes (Wintergerst et al. 2007).

On the other hand, excess Se can cause acute and chronic toxicity, and common symptoms are nausea, vomiting, diarrhoea, hair loss, infertility, skin rash and nervous system disorders (Kieliszek and Błażejak 2016; MacFarquhar et al. 2010). Although rare, Se overdose in humans can have detrimental effects, and can even lead to fatality. An animal study was carried out to determine the effect of excess Se supplementation, and it was observed that immune responses were suppressed where the mRNA and concentrations of IL-2 and IFN-gamma in chicken serum and thymus were significantly decreased (Wang et al. 2016). Apart from a decrease in immunity, other observed effects were an increase in oxidative damage and a series of clinical pathology changes such as cortex drop, incrassation of the medulla and degeneration of the reticular cells (Wang et al. 2016).

6.3.2 Iron (Fe)

Iron is the most abundant transition metal in vertebrates, including humans. Fe is an essential co-factor for various biological functions such as oxygen transport, respiration, amino acid and lipid metabolism, and redox reactions. Dietary Fe sources are divided into two: food containing haem proteins, such as myoglobin, haemoglobin and cytochromes, and non-haem Fe sources, which contain ferrous and ferric Fe instead. Muscle meats, shellfish and liver are high in haem Fe while legumes, spinach, grains and nuts are rich in non-haem Fe. However, some of these plants contain phytate that could inhibit Fe absorption by the intestine. Ascorbic acid can overcome this effect when present in a sufficiently high amount (Davidsson 2003). The RDI of Fe in adults ranges from 8 to 18 mg, while pregnant women require as much as 27 mg of Fe per day. There are about 3–5 g of Fe in the human body and most of it is in the blood, contained within haemoglobin, some in plasma bound to transferrin protein, and other organs such as the liver, bone marrow and muscle.

Fe is involved in immune cell proliferation and maturation, particularly of naive lymphocytes as well as in cytokine production and mechanism of action (Alpert 2017; Calder 2020; Wintergerst et al. 2007). For B-cell proliferation, it has been shown that the process is also reliant on the uptake of transferrin Fe (Beck 1999). Transferrin Fe is needed for the clonal expansion of lymphocytes. Activation of T lymphocytes by IL-2 and expression of transferrin receptor CD71 must occur for Fe uptake to precede DNA synthesis (Beck 1999). Pure Fe deficiency can also lead to a change in the helper/suppressor CD4/CD8 T-cell ratio (Spallholz and Stewart 1989). However, Fe does not have a marked effect on humoral immunity, as serum immunoglobulin production and the complement system are not greatly affected by Fe deficiency (Beck 1999; Spallholz and Stewart 1989).

Homeostasis of Fe is unique compared to other trace elements because regulation to maintain Fe in the normal range happens through the absorption mechanism and not excretion (Bhattacharya et al. 2016). Most Fe-containing proteins are too big to pass via glomerular filtration and therefore Fe loss in urine is very minimal (Kohlmeier 2015). Alteration to cellular Fe homeostasis can lead to detrimental consequences and impair the overall host immune function. Deficiency in Fe can result in spleen and thymus atrophy and reduce the activity of natural killer cells. Fe overload can lead to damaging inflammatory effects, assists the invasion of tumour cells and facilitates the development of infection by promoting microbial growth (Alpert 2017; Beck 1999; Kieffer and Schneider 1991).

Excess of Fe affects cellular immunity by increasing the body's susceptibility to infection, although the exact mechanisms involved remain poorly understood (Calder 2020). Micro-organisms that rely on Fe for their metabolism can flourish and become pathogenic in the presence of excess Fe. The body reacts to excess Fe intake by binding the Fe with proteins such as transferrin and lactoferrin to reduce this effect (Alpert 2017). Therefore, serum levels of Fe may decline during inflammation and infection.

6.3.3 Manganese (Mn)

Manganese is a co-factor used in a diverse array of important enzymes involved in carbohydrate, protein and lipid metabolisms. This transition metal is commonly found in black tea, grains, sweet potato, spinach, rice and nuts. Daily intake levels of 1.8 mg for women and 2.3 mg for men are thought to be safe and adequate (Kohlmeier 2015). In mammalians, the levels of Mn range from 0.3 to 2.9 µg Mn/g wet tissue weight and are mostly concentrated in the mitochondria of metabolically active organs like bone, liver, pancreas and kidney (Kehl-Fie and Skaar 2010; Kohlmeier 2015; Nawi et al. 2019).

Although the principal source of Mn is diet, inhalation exposure may occur in some occupational cohorts. A study was carried out to investigate the effects of Mn on the cellular and humoral system in welders exposed to Mn fume (Nakata et al. 2006) where B lymphocytes (CD19$^+$), T-lymphocyte subpopulations, natural killer cells and total lymphocytes CD3$^+$ as well as serum immunoglobulin (IgG, IgA and IgM) were analysed. It was found that T lymphocytes, particularly CD8$^+$ and CD4$^+$CD45RA$^+$, and CD19$^+$ B lymphocytes were significantly affected by exposure to the fume, but not the serum immunoglobulins. It was also suggested that cellular and humoral immune systems are independently affected upon exposure to Mn.

Studies on Mn deficiency or toxicity in humans are scarce. Mn is considered an important trace element in the innate immune sensing of tumours, and it can also enhance the adaptive immune response against tumours (Lv et al. 2020). It was found that a low level of Mn significantly enhanced tumour growth and metastasis, and reduced tumour-infiltrating CD8$^+$ T cells. The same experiment also demonstrated that Mn could significantly promote dendritic cells and macrophage maturation and antigen presentation, augmented CD8$^+$ T cells and natural killer cell activation, and increased the number of CD44hiCD8$^+$ T cells via the cGAS-STING pathway, a component of the innate immune system (Lv et al. 2020). High supplementation of Mn, on the other hand, significantly reduced the lymphocytes' proliferative responses but greatly enhanced natural killer cell activity in rats exposed to lipopolysaccharide as a mitogen (Son et al. 2007). These findings suggest that a high dose of Mn may exert a differential effect on the function of each immune cell.

The body maintains tight homeostatic control on both the absorption and excretion of Mn. About 1–5% of the ingested amount is normally absorbed and biliary secretion is the main pathway for its excretion. Pancreatic or urinary excretion is generally very minimal.

6.3.4 Copper (Cu)

Copper is an essential catalytic co-factor for redox chemistry and its enzymes regulate physiological pathways such as energy production, Fe metabolism, connective tissue maturation and neurotransmission (Alpert 2017; Spallholz and Stewart 1989). Copper can be found in seeds, grains, beans, nuts, shellfish and organ meats. In living organisms, this trace element exists in both oxidised cupric ions (Cu^{2+}) and reduced cuprous ions (Cu$^+$). Average intake of Cu in adult humans ranges from 0.6 to 1.6 mg/dl (Tapiero et al. 2003).

Cu is involved in both humoral and cell-mediated immunity systems. Cu deficiency has been shown to reduce B-cell activity in mice subjected to various experimental conditions involving exposure to antigens (Beck 1999). In healthy male adult humans fed with low dietary Cu, it was found that the lymphoproliferative responses to mitogen and the secretion of IL-2 were reduced, but the low Cu diet did not affect the numbers of CD3$^+$, CD4$^+$ and CH8$^+$ T cells, or neutrophil phagocytic function (Kelley et al. 1995). Interestingly, in malignant tissues, it was observed that Cu increased production of IL-2 by the activated lymphocytic cells and these tissues exhibited a higher concentration of Cu than normal healthy tissues (Tapiero et al. 2003).

In mild cases of Cu deficiency, the production of IL-2 and T-cell proliferation were reduced, and in severe cases, the neutrophils count was diminished (Alpert 2017). Unlike serum Fe, in the events of inflammation, infection and cancer, serum Cu levels will be elevated (Gupta et al. 1991; Tapiero et al. 2003). However, the mechanism behind Cu elevation in malignancies remains unclear. It is postulated that it could be due to the destruction and necrosis of the malignant tissues leading to the release of Cu into the circulation (Gupta et al. 1991).

The level of Cu needs to be precisely regulated to prevent the accumulation of Cu ions which will lead to cytotoxicity. The main regulatory mechanism controlling the homeostasis of Cu is excretion, where excess Cu will be returned to the liver by carrier plasma proteins, namely transcuprein, albumin and caeruloplasmin (Tapiero et al. 2003). Formation and storage as a complex with metallothionein also contribute to the maintenance of homeostasis (Kohlmeier 2015). The transcription of metallothionein is induced by Cu, Zn, Cd, glucocorticoid and IL-6. Cu deficiency is rare but in children with Menkes syndrome, an X-linked recessive disorder, a mutation to the ATP7A gene affects the Cu transport system and impairs Cu absorption by the body (Beck 1999).

6.3.5 Zinc (Zn)

Zinc is critically important for vertebrates, as it can affect both innate and adaptive immune functions. It is the second most abundant transition metal in humans following Fe. Meat, milk and fish contain considerable amounts of zinc, but the bioavailability of Zn in vegetables is low. The RDI for Zn is 15 mg, and pregnant and lactating women need more Zn than adults and children. The serum has 0.8 µg/g of Zn, and the amounts are higher in the spleen, liver and kidney, which ranges from 100 to 200 µg/g (Kehl-Fie and Skaar 2010).

Many studies have been carried out in recent decades concerning the role of Zn in humoral immunity and cellular immunity (Alpert 2017; Beck 1999; Dardenne 2002; Wu et al. 2018). Zn increases cellular components of innate immunity, antibody response and cytotoxic CD8$^+$ T-cell count (Alpert 2017). Zn also affects Zn-dependent enzymes – its deficiency has marked effects on immunological responses involving thymic involution and T-cell immunity, particularly CD4$^+$ helper T cells and CD8$^+$ killer T cells (Spallholz and Stewart 1989). A genetic disorder called acrodermatitis enteropathica, which causes intestinal Zn malabsorption due to mutation to a gene encoded for the Zn transporter ZIP-4, is known to exhibit abnormalities in cellular immunity. Patients with this disorder are prone to infection and suffer from thymic atrophy, reduced lymphocyte proliferative response towards mitogen and decreased CD4$^+$ cells (Dardenne 2002; Prasad 2014).

In reviews by Prasad and Wu and colleagues, even mild Zn deficiency could result in severe impairments of the body's clinical, biochemical and immunological functions, including neutrophil functions, lymphocyte proliferation, decreased IL-2 as well as serum thymulin, macrophage phagocytic and natural killer cell lytic activities (Prasad 2014; Wu et al. 2018). However, these impairments, including the T-cell-mediated immune dysfunction, can be reversed with Zn supplementation.

It is interesting to note that the immune system can be either stimulated or suppressed depending on the type of immune stimulus and/or level of Zn present in the system (Beck 1999). The extracellular Zn level can be altered in response to microbial infection. In an abscessed tissue caused by *Staphylococcus aureus* infection, no detectable level of Zn is observed, compared to the surrounding healthy tissue which has a high level of Zn (Corbin et al. 2008). The factor responsible for this effect is still unknown, but the localisation effect is thought to be a representation of its immunological strategy to control infection (Kehl-Fie and Skaar 2010). Cellular Zn concentration exhibits a similar response against intracellular pathogens. Activation of T cells and dendritic antigen-presenting cells reduces the lysosomal and cytoplasmic Zn levels respectively, as mechanisms to disrupt Zn-dependent bacterial processes, particularly those involving the Zn transporters (Kehl-Fie and Skaar 2010).

Cellular Zn concentration relies on the relative activities of influx and efflux transporters. Similar to Cu homeostasis, controlling the expression of metallothionein is the most prominent mechanism in maintaining overall Zn concentration. Zn can be excreted from the body via sweat, skin, hair, faeces and urine. Excretion in urine is very minimal, as almost all Zn in the blood will form complexes with larger proteins such as albumin and alpha-2-macroglobulin and not be able to be reabsorbed by the renal tubule (Kohlmeier 2015).

6.3.6 Fluoride (F)

Fluorine, which falls in the halogen group, is one of the most abundant elements in nature and its ionic form is known as fluoride ion. Fluoride can be found in water, foods, soil and in several salts such as fluorite and fluorapatite, the main inorganic component that gives the skeletal framework to hard tissues. Due to its reactivity, it naturally exists as a compound in combination with other elements. Water, food, industrial exposure and drugs are usually the routes by which F enters the human body and the environment. The contribution of F to body weight is often considered negligible, but its action is exerted in a concentration-dependent manner.

The effects of F exposure on human body tissues can be both beneficial and detrimental. F is incorporated into the structures of oral hard tissue during the mineralisation phase of tooth formation. Thus, F is involved in strengthening teeth and bones, which also contributes to the prevention of osteoporosis. Excessive F intake, especially during the early phase of tooth formation, may result in dental fluorosis and continuous exposure either from a single source or in combination with other sources such as fluoridated milk or fluoridated salt can lead to adverse effects such as skeletal and non-skeletal fluorosis, which includes cardiac fluorosis. Damage to the cardiovascular system and other soft tissues is mainly due to its action in inhibiting numerous enzymes, forming free radicals which later lead to oxidative stress (Basha and Sujitha 2011).

In 2019, Yan and colleagues reported a significantly decreased amount of mRNA and protein levels of IL-1, IL-6 and IL-10 in the heart tissue of rats with chronic fluorosis, exposed to low and high levels of sodium F. The damage induced by fluorosis to the heart tissue was concluded to be an immune response to oxidative stress and myocardial apoptosis (Cheng et al. 2013). In another study, the spleens of mice were found to be damaged following superfluous intake of sodium F (Li et al. 2021). The immune response to the induced injury was investigated and it was postulated that F caused an imbalance in the proportion of Type 1 and Type 2 helper T cells. The levels of mRNA expression of IL-2, IFN-gamma and tumour growth factor (TGF)-beta were also found to be decreased. On the other hand, the levels of certain cytokines, namely IL-4, IL-6 and IL-10 were found to be increased (Li et al. 2021).

6.4 Trace Elements and Immunity of the Oral Cavity

The relationship between trace elements and oral health has long been documented (Apon and Kamble 2019; Gaur and Agnihotri 2017; Najeeb et al. 2016; Nizam et al. 2014). According to a study by Ghadimi and colleagues (2013), a total of 19 trace elements were detected in human enamel via inductively coupled plasma-optical emission spectroscopy, namely Se, aluminium, potassium, magnesium, sulfur, sodium, Zn, silicon, boron, cobalt, chromium, Cu, Fe, Mn, molybdenum, nickel, plumbum, antimony and titanium. The presence of these trace elements in enamel was suggested to be associated with its physicochemical properties. The source of these elements was deduced to be saliva, dental prosthesis or dental porcelain, where the trace elements may be incorporated into the enamel crystal lattice.

Between the different dental hard tissues, namely enamel and dentine, the distribution of trace elements was found to be varied. The amounts of certain trace elements such as Cu, plumbum, cobalt, aluminium, iodine, strontium, Se, nickel and Mn were found to be higher in enamel than dentine (Derise and Ritchey 1974; Ghadimi et al. 2013; Lappalainen and Knuuttila 1981). On the other hand, the amount of Fe and fluorine was higher in dentine than in enamel. The amount of trace elements embedded in the different layers of the enamel crystal lattice also varies, suggesting that trace elements originate from the environment, and are incorporated during the mineralisation stage of amelogenesis (Ghadimi et al. 2013).

A considerable amount of evidence confirms that poor oral health is associated not only with infectious diseases such as gingivitis, periodontitis and caries, but also non-communicable diseases such as malignancy, heart disease, diabetes mellitus, rheumatoid arthritis and inflammatory bowel diseases (Vasovic et al. 2016). Having an underlying health condition may cause poor oral health and increase the severity of other diseases. The levels of various trace elements in non-malignant oral diseases, which include periodontal disease and caries, are summarised in Table 6.3.

6.4.1 Trace Elements in Periodontal Disease

Periodontal disease is an inflammatory condition which begins with the development of gingivitis, the mildest form of periodontal disease. Gingivitis is an inflammation of the gingiva which may cause it to be swollen and to bleed easily. If it persists, this reversible condition may progress to irreversible periodontitis, where the inflammation spreads to the periodontium. It is characterised by the apical migration of junctional epithelium, forming pocket epithelium. Consequently, these conditions will cause resorption of bone at the alveolar crest, leading to the destruction of the periodontium.

The aetiology of periodontal disease is thought to be associated with multiple factors, including genetics, microbial dysbiosis and environmental factors. The interactions between supragingival and subgingival polymicrobial biofilms with the host immune response are deemed to be a vital point in the progression of periodontal disease. Both innate and adaptive immune responses are associated with the disease. However, damage to the periodontal tissue is not directly caused by periodontal pathogens. Instead, breakdown of the tissue is caused by the subversion of host immune responses that involve neutrophils, the complement system and reactive oxygen species (ROS) (Hajishengallis 2015).

Reactive oxygen species are important signalling molecules involved in various cellular activities and processes such as cellular differentiation, apoptosis and phagocytosis. Oxidative stress caused by the increased production of ROS is involved

Table 6.3 Trace elements in non-malignant oral diseases.

Trace element	Oral disease	Sample	Level compared to healthy control	References
Selenium	Periodontitis	Serum	↓	(Thomas et al. 2013)
	Chronic and aggressive periodontitis, gingivitis	Saliva	↑	(Inonu et al. 2020)
	Caries	Urine	↑	(Hadjimarkos et al. 1952)
	Caries	Saliva	↓	(Nireeksha 2020)
	Caries	Teeth	↑	(Amin et al. 2016)
Iron	Chronic and aggressive periodontitis, gingivitis	Saliva	↑	(Inonu et al. 2020)
	Plummer–Vinson syndrome		↓	(Bhattacharya et al. 2016)
Manganese	Periodontal disease	Plasma	↓	(Kim et al. 2014)
	Chronic periodontitis	Saliva	↑	(Talal et al. 2017)
	Caries	Teeth	↑	(Amin et al. 2016)
Magnesium	Chronic and aggressive periodontitis, gingivitis	Saliva	↑	(Inonu et al. 2020)
	Chronic and aggressive periodontitis	Plasma	↑	(Dannan and Hanno 2018)
Cadmium	Chronic periodontitis	Saliva	↑	(Talal et al. 2017)
Copper	Chronic periodontitis	Serum	↑	(Thomas et al. 2013)
	Aggressive periodontitis; chronic and acute gingivitis	Plasma	↑	(Dannan and Hanno 2018)
Zinc	Chronic periodontitis	Serum	↓	(Thomas et al. 2013)
Fluoride	Dental fluorosis	Salivary	↑	(Singam et al. 2014)
Aluminium	Caries	Teeth	↑	(Amin et al. 2016)

in the pathogenesis of numerous diseases, including periodontitis (Baltacioglu et al. 2014). High concentrations of ROS cause cytotoxic effects on periodontal tissues, and ROS have been suggested to play a crucial role in determining the fate of periodontal cells by inducing either autophagy or apoptosis (Liu C.C. et al. 2017).

The effects of ROS are not always detrimental; the role of ROS in periodontal disease has been dubbed a 'double-edged sword' (Liu C.C. et al. 2017). In a review by Liu C.C. et al. (2017), low concentrations of ROS have positive effects in vitro, where they can stimulate the proliferation and differentiation of human periodontal ligament fibroblasts. High concentrations of ROS may attack pathogens, either directly or indirectly (Liu C.C. et al. 2017). The direct elimination of pathogens occurs via the results of oxidative damage to biocompounds and indirect effects occur via non-oxidative mechanisms such as pattern recognition receptor signalling, autophagy, neutrophil extracellular trap formation and T-lymphocyte responses (Paiva and Bozza 2014). Therefore, a delicate balance must be maintained to ensure the periodontal tissue can receive the benefits granted by ROS.

Excessive generation of highly reactive molecules such as ROS needs to be neutralised by antioxidant systems, as failure will result in significant damage to DNA, proteins and lipids. Many trace elements, such as Se, Cu, Zn, Mn and Fe, act as co-factors of antioxidant enzymes and the amounts of these trace elements have significant effects on the activity of these enzymes. For example, Se, in the form of selenocysteine, is an integral component of the active site of glutathione peroxidase. Zn, Cu and Mn form parts of superoxide dismutase enzymes, and the Fe ion is an important component of the catalase enzyme.

6.4.1.1 Selenium (Se)

The positive nutritional effects of Se on periodontium are mainly attributed to its antioxidant properties (Apon and Kamble 2019; Gaur and Agnihotri 2017). A combination of Se and alpha-tocopherol exhibited possible synergistic effects on the proliferation and wound healing rates of human gingival fibroblast and periodontal ligament fibroblast cells, in vitro (Nizam et al. 2014). These two micronutrients were discovered to enhance the production of basic fibroblast growth factor in both types of cells and increase the synthesis of collagen type I in the periodontal ligament fibroblast cells (Nizam et al. 2014).

Serum levels of Se, along with glutathione and catalase, were significantly decreased in periodontitis patients with and without type 2 diabetes mellitus, suggesting that reduced levels of these three antioxidant parameters indicated an imbalance of the host response (Thomas et al. 2013). This then triggered an increase in the production of ROS, leading to the destruction of the periodontal tissue (Thomas et al. 2013).

In a study by Inonu and colleagues (2020), increased salivary levels of Se, along with Mg, Fe and calcium, were found to be significantly correlated with severity of periodontal disease (Inonu et al. 2020). The levels of Se in the saliva collected from subjects with chronic and aggressive periodontitis were higher compared to levels observed in gingivitis and systemically healthy subjects. The higher levels were attributed to the increased need for Se by the host to form the antioxidant enzyme glutathione peroxidase to neutralise the excessive ROS formed by the severe condition, as a form of gingival antioxidant defence mechanism.

Although a majority of research findings agreed that Se may affect periodontal status by dysregulation of the host immune response, Saxen et al. (1983) did not. This study also discovered that a high dose of Se did not cause periodontitis and caries. This conclusion was made based on a study investigating the outcome when sodium selenite supplements were used to treat children with Spielmeyer–Sjogren disease (Saxen et al. 1983).

6.4.1.2 Iron (Fe)

Several oral manifestations, namely angular cheilitis, atrophic glossitis, generalised oral mucosal atrophy, candidiasis, pallor and stomatitis, can be caused by Fe deficiency anaemia resulting from the lack of serum Fe (Bhattacharya et al. 2016). The triad combination of Fe deficiency anaemia, postcricoid dysphagia and upper oesophageal webs is the classic presentation of a rare premalignant condition termed Plummer–Vinson syndrome, which is associated with an increased incidence of postcricoid carcinoma (Bhattacharya et al. 2016). Reduction in total serum Fe was also observed in patients with oral squamous cell carcinoma, but not in premalignant oral leucoplakia, suggesting the difference was due to the tumour burden that eventually led to malnutrition (Jayadeep et al. 1997).

Ferritin, a protein that stores Fe, was found to be upregulated in periodontal tissues with periodontitis, induced by the production of proinflammatory cytokines IL-6 and TNF-alpha, suggesting involvement of ferritin in the development of periodontitis (Huang et al. 2019). An association between Fe overload and the progress of periodontitis was observed in 123 patients with homozygous sickle cell anaemia, as demonstrated by an increase in the level of serum transferrin saturation (Costa et al. 2020). However, the serum ferritin level was not significantly associated with periodontal status, as opposed to the findings by Huang et. al. (2019) and Davidopoulou et al. (2021).

Salivary Fe content was found to be significantly increased in chronic periodontitis and generalised aggressive periodontitis patients, compared to subjects with healthy periodontium (Inonu et al. 2020). The increase in the concentration was attributed to the increased haemoglobin concentration in inflamed periodontal tissue and/or the presence of subgingival biofilm. Like Se, an imbalance in Fe level may cause the production of ROS, which will destroy periodontal tissue. Fe overload catalyses the Fenton reactions which convert the hydrogen peroxide to hydroxy radicals and hydroxyl ions (Apon and Kamble 2019).

6.4.1.3 Manganese (Mn)

The level of Mn in plasma was found to have a significant inverse association with periodontal status, following adjustments for sociodemographic variables, oral and general health behaviour, oral health status and systemic conditions (Kim et al. 2014). A significant association is strongly exhibited in males compared to females. The presence of oestrogen in women might have a protective role against oxidative stress (Kim et al. 2014). Conversely, the levels of salivary Mn, along with cadmium, were found to be significantly increased in patients with chronic periodontitis (Talal et al. 2017).

6.4.1.4 Copper (Cu)

The serum level of Cu was found to be significantly increased in patients with type 2 diabetes mellitus suffering from chronic periodontitis (Thomas et al. 2013). The level of Cu in plasma from patients with periodontal diseases was significantly increased, particularly in patients with aggressive periodontitis (Dannan and Hanno 2018). The plasma levels of this trace element were also found to be increased in patients with chronic and acute gingivitis (Dannan and Hanno 2018).

It was postulated that the change was due to the occurrence of an inflammatory reaction, where caeruloplasmin, a major carrier protein of Cu, could be involved in the process. Caeruloplasmin is also known as an acute-phase reactant and this protein inhibits the Cu ion-stimulated formation of reactive oxidants and scavenges hydrogen peroxide and superoxide, resulting in the protection of host tissues against the toxic oxygen metabolites released from phagocytic cells during an acute-phase response (Dannan and Hanno 2018; Pang et al. 2010).

6.4.1.5 Zinc (Zn)

The serum level of Zn was found to be significantly decreased in patients with type 2 diabetes mellitus and chronic periodontitis (Thomas et al. 2013). Zn is essential for DNA and protein synthesis because it acts as a co-factor in DNA polymerase and RNA polymerase, and therefore the study suggested that Zn deficiency may reduce cellular proliferation and regenerative capacity. Apart from that, the deficiency may also lower the immune response and increase oxidative stress, and these factors are known to contribute to the development of periodontal diseases (Thomas et al. 2013).

6.4.1.6 Magnesium (Mg)

Plasma magnesium levels were significantly associated with the different types of periodontal disease (Dannan and Hanno 2018). The level was lower in patients suffering from chronic periodontitis compared to those with aggressive periodontitis, but both conditions showed significantly higher levels compared to healthy subjects. An increase in magnesium concentrations was also observed in plasma taken from patients with acute gingivitis and chronic gingivitis (Dannan and Hanno 2018). Similarly, the concentrations of salivary Mg were found to be higher in patients with gingivitis, chronic periodontitis and generalised aggressive periodontitis, compared to healthy controls (Inonu et al. 2020).

Mg is a calcium channel blocker, and its deficiency can change the function of calcium in inflammatory and oxidative stress, affecting these processes and aggravating the progress of the periodontal disease (Inonu et al. 2020; Meisel et al. 2005). Therefore, analysis of the serum Mg/calcium ratio was suggested to be more relevant in assessing periodontal health status and the risk of tooth loss, according to a cross-sectional study done with five-year follow-up data (Meisel et al. 2016).

6.4.1.7 Cadmium (Cd)

Cadmium is toxic in moderate doses, but this trace element is believed to have physiological roles in humans. It is also an antagonist of certain trace elements such as Fe, Cu and Zn, as well as calcium. The levels of salivary cadmium, along with Mn, were found to be significantly increased in patients with chronic periodontitis (Talal et al. 2017). It was suggested that the increase in Cd level was due to its release from intraoral alloys in the patients. Cd is considered a potentially toxic trace element by the WHO, and exposure to this element may cause the release of inflammatory mediators leading to the destruction of periodontal tissue (Talal et al. 2017).

6.4.1.8 Fluoride (F)

Fluoride is known to have an anticariogenic effect due to its ability to be incorporated into tooth enamel during remineralisation. However, this trace element also has antimicrobial properties. Evidence shows that a low daily dose of F may affect the metabolism of bacteria associated with the initiation and progression of bacteria-related oral diseases, by inhibiting their enzyme activities (Nicholson and Czarnecka 2008). Acidification of the bacterial cytoplasm through the formation of H^+ and F^- ions from hydrogen F and disruption of the bacterial metabolism by inhibition of vital bacterial enzymes such as proton-releasing adenosine triphosphatase and enolase contribute to the antibacterial action of F ion. A reduction in IgA protease synthesis, which is an example of enzyme inhibition, and a reduction in extracellular polysaccharide production play an important role in decreasing bacterial adherence to dental hard tissues (Ullah and Zafar 2015).

Studies on the effects of F on periodontal disease status are scarce. In 2014, Singam and colleagues estimated the levels of salivary and serum F in subjects diagnosed with periodontitis and dental fluorosis. It was found that there was no correlation between F levels and severity of periodontal disease (Singam et al. 2014). Nevertheless, salivary F levels were found to have a significant influence on the severity of dental fluorosis.

6.4.2 Trace Elements in Caries

Caries is a multifactorial chronic infectious disease caused by a complex microbiological interaction between cariogenic (acidogenic and aciduric) bacteria and fermentable carbohydrates, leading to the production of organic acids that will subsequently cause demineralisation of the enamel. Unlike gingivitis and periodontitis, caries is not an inflammatory disease, but an immune response is vital to provide resistance against the cariogenic bacteria. Healthy dental pulp and oral environment are crucial in preserving the integrity of the oral hard tissues. There are many studies investigating the roles of trace elements in the prevention of caries.

In a cariogenic environment, the buffering capacity of saliva provided by the presence of bicarbonate ions can control the equilibrium between the demineralisation and remineralisation properties of saliva, which is attributed to the presence of calcium and phosphate ions. Along with other non-specific defence mechanisms provided by the saliva, such as its lubrication and cleansing actions, the presence of a non-specific immune response offered by salivary antimicrobial proteins such as histatin and lactoferrin is also relevant to preserve oral health. Histatin is an enzyme composed of Cu and is known to have antifungal activity against *Candida albicans*. Lactoferrin, a protein whose main physiological activity is to bind Fe, also exhibited antibacterial, antiviral, antifungal and antiparasitic properties (Jenssen and Hancock 2009).

The effects of trace elements on dental caries are still being discussed by scholars around the world. In a systemic review by Pathak and colleagues (Pathak et al. 2015), molybdenum, vanadium, F, strontium and lithium were categorised as cariostatic elements, while Se, Cd, lead, Mn, Cu and Zn were categorised as caries-promoting elements.

One of the most widely studied trace elements in the prevalence of caries in the human population is Se which can be traced back to as early as the 1950s (Hadjimarkos et al. 1952). This study revealed that there was a significant direct association between the degree of caries susceptibility and the amount of Se found in the urine of school children from two counties in Oregon (Clatsop and Klamath) where Se is not known to be present (Hadjimarkos et al. 1952). Higher urinary Se was detected in those living in Clatsop, who had a higher prevalence of caries, indicated by a Decayed, Missing, Filled (DMF) index of 14.4, than those living in Klamath (DMF index = 9.0). However, the mechanism was still debated until eight years later. In 1960, it was demonstrated that Se could suppress the protective effect of F in reducing dental caries in permanent teeth of children who consumed highly fluoridated water (0.6–2.6 ppm) in the seleniferous area (Tank and Storvick 1960). The study also discovered that the rates of enamel hypoplasia and malocclusion were increased in the seleniferous areas (Tank and Storvick 1960).

Contrary to the above findings, Se has been reported to have an anticariogenic effect and Se nanoparticles made from broccoli (*Brassica oleracea*) were developed to assess its antioxidant and antimicrobial properties against cariogenic microorganisms (Dhanraj and Rajeshkumar 2021). It has been reported before that salivary Se was significantly higher in the caries-free group, suggesting the protective role of Se on the tooth surface by the attachment of this element to the apatite structure, therefore decreasing the solubility of the tooth enamel (Nireeksha 2020). However, in a study conducted by Amin et. al. (2016), it was found that the concentration of several elements, i.e. aluminium, Mn and Se, in carious teeth were significantly higher than in sound teeth. It was postulated that the incorporation of these elements into apatite microcrystals following localised dissolution by the acids from bacterial metabolism would alter the apatite's properties, especially its solubility, rendering it susceptible to further dissolution (Amin et al. 2016; Davies and Anderson 1987). Se settles in the enamel's microcrystal structure at the start of decay, making it more susceptible to dissolution (Qamar et al. 2017). The incorporation of Se in tooth enamel was found to exhibit a positive correlation with the cell lattice parameters along the a-axis and c-axis, because the ionic radius of Se^{4+} is larger than that of P^{5+}, and the substitution of Se in synthetic hydroxyapatite would increase the lattice parameters (Ghadimi et al. 2013).

F ion promotes remineralisation by forming fluorapatite mineral ($Ca_{10}(PO_4)_6F_2$) which is more resistant to demineralisation and acid dissolution by bacteria, compared to hydroxyapatite ($Ca_{10}(PO_4)_6(OH)_2$). Instead of a hydroxyl ion, F claims the central position in the apatite crystal lattice, hence forming the fluorapatite. Having a lower solubility product, F reduces the dissolving power of saliva towards the tooth mineral, decreases the solubility of the apatite, and improves the crystallisation kinetics of the mineralisation process.

It must be emphasised that these studies attributed the anticariogenic effect of the above trace elements to their physicochemical properties, not a reaction by the host's immune response per se. However, there is research trying to prevent the occurrence of caries by eliciting the host immune response against the cariogenic micro-organisms (Gambhir et al. 2012; Babu et al. 2016). Given the multitude of beneficial effects presented by trace elements in the oral immune system, this provides avenues to expand the research on trace elements in preventing dental caries.

6.4.3 Trace Elements in Oral Malignancy

The most common causes of oral malignancy include heavy tobacco and alcohol use, excessive sun exposure, human papillomavirus and a compromised immune system. The levels of trace elements in various types of premalignant and malignant conditions of the oral cavity vary (Table 6.4).

Table 6.4 Trace elements in oral premalignant and malignant conditions.

Trace element	Oral premalignant/ malignant condition	Sample	Level compared to healthy control	References
Selenium	Oral squamous cell carcinoma	Serum	↓	(Khanna and Karjodkar 2006)
	Squamous cell carcinoma of the oral cavity or oropharynx	Erythrocyte	↓	(Goodwin et al. 1983)
		Plasma	↑	(Goodwin et al. 1983)
Iron	Oral squamous cell carcinoma	Serum	↓	(Jayadeep et al. 1997; Khanna and Karjodkar 2006)
	Oral submucous fibrosis	Saliva	↓	(Bagewadi et al. 2022)
Copper	Oral submucous fibrosis, oral leucoplakia, oral squamous cell carcinoma	Serum	↑	(Khanna and Karjodkar 2006)
	Oral submucous fibrosis, oral leucoplakia, oral cancer	Serum	↓	(Varghese et al. 1987)
	Oral submucous fibrosis, oral leucoplakia, oral lichen planus	Saliva	↑	(Ayinampudi and Narsimhan 2012)
	Oral squamous cell carcinoma	Saliva	↑	(Ayinampudi and Narsimhan 2012)
	Oral submucous fibrosis	Buccal mucosal biopsies	↑	(Trivedy et al. 2000)
	Oral submucous fibrosis	Saliva	↑	(Bagewadi et al. 2022)
Zinc	Oral submucous fibrosis, oral leucoplakia, oral cancer	Serum	↓	(Varghese et al. 1987)
	Oral submucous fibrosis, oral leucoplakia, oral lichen planus	Saliva	↑	(Ayinampudi and Narsimhan 2012)
	Oral squamous cell carcinoma	Saliva	↑	(Ayinampudi and Narsimhan 2012)
	Oral submucous fibrosis	Saliva	↓	(Bagewadi et al. 2022)

Research investigating the involvement of trace elements and cancer often addresses the role of host immune responses (Khanna and Karjodkar 2006; Kiremidjian-Schumacher et al. 2000). Serum Cu levels were shown to have a gradual increase in patients from precancer conditions to cancerous conditions, i.e. from oral submucous fibrosis and oral leucoplakia to oral squamous cell carcinoma (Khanna and Karjodkar 2006). In contrast, serum Fe and Se levels were significantly decreased in oral carcinoma patients. Circulating immune complexes merely represent the host's physiological and immune response in producing specific antibodies to the antigenic substance (Khanna and Karjodkar 2006).

Se is one of the most studied trace elements in terms of its chemopreventive activities. It was hypothesised that the molecular mechanism in the reduction of cancer risk by Se is linked with its abilities to induce apoptosis. Such a hypothesis is based on the involvement of the Fas ligand, a mediator of apoptosis, and stress kinase pathways, along with the Se inhibitory effect (Fleming et al. 2001). However, this trace element is also reported to cause oxidative stress and redox changes in primary cultures of oral carcinoma biopsies (Fleming et al. 2001).

Se supplementation, in a form of sodium selenite, during the treatment of squamous cell carcinoma of the head and neck markedly enhanced the cell-mediated immune response. Se supplements seem to activate the lymphocytes to respond to stimulation by mitogens to generate cytotoxic lymphocytes and destroy tumour cells (Kiremidjian-Schumacher et al. 2000).

Oral administration of Cu and resveratrol, a plant polyphenol known for its antioxidant activity, to advanced squamous cell carcinoma patients resulted in the deactivation of cell-free chromatin particles, the instigators of cancer hallmarks and immune checkpoints, released by the dying cancer cells (Pilankar et al. 2022). The treatment resulted in the downregulation of 23 biomarkers for cancer hallmarks and five immune checkpoints: PDL-1, PD-1, CTLA-4, TIM-3 and NKG2A. This led to the prospect of using the pro-oxidant combination of Cu and resveratrol as a novel non-toxic form of cancer treatment, where instead of killing the cancer cells, they could heal the cells based on their effects on the hallmarks of cancers and immune checkpoints, which are also the hallmarks of wound healing (Pilankar et al. 2022).

6.5 Conclusion

Trace elements are vital for the host immune response to function optimally. The delicate balance must be maintained to ensure no detrimental effect arises from insufficient or excessive intake. It is now well established that treatment approaches involving micronutrient supplements, including antioxidants, as a possible adjunct therapy to oral diseases, particularly caries and periodontal disease, have a better prognosis (Dommisch et al. 2018; Gaur and Agnihotri 2017; Kaur et al. 2019; Manjunath 2011). It is well known that trace elements play major roles in both innate and adaptive immune response, so they are important in the prevention and management of oral diseases. It is predicted that trace elements will continue to be important in oral health care and oral immunology research.

References

Alpert, P.T. (2017). The role of vitamins and minerals on the immune system. *Home Health Care Manage. Pract.* 29 (3): 199–202.

Amin, W., Almimar, F. and Alawi, D. M. (2016). Quantitative analysis of trace elements in sound and carious enamel of primary and permanent dentitions. *Br. J. Med. Med. Res.* 11: 1–10.

Apon, A. and Kamble, P. (2019). Role of trace mineral in periodontal health: a review. *Clin. Trials Degen. Dis.* 4 (2): 30–36.

Avery, J.C. and Hoffmann, P.R. (2018). Selenium, selenoproteins, and immunity. *Nutrients* 10 (9).

Ayinampudi, B.K. and Narsimhan, M. (2012). Salivary copper and zinc levels in oral pre-malignant and malignant lesions. *J. Oral Maxillofac. Pathol.* 16 (2): 178–182.

Babu, A., Malathi, L., Karthick, R. and Sankari, S.L. (2016). Immunology of dental caries. *Biomed. Pharmacol. J.* 9 (2).

Bagewadi, S.B., Hirpara, D.R., Paliwal, A. et al. (2022). Estimation of salivary copper, zinc, iron, and copper-to-zinc ratio in oral submucous fibrosis patients: a case-control study. *J. Contemp. Dent. Pract.* 23 (3): 303–306.

Baltacioglu, E., Kehribar, M. A., Yuva, P. et al. (2014). Total oxidant status and bone resorption biomarkers in serum and gingival crevicular fluid of patients with periodontitis. *J. Periodontol.* 85 (2): 317–326.

Basha, M.P. and Sujitha, N.S. (2011). Chronic fluoride toxicity and myocardial damage: antioxidant offered protection in second generation rats. *Toxicol. Int.* 18 (2): 99–104.

Beck, M.A. (1999). Trace minerals, immune function, and viral evolution. In: *Military Strategies for Sustainment of Nutrition and Immune Function in the Field*, 337–360. Washington, DC: National Academies Press.

Bhattacharya, P.T., Misra, S.R. and Hussain, M. (2016). Nutritional aspects of essential trace elements in oral health and disease: an extensive review. *Scientifica* 2016: 5464373.

Böck, A. (2013). Selenoprotein synthesis. In: *Encyclopedia of Biological Chemistry*, 2e (eds W.J. Lennarz and M.D. Lane), 210–213. New York: Academic Press.

Broome, C.S., McArdle, F., Kyle, J.A. (2004). An increase in selenium intake improves immune function and poliovirus handling in adults with marginal selenium status. *Am. J. Clin. Nutr.* 80 (1): 154–162.

Calder, P.C. (2020). Nutrition, immunity and COVID-19. *BMJ Nutr. Prev. Health* 3 (1): 74–92.

Campos, R.D., de Jesus, L.M., Morais, D.A. et al. (2021). Low urinary selenium levels are associated with iodine deficiency in Brazilian schoolchildren and adolescents. *Endocrine* 73 (3): 609–616.

Cheng, R.Y., Nie, Q.L., Sun, H.F. et al. (2013). Fluoride-induced oxidative stress in rat myocardium through the Bax/Bcl-2 signalling pathway. *Fluoride* 46 (4): 198–203.

Corbin, B.D., Seeley, E.H., Raab, A. et al. (2008). Metal chelation and inhibition of bacterial growth in tissue abscesses. *Science* 319 (5865): 962–965.

Costa, S.A., Moreira, A.R.O., Costa, C.P.S. and Souza, S.D.C. (2020). Iron overload and periodontal status in patients with sickle cell anaemia: a case series. *J. Clin. Periodontol.* 47 (6): 668–675.

Dannan, A. and Hanno, Y. (2018). The relationship between periodontal diseases and plasma level of copper and magnesium. *Dentistry* 8: 2.

Dardenne, M. (2002). Zinc and immune function. *Eur. J. Clin. Nutr.* 56 (Suppl 3): S20–23.

Davidopoulou, S., Pikilidou, M., Yavropoulou, M.P., Kalogirou, T.E., Zebekakis, P. and Kalfas, S. (2021). Aggravated dental and periodontal status in patients with sickle cell disease and its association with serum ferritin. *J. Contemp. Dent. Pract.* 22 (9): 991–997.

Davidsson, L. (2003). Approaches to improve iron bioavailability from complementary foods. *J. Nutr.* 133 (5 Suppl 1): 1560s–1562s.

Davies, B.E. and Anderson, R.J. (1987). The epidemiology of dental-caries in relation to environmental trace-elements. *Experientia* 43 (1): 87–92.

Derise, N.L. and Ritchey, S.J. (1974). Mineral composition of normal human enamel and dentin and the relation of composition to dental caries. II. Microminerals. *J. Dent. Res.* 53 (4): 853–858.

Dhanraj, G. and Rajeshkumar, S. (2021). Anticariogenic effect of selenium nanoparticles synthesized using Brassica oleracea. *J. Nanomaterials* 11: 1–9.

Dommisch, H., Kuzmanova, D., Jonsson, D., Grant, M. and Chapple, I. (2018). Effect of micronutrient malnutrition on periodontal disease and periodontal therapy. *Periodontology 2000* 78 (1): 129–153.

dos Santos, M., Veneziani, Y., Muccillo-Baisch, A L. and Da Silva, F.M.R. (2019). Global survey of urinary selenium in children: a systematic review. *J. Trace Elements Med. Biol.* 56: 1–5.

Fleming, J., Ghose, A. and Harrison, P.R. (2001). Molecular mechanisms of cancer prevention by selenium compounds. *Nutrition Cancer* 40 (1): 42–49.

Frieden, E. (1974). The evolution of metals as essential elements (with special reference to iron and copper). *Adv. Exp. Med. Biol.* 48 (0): 1–29.

Frieden, E. (1985). New perspectives on the essential trace-elements. *J. Chem. Educ.* 62 (11): 917–923.

Gambhir, R., Kapoor, V. and Setia, S. (2012). Immunology in prevention of dental caries. *Universal Res. J. Dent.* 2: 58.

Gaur, S. and Agnihotri, R. (2017). Trace mineral micronutrients and chronic periodontitis – a review. *Biol. Trace Element Res.* 176 (2): 225–238.

Ghadimi, E., Eimar, H., Marelli, B. et al. (2013). Trace elements can influence the physical properties of tooth enamel. *Springerplus* 2: 499.

Goodwin, W.J., Lane, H.W., Bradford, K. (1983). Selenium and glutathione-peroxidase levels in patients with epidermoid carcinoma of the oral cavity and oropharynx. *Cancer* 51 (1): 110–115.

Grochowski, C., Blicharska, E., Krukow, P. et al. (2019). Analysis of trace elements in human brain: its aim, methods, and concentration levels. *Front. Chem.* 7: 115.

Gupta, S.K., Shukla, V.K., Vaidya, M.P., Roy, S.K. and Gupta, S. (1991). Serum trace elements and Cu/Zn ratio in breast cancer patients. *J. Surg. Oncol.* 46 (3): 178–181.

Hadjimarkos, D.M., Storvick, C.A. and Remmert, L.F. (1952). Selenium and dental caries; an investigation among school children of Oregon. *J. Pediatr.* 40 (4): 451–455.

Hajishengallis, G. (2015). Periodontitis: from microbial immune subversion to systemic inflammation. *Nat. Rev. Immunol.* 15 (1): 30–44.

Hoffmann, P.R. and Berry, M.J. (2008). The influence of selenium on immune responses. *Mol. Nutr. Food Res.* 52 (11): 1273–1280.

Huang, W., Zhan, Y., Zheng, Y., Han, Y., Hu, W. and Hou, J. (2019). Up-regulated ferritin in periodontitis promotes inflammatory cytokine expression in human periodontal ligament cells through transferrin receptor via ERK/P38 MAPK pathways. *Clin. Sci.* 133 (1): 135–148.

Huang, Z., Rose, A.H. and Hoffmann, P.R. (2012). The role of selenium in inflammation and immunity: from molecular mechanisms to therapeutic opportunities. *Antioxid. Redox Signal.* 16 (7): 705–743.

Inonu, E., Hakki, S.S., Kayis, S.A. and Nielsen, F.H. (2020). The association between some macro and trace elements in saliva and periodontal status. *Biol. Trace Element Res.* 197 (1): 35–42.

Jayadeep, A., Raveendran Pillai, K., Kannan, S. et al. (1997). Serum levels of copper, zinc, iron and ceruplasmin in oral leukoplakia and squamous cell carcinoma. *J. Exp. Clin. Cancer Res.* 16 (3): 295–300.

Jenssen, H. and Hancock, R.E.W. (2009). Antimicrobial properties of lactoferrin. *Biochimie* 91 (1): 19–29.

Kamwesiga, J., Mutabazi, V., Kayumba, J. et al. (2015). Effect of selenium supplementation on CD4+ T-cell recovery, viral suppression and morbidity of HIV-infected patients in Rwanda: a randomized controlled trial. *Aids* 29 (9): 1045–1052.

Karacabey, K. and Ozdemir, N. (2012). The effect of nutritional elements on the immune system. *J. Obes. Wt Loss Ther.* 2: 152.

Kaur, K., Sculley, D., Wallace, J. et al. (2019). Micronutrients and bioactive compounds in oral inflammatory diseases. *J. Nutr. Intermed. Metab.* 18: 100105.

Kehl-Fie, T.E. and Skaar, E.P. (2010). Nutritional immunity beyond iron: a role for manganese and zinc. *Curr. Opin. Chem. Biol.* 14 (2): 218–224.

Kelley, D.S., Daudu, P.A., Taylor, P.C., Mackey, B.E. and Turnlund, J.R. (1995). Effects of low-copper diets on human immune response. *Am. J. Clin. Nutr.* 62(2): 412–416.

Khanna, S.S. and Karjodkar, F.R. (2006). Circulating immune complexes and trace elements (copper, iron and selenium) as markers in oral precancer and cancer: a randomised, controlled clinical trial. *Head Face Med.* 2: 33.

Kieffer, F. and Schneider, H. (1991). Minerals and trace elements in the immune system. *Nutrition Food Sci.* 91 (3): 7–9.

Kieliszek, M. and Błażejak, S. (2016). Current knowledge on the importance of selenium in food for living organisms: a review. *Molecules* 21 (5):609.

Kim, H.S., Park, J.A., Na, J.S., Lee, K.H. and Bae, K.H. (2014). Association between plasma levels of manganese and periodontal status: a study based on the Fourth Korean National Health and Nutrition Examination Survey. *J. Periodontol.* 85 (12): 1748–1754. 140250

Kiremidjian-Schumacher, L., Roy, M., Glickman, R. et al. (2000). Selenium and immunocompetence in patients with head and neck cancer. *Biol. Trace Element Res.* 73 (2): 97–111.

Kohlmeier, M. (2015). Minerals and trace elements. In: Nutrient Metabolism, 2e, 673–807. New York: Academic Press.

Lappalainen, R. and Knuuttila, M. (1981). X-ray diffraction patterns in human dentin, enamel and synthetic apatites related to Zn concentration. *Scand. J. Dent. Res.* 89 (6): 437–444.

Laur, N., Kinscherf, R., Pomytkin, K., Kaiser, L., Knes, O. and Deigner, H.P. (2020). ICP-MS trace element analysis in serum and whole blood. *PLoS One* 15 (5): e0233357.

Li, Y.Y., Du, X.P., Zhao, Y.F., Wang, J.M. and Wang, J.D. (2021). Fluoride can damage the spleen of mice by perturbing Th1/Th2 cell balance. *Biol. Trace Element Res.* 199 (4): 1493–1500.

Liu, C.C., Mo, L Y., Niu, Y.L., Li, X., Zhou, X.D. and Xu, X. (2017). The role of reactive oxygen species and autophagy in periodontitis and their potential linkage. *Front. Physiol.* 8: 439.

Liu, Zhang, Y., Piao, J.H. et al. (2017). Reference values of 14 serum trace elements for pregnant Chinese women: a cross-sectional study in the China Nutrition and Health Survey 2010–2012. *Nutrients* 9(3): 309.

Lv, M., Chen, M., Zhang, R. et al. (2020). Manganese is critical for antitumor immune responses via cGAS-STING and improves the efficacy of clinical immunotherapy. *Cell Res.* 30 (11): 966–979.

MacFarquhar, J.K., Broussard, D.L., Melstrom, P. et al. (2010). Acute selenium toxicity associated with a dietary supplement. *Arch. Intern. Med.* 170 (3): 256–261.

Maggini, S., Wintergerst, E.S., Beveridge, S. and Hornig, D.H. (2007). Selected vitamins and trace elements support immune function by strengthening epithelial barriers and cellular and humoral immune responses. *Br. J. Nutr.* 98 (Suppl 1): S29–35.

Manjunath, R.S. (2011). Role of antioxidants as an adjunct in periodontal therapy. *J. Adv. Oral Res.* 2 (2): 9–16.

Mehmet Sinan, D. (2018). Relation of trace elements on dental health. In: *Trace Elements* (eds M.S. Hosam El-Din and E.-A. Eithar). London: IntechOpen.

Mehri, A. (2020). Trace elements in human nutrition (II) – an update. *Int. J. Prev. Med.* 11: 2.

Meisel, P., Schwahn, C., Luedemann, J., John, U., Kroemer, H.K. and Kocher, T. (2005). Magnesium deficiency is associated with periodontal disease. *J. Dent. Res.* 84 (10): 937–941.

Meisel, P., Pink, C., Nauck, M., Jablonowski, L., Voelzke, H. and Kocher, T. (2016). Magnesium/calcium ratio in serum predicts periodontitis and tooth loss in a 5-year follow-up. *JDR Clin. Trans. Res.* 1 (3): 266–274.

Najeeb, S., Zafar, M.S., Khurshid, Z., Zohaib, S. and Almas, K. (2016). The role of nutrition in periodontal health: an update. *Nutrients* 8 (9): 530.

Nakata, A., Araki, S., Park, S.H. et al. (2006). Decreases in CD8+ T, naive (CD4+CD45RA+) T, and B (CD19+) lymphocytes by exposure to manganese fume. *Ind. Health* 44 (4): 592–597.

Nawi, A.M., Chin, S.F., Azhar Shah, S. and Jamal, R. (2019). Tissue and serum trace elements concentration among colorectal patients: a systematic review of case-control studies. *Iran J. Public Health* 48 (4): 632–643.

Nicholson, J.W. and Czarnecka, B. (2008). Fluoride in dentistry and dental restoratives. In: *Fluorine and Health: Molecular Imaging, Biomedical Materials and Pharmaceuticals* (ed. A. Tressaud), 333–378. St Louis, MO: Elsevier.

Nickel, E.H. (1995). Definition of a mineral. *Mineralogical Magazine* 59 (397): 767–768.

Nireeksha, Hegde, M., Kumari, S., Sharmila and Roopa (2020). Salivary selenium levels in dental caries. *Indian J. Public Health Res. Dev.* 11 (6): 1141–1145.

Nizam, N., Discioglu, F., Saygun, I. et al. (2014). The effect of α-tocopherol and selenium on human gingival fibroblasts and periodontal ligament fibroblasts in vitro. *J. Periodontol.* 85 (4): 636–644.

Pagmantidis, V., Méplan, C., van Schothorst, E.M., Keijer, J. and Hesketh, J.E. (2008). Supplementation of healthy volunteers with nutritionally relevant amounts of selenium increases the expression of lymphocyte protein biosynthesis genes. *Am. J. Clin. Nutr.* 87 (1): 181–189.

Paiva, C.N. and Bozza, M.T. (2014). Are reactive oxygen species always detrimental to pathogens? *Antiox. Redox Signal.* 20 (6): 1000–1037.

Pang, W.W., Abdul-Rahman, P.S., Wan-Ibrahim, W.I. and Hashim, O.H. (2010). Can the acute-phase reactant proteins be used as cancer biomarkers? *Int. J. Biol. Markers* 25 (1): 1–11.

Pathak, M., Shetty, V. and Kalra, D. (2015). Trace elements and oral health: a systematic review. *J. Adv. Oral Res.* 7 (2).

Pilankar, A., Singhavi, H., Raghuram, G.V. et al. (2022). A pro-oxidant combination of resveratrol and copper down-regulates hallmarks of cancer and immune checkpoints in patients with advanced oral cancer: results of an exploratory study (RESCU 004). *Front. Oncol.* 12: 1000957.

Prasad, A.S. (2014). Zinc is an antioxidant and anti-inflammatory agent: its role in human health. *Front. Nutr.* 1: 14.

Qamar, Z., Rahim, Z.B.H.A., Chew, H.P. and Fatima, T. (2017). Influence of trace elements on dental enamel properties: a review. *J. Pakistan Med. Assoc.* 67 (1): 116–120.

Ruiz Roca, J., Maria, L., Mi, R., Asta, T., Pons-Fuster, E. and Lopez Jornet, P. (2019). Oral health status and trace elements in saliva of children and teenagers with intellectual disabilities: a preliminary study. *Oral Health Care* 4.

Saxen, L., Viljanen, T. and Westermarck, T. (1983). Occurrence of caries and periodontal disease in selenium-treated patients with Spielmeyer-Sjogren's disease. *Scand. J. Dent. Res.* 91 (5): 356–359.

Singam, H., Akula, U., Palakuru, S., Palaparthi, R., Sisinty, V. and Guntakalla, V. (2014). Evaluation of the influence of serum and salivary fluoride levels on periodontal disease status in endemic fluorosis patients. *J. Dr. NTR University of Health Sciences* 3 (5): 9–12.

Son, E.W., Lee, S.R., Choi, H.S. et al. (2007). Effects of supplementation with higher levels of manganese and magnesium on immune function. *Arch. Pharm. Res.* 30 (6): 743–749.

Spallholz, J.E. and Stewart, J.R. (1989). Advances in the role of minerals in immunobiology. *Biol. Trace Elements Res.* 19 (3): 129–151.

Spallholz, J.E., Boylan, L.M. and Larsen, H.S. (1990). Advances in understanding selenium's role in the immune system. *Ann. N Y Acad. Sci.* 587: 123–139.

Stone, C.A., Kawai, K., Kupka, R. and Fawzi, W.W. (2010). Role of selenium in HIV infection. *Nutr. Rev.* 68 (11): 671–681.

Talal, S., Abdulla, W., Abdul Ameer, L., Raheem, Z. and Jabor, A. (2017). Estimation of salivary cadmium, calcium and manganese level in periodontal disease patients. *Int. J. Sci. Res.* 6: 949–952.

Tank, G. and Storvick, C.A. (1960). Effect of naturally occurring selenium and vanadium on dental caries. *J. Dent. Res.* 39: 473–488.

Tapiero, H., Townsend, D.M. and Tew, K.D. (2003). Trace elements in human physiology and pathology. *Copper. Biomed. Pharmacother.* 57 (9): 386–398.

Thomas, B., Ramesh, A., Suresh, S. and Prasad, B.R. (2013). A comparative evaluation of antioxidant enzymes and selenium in the serum of periodontitis patients with diabetes mellitus type 2. *Contemp. Clin. Dent.* 4 (2): 176–180.

Trivedy, C.R., Warnakulasuriya, K.A.A.S., Peters, T.J., Senkus, R., Hazarey, V.K. and Johnson, N.W. (2000). Raised tissue copper levels in oral submucous fibrosis. *J. Oral Pathol. Med.* 29 (6): 241–248.

Ullah, R. and Zafar, M.S. (2015). Oral and dental delivery of fluoride: a review. *Fluoride* 48 (3): 195–204.

Varghese, I., Sugathan, C.K., Balasubramoniyan, G. and Vijayakumar, T. (1987). Serum copper and zinc levels in premalignant and malignant lesions of the oral cavity. *Oncology* 44 (4): 224–227.

Vasovic, M., Gajovic, N., Brajkovic, D., Jovanovic, M., Zdravkovic, N. and Kanjevac, T. (2016). The relationship between the immune system and oral manifestations of inflammatory bowel disease: a review. *Centr. Eur. J. Immunol.* 41 (3): 302–310.

Wang, Y., Jiang, L., Li, Y., Luo, X. and He, J. (2016). Effect of different selenium supplementation levels on oxidative stress, cytokines, and immunotoxicity in chicken thymus. *Biol. Trace Elements Res.* 172 (2): 488–495.

Wintergerst, E.S., Maggini, S. and Hornig, D.H. (2007). Contribution of selected vitamins and trace elements to immune function. *Ann. Nutr. Metab.* 51(4): 301–323.

World Health Organization (WHO) (1996). *Trace Elements in Human Nutrition and Health*. Geneva: World Health Organization.

Wu, D., Lewis, E.D., Pae, M. and Meydani, S.N. (2018). Nutritional modulation of immune function: analysis of evidence, mechanisms, and clinical relevance. *Front. Immunol.* 9: 3160.

Yan, X.Y., Dong, N., Hao, X.H. et al. (2019). Comparative transcriptomics reveals the role of the toll-like receptor signaling pathway in fluoride-induced cardiotoxicity. *J. Agric. Food. Chem.* 67 (17): 5033–5042.

Yu, Q., Sun, X., Zhao, J. et al. (2019). The effects of zinc deficiency on homeostasis of twelve minerals and trace elements in the serum, feces, urine and liver of rats. *Nutr. Metab* 16: 73.

Zheng, W. and Monnot, A.D. (2012). Regulation of brain iron and copper homeostasis by brain barrier systems: implication in neurodegenerative diseases. *Pharmacol. Ther.* 133 (2): 177–188.

7

Oral Microbiome and Oral Cancer

Manosha Perera[1], Irosha Perera[2] and W.M. Tilakaratne[3]

[1] Department of Medical Laboratory Sciences, Faculty of Allied Health Sciences, General Sir John Kotelawala Defence University, Dehiwala-Mount Lavinia, Sri Lanka
[2] Preventive Oral Health Unit, National Dental Hospital (Teaching), Colombo, Sri Lanka
[3] Department of Oral and Maxillofacail Clinical Sciences, Faculty of Dentistry, University of Malaya, Kuala Lumpur, Malaysia

7.1 Definition of the Oral Microbiome

The oral cavity is the major gateway to the human body as it connects with the gastrointestinal tract, respiratory tract and sinuses. It consists of anatomical components such as the soft tissues (gingival sulcus, attached gingiva, tongue, cheek, lip and soft palate), hard tissues (hard palate and teeth) and the saliva. From a microbial ecology point of view, each component can be considered as a distinct niche/microhabitat whilst the oral cavity harbours the most diverse microbiota second to the gastrointestinal tract (Caselli et al. 2020; Verma et al. 2018; Kilian et al. 2016). Numerous factors such as nutrient availability, pH, attachment ligands, availability of oxygen and immune elements govern the composition of microbial communities in different microhabitats. Thus, each microhabitat maintains a unique ecosystem that provides a setting for symbiotic interactions among the various microbes within that ecosystem and the host.

The warm and moist environment of the oral cavity facilitates the growth of inhabiting microbes, by providing host-derived nutrients available in saliva and gingival crevicular fluid in the form of carbohydrates, amino acids, proteins, glycoproteins, peptides, and vitamins. Thus, the human oral cavity is a highly heterogeneous ecosystem with significantly different microbial communities, forming a unique 'normobiotic meta community' which maintains homeostasis with the host in health (*normobiosis*) (Caselli et al. 2020; Verma et al. 2018; Kilian et al. 2016).

Oral microbes need to become attached to oral surfaces if they are to remain in the mouth. Thus, microbes grow as interactive communities on mucosal and dental surfaces, in the form of structurally as well as functionally organised biofilms. All micro-organisms, their metagenome, metatranscriptome, metaproteome, metabolome and the microenvironments they inhabit in the oral cavity, are collectively referred to as the 'oral microbiome' (Caselli et al. 2020: Verma et al. 2018; Kilian et al. 2016). This oral microbiome consists mainly of bacteria followed by fungi dominated by *Candida*, viruses, methanogenic archaea and parasite species (*Trichomonas tenax* and *Entamoeba gingivalis*). In healthy conditions, the oral microbiome resists colonisation by pathogens by competition for attachment sites, nutrition, lysis by bacteriocins and promoting host defence mechanisms (Caselli et al. 2020; Verma et al. 2018; Kilian et al. 2016).

7.2 Biological Evolution of the Oral Microbiome

The oral microbiome has been subjected to compositional changes throughout human civilization, from the Neolithic era through to the Industrial Revolution to the modern era of Evidence Based Medicine. The contributing human factors in that progressive compositional change include the use of fire, the food consumed in the Agricultural Revolution, the upsurge in consumption of refined sugar after the Industrial Revolution, oral hygiene practices and the arrival of antimicrobial therapies (Gillings et al. 2015; Weyrich 2021).

Temporal changes in the oral microbiome have been observed in archaeological dental calculus from hunter-gatherers of the Neolithic societies and the Industrial Revolution. There was a trend towards reduced species diversity in each of these evolutionary milestones. The introduction of refined sugar to the diet is reported to have occurred in the early Industrial Revolution. Acid-tolerant bacterial species were able to thrive in the oral cavity by evolving their metabolism involving the metagenome to adapt to 'postagricultural' changes in the diet. Defence and resistance mechanisms were developed against elevated oxidative stress and acidic by-products respectively to achieve an efficient carbohydrate metabolism. Hence, aciduric and acidogenic bacterial species thrive better than those which did not adopt metabolically, and *Streptococcus mutans* provides a classic example in this regard (Gillings et al. 2015).

Since in the Industrial Revolution humans were exposed to heavy metals, disinfectants, biocides and antibiotics, it is assumed that microbes equipped with resistance determinants for antimicrobials became more dominant.

In the nineteenth century worldwide access to standard oral hygiene practices started. Epidemiological evidence has shown a significant association between the oral microbiome and tooth brushing and flossing – a phenomenon later confirmed by empirical evidence (Gillings et al. 2015; Weyrich 2021). Laboratory evidence also confirmed that lifestyle-related risk habits such as smoking, betel nut chewing and alcohol consumption have been causing compositional and functional changes in the oral microbiome (Al-Marzooq et al. 2022; Uehara et al. 2021; Jia et al. 2021; Fan et al. 2018). Interestingly, there is emerging evidence to suggest co-evolution of microbiomes in mammals as well as in humans, thus sharing many similarities in their composition and organisation (Groussin et al. 2017, 2020).

7.3 Acquiring the Oral Microbiome

The presence of bacteria in the placenta, umbilical cord blood, amniotic fluid and meconium in full-term pregnancies without overt infection has been reported (Markéta et al. 2021; Kaan et al. 2021; Deo and Deshmukh 2019). This indicates the possibility of migration of maternal bacteria via the placenta. Evidence supports the higher resemblance of the placental microbiome with the pregnant mother's oral microbiome (Gomez-Arango et al. 2017). Hence the initial acquisition of the oral microbiome takes place at the fetal stage. However, practically it is not easy to assess the microbial flora of the fetal mouth due to inherent limitations in taking specimens of the fetus for laboratory investigations.

After birth, the oral microbiome is further shaped by vertical and horizontal transmissions during the postnatal period. Vertical transmission is related to the mode of delivery and the method of feeding (Coelho et al. 2021; Li et al. 2021; Sulyanto et al. 2019). A significant number of these initial bacterial colonisers are of maternal origin. In addition, a newborn can acquire bacteria by breathing and contact with parents and care givers. This method of acquisition is termed 'horizontal transmission' (Xiao et al. 2020). In line with this observation, *Lactobacillus*, *Prevotella* and *Sneathia* are the major bacterial genera among the initial colonisers of the oral microbiome of babies born by vaginal birth that are similar to the mother's major vaginal bacterial genera (Kaan et al. 2021; Mukherjee et al. 2021; Dominguez-Bello et al. 2010). In contrast, *Staphylococcus*, *Corynebacterium* and *Propionibacterium* are the predominant initial colonisers of babies born by caesarean section, which are similar to the main genera of the mother's skin. Hence, vaginally born babies harbour a higher number of taxa three months after birth compared with babies born by caesarean section. Breastfed infants (three months old) showed higher colonisation with oral lactobacilli than formula-fed infants (Kaan et al. 2021; Mukherjee et al. 2021; Dominguez-Bello et al. 2010).

Inoculum dose and the status of immune tolerance of the newborn are the main factors that govern this initial colonisation process (Kaan et al. 2021; Mukherjee et al. 2021; Dominguez-Bello et al. 2010). Again, the primary colonisers or pioneers facilitate the colonisation of secondary colonisers of the oral cavity by changing the environment via their metabolism. Thus, *Streptococcus* and *Staphylococcus* are frequent colonizers after just 24 hours from birth. *Streptococcus salivarius*, a pioneer of newborns, can produce extracellular adhesin to facilitate the attachment of *Actinomyces* to oral epithelial cells. The formation of a more diverse stable microbial community is the main outcome of this microbial succession process (Kaan et al. 2021; Mukherjee et al. 2021; Dominguez-Bello et al. 2010).

The microbial communities evolve with the growth of the baby. A distinct oral microbial profile of the baby is observed five months after birth and is attributed to maternal inheritance and environmental exposure (Kaan et al. 2021; Mukherjee et al. 2021; Dominguez-Bello et al. 2010). Environmental exposure is mainly facilitated by ingestion of food contact with other adults (parents and care givers) and children (siblings) (Kaan et al. 2021; Mukherjee et al. 2021; Dominguez-Bello et al. 2010).

Further changes in the oral microbiome occur during the period of tooth eruption, the first major ecological event in the mouth (Xu et al. 2022; Xiao et al. 2020). A complex composition of the oral microbiome starts to appear by the age of three while complexity increases with age. Changes in oral habitat with the replacement of deciduous teeth by secondary teeth is the second major ecological event that also contributes to the composition of the oral microbiome (Kaan et al. 2021; Mukherjee et al. 2021; Dominguez-Bello et al. 2010; Xiao et al. 2020). After this period, the microbiome consists mainly of bacteria, including the six phyla: *Firmicutes, Proteobacteria, Actinobacteria, Bacteroidetes, Fusobacteria* and *Spirochaetes*. The most prevalent genera are *Streptococcus, Haemophilus, Neisseria* and *Veillonella*. Even at the age of three, the salivary microbiome is a complex entity, but the maturation process of the oral microbiome continues until adulthood.

7.4 Oral Biofilm or Dental Plaque

Micro-organisms grow as interactive communities on mucosal and dental surfaces, in the form of structurally as well as functionally organised biofilms. Biofilm formation is an ecological event of microbial community succession with time as the structure and function of a community are being subjected to temporal changes. The development of biofilms occurs in three successional phases: *initiation, progression* and *establishment*. The total biomass keeps on increasing with time in all three phases (Marsh and Bradshaw 1995; O'Toole et al. 2000; Berger et al. 2018).

7.4.1 Initiation Phase of Oral Biofilm Formation

In the *initiation phase*, the substrate is freely available to primary colonisers having no specific nutritional requirements. The entire surface of the mouth is covered by a layer of adsorbed molecules of salivary and bacterial origin, which is known as an acquired pellicle. The competition among community members for attachment sites and nutrients is largely absent at this stage. Nevertheless, most vulnerable competitors can be eliminated due to competition and antagonism among them (Marsh and Bradshaw 1995; O'Toole et al. 2000; Berger et al. 2018).

In an immature biofilm, primary colonisers may form reversible as well as irreversible attachments. They use prolonged weak physicochemical interactions between charged molecules on their cell walls and oral surfaces as reversible attachments, with the possibility of detachment. These pioneers also utilise strong short-range stereochemical interactions between adhesions on the bacterium and complementary receptors in the acquired pellicle, to become permanent members. Streptococci are the classic example of pioneers who modify the local environment by their metabolic activities to facilitate the subsequent colonisation of more fastidious successors. Secondary colonisers make use of this situation to make co-adhesions to attach to receptors on primary colonisers. Subsequently, they increase in numbers. This structurally and functionally organised entity increases its complexity during development.

The formation of a biofilm matrix is achieved by extracellular polymers synthesised by attached bacteria. This matrix acts as a structural scaffold and biologically active entity by retaining numerous molecules consisting of enzymes. In this phase, community diversity increases rapidly before dropping into an intermediate state due to the extinction of some of these pioneering colonisers (Marsh and Bradshaw 1995; O'Toole et al. 2000; Berger et al. 2018).

7.4.2 Progression Phase of Oral Biofilm Formation

In the *progression* phase, the resident bacteria interact both synergistically and antagonistically. Metabolic forces among them operate synergistically to break down complex host macromolecules such as mucin to obtain nutrients. Subsequently, cascades of food chains manifest in the biofilm where the metabolic product of one organism becomes a primary nutrient for another. Furthermore, bacterial cells communicate by signalling with each other, using a range of diffusible molecules which facilitate the co-ordination of gene expression among members of the microbial community. Peptides are used for communication between Gram-positive bacteria. In contrast, autoinducer 2 is employed by many Gram-negative species to communicate among them (Marsh and Bradshaw 1995; O'Toole et al. 2000; Berger et al. 2018).

7.4.3 Establishment Phase of Oral Biofilm Formation

In the *biofilm establishment* phase, the community matures and thickens with spatial heterogeneity. Inferior competitors (bacterial species which do not possess superior qualities of adaptation for better adherence such as having specific receptors) may find opportunities to re-establish and to form a stabilised biofilm with the high species richness and diversity. In this stage, biofilm members are found to be well equipped with biological properties for better survival as a consortium than a single species. They also exhibit improved resistance to antimicrobial agents and the host's defence mechanisms.

Once stabilised, the composition of microbial communities in a biofilm remains relatively constant over time (Marsh and Bradshaw 1995; O'Toole et al. 2000; Berger et al. 2018).

7.4.4 Microbial Diversity of Oral Biofilms

The microbial diversity of biofilms varies between different surfaces of the mouth. Biofilms with high microbial diversity are found on the highly papillated surfaces of the tongue (Heller et al. 2016). The microbial load at mucosal sites is relatively low due to desquamation. Teeth are non-shedding surfaces and the highest amount of biomass in the mouth can be seen on them. The largest numbers and diversity of the oral microbiota are found at sites such as the gingival crevice, with subgingival plaque which could be identified as stagnant sites which provide protection against oral removal forces. Fissures on occlusal surfaces are colonised with high numbers of aerobic and facultatively anaerobic, saccharolytic Gram-positive bacteria, predominantly streptococci, and few anaerobes or Gram-negative bacteria. In contrast, high proportions of proteolytic and many Gram-negative obligate anaerobes are present in the gingival crevice.

The recent advancements in 'omics' and matrix biology technologies have provided an extraordinary opportunity to study the structure and function of species in oral biofilms (Kilian et al. 2016). Epidemiological evidence has suggested the possible roles played by them in health and disease. Decades of laboratory investigations have provided information on some virulence mechanisms. Hence, there is a wealth of information on pathobiont-induced oral inflammatory diseases. Dental caries and periodontitis are classic examples of pathobiont-induced oral inflammatory diseases that cause the destruction of enamel and dentine and infection and inflammation of the pulp tissues (with regard to dental caries) and the tooth-supporting structures such as gingiva and periodontal ligament and alveolar bone in the case of progressive periodontitis (Seneviratne et al. 2011).

7.5 Oral Cancer

Oral cancer is a subgroup of head and neck cancers (HNCs) which is a biologically heterogeneous group of neoplasms involving several distinct anatomical sites within the head and neck (Johnson et al. 2018). Furthermore, oral cancer consists of malignant neoplasms, mainly oral squamous cell carcinoma (OSCC) evolving from the lining epithelium of mucous membranes (*International Classification of Disease*, 10th revision [ICD-10]): lips (C00), base of the tongue (C01), oral cavity including the anterior two-thirds of the tongue (C02–C06) respectively (Figure 7.1) (Johnson et al. 2018). Furthermore, oral cancer is a multifactorial disease that is causally linked to a variety of environmental, genetic and epigenetic factors and demonstrates population as well as geographic location specificity (Sarode et al. 2020; Johnson et al. 2018).

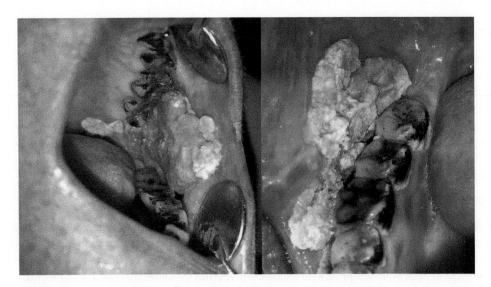

Figure 7.1 Clinical appearance of oral cancer (oral squamous cell carcinoma).

7.5.1 Oral Carcinogenesis in Brief

In normal conditions, the equilibrium between cell proliferation and cell death of oral epithelium is kept under tight regulation. This is governed by specific genes that are broadly categorised as either proto-oncogenes or tumour suppressor genes. Regulated expression of those gene products (polypeptides) governs cell division, growth, survival and apoptosis. These gene products generate specific excitatory as well as inhibitory signals to maintain the equilibrium between cell proliferation and cell death. Proto-oncogenes encode classes of proteins such as epidermal growth factor receptor (EGFR) and cell signalling molecules such as cyclins which facilitate DNA replication, cell division and inhibition of apoptosis. In contrast, the tumour suppressor gene products inhibit cellular proliferation and growth and promote apoptosis.

Oral carcinogenesis is a complex, complicated multistage process comprising an array of molecular events, which occurs when the oral squamous epithelium is affected by a series of genetic and epigenetic as well as histological changes via multiple pathways (Mascolo et al. 2012; Dumache et al. 2015; Perera et al. 2018; Farah et al. 2019).

Genetic changes are caused by known oral carcinogens. There are specific genes that encode specific enzymes to metabolise these carcinogens. Single nucleotide polymorphisms (SNP) are the most abundant form of genetic variation that can enhance oral carcinogenesis by defective metabolism of carcinogens by altering carcinogen metabolising enzyme functions. Moreover, the genetic changes of oral carcinogenesis include several critical mutations/aberrations resulting in defective ability to repair genetic damage caused by carcinogens, enhanced function of several proto-oncogenes, oncogenes and/or the deactivation of tumour suppressor genes. This gives rise to overactivity of growth factors and its cell surface receptors, which could enhance intracellular messenger signalling, resulting in increased production of transcription factors (Mascolo et al. 2012; Dumache et al. 2015; Farah et al. 2019).

Epigenetic changes consist of DNA methylation, histone posttranslational modifications and non-coding RNAs (ncRNAs). These changes can convert proto-oncogenes into oncogenes. Activation of growth factor receptors in human tumours includes mutations, gene rearrangements and overexpression. Aberrant expression of several oncogenes, including epidermal growth factor receptor (EGFR/c-erb 1), members of the Ras gene family, c-myc, int-2, hst-1, PRAD-1 and bcl-1 as well as inactivation of tumour suppressor genes (TSGs) such as p14, ARF, p15 INK4B, p 16 INK4A and p53 play a crucial role in the initiation of oral carcinogenesis, transforming normal cells to neoplastic cells. Furthermore, mutations and altered expression of other important TSGs such as *NOTCH1* have been suggested by drivers of cancer progression. In addition, *MDM2*, which is a proto-oncogene promoting tumour formation by targeting tumour suppressor proteins such as p53, is amplified in 25–40% of cancers. Accordingly, the co-expression of p53/*MDM2* proteins has gained recognition as an indicator of tumour aggressiveness in OSCC (Mascolo et al. 2012; Dumache et al. 2015; Farah et al. 2019).

However, there are DNA repair genes to rectify the altered genes. These genes function in a diverse set of pathways that involve the recognition and removal of DNA lesions, tolerance to DNA damage, and protection from errors of incorporation made during DNA replication. Mutations in these genes can paralyse DNA repair pathways. The two forces (mutation and repair) counteract but the balance is shifted a little on the mutational side of the interaction so some mutations will become permanent and carcinogenesis is initiated. Consequently, neoplastic cells divide more rapidly by uncontrolled cell proliferation due to the acquisition of growth signalling autonomy which means independence in cell growth. This will lead to evasion of apoptosis, cellular immortalisation and angiogenesis. Finally, neoplastic cells become functionally independent from their normal oral keratinocyte neighbours with the capacity for migration and reprogramming their energy metabolism (Mascolo et al. 2012; Dumache et al. 2015; Farah et al. 2019).

At the same time, an immunological surveillance/immuno-editing process is provided by the host's immune system to detect and destroy neoplastically transformed cells. These neoplastic cells use strategies to evade the immune system; the expression of immune inhibitory molecules is one of them. Using this strategy, neoplastic cells escape from elimination by immune cells, causing immune suppression. Consequently, carcinogenesis keeps on progressing while invading normal tissues at local or distant sites, which is called metastasis (Chakraborty et al. 2018).

Histopathological changes in tissues include loss of maturation, architectural disorganisation and various features of cytological atypia (Odell et al. 2021). Invasive carcinomas can be divided into keratinising and non-keratinising carcinomas. Furthermore, the degree of differentiation is expressed as poorly, moderately and well differentiated (Figure 7.2).

7.5.2 Global Burden of Oral Cancer

The most frequently encountered oral cancers are the oral squamous cell carcinomas. Oral cancer is ranked as the eighteenth most common cancer type globally, demonstrating an estimated 354 564 cases and 177 384 deaths annually

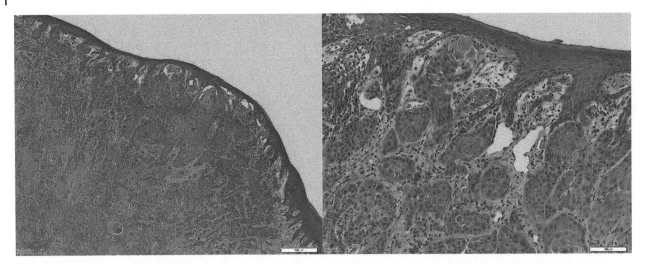

Figure 7.2 Histopathological features of oral squamous cell carcinoma. Tumour islands invading into connective tissue.

(Bray et al. 2018). Two-thirds of all cases are recorded in countries with transitioning economies. Oral cancer demonstrates a predilection for males. Furthermore, the majority of disease burden is carried by socially disadvantaged population groups in developing countries as well as minority ethnic groups in developed countries. Papua New Guinea, Bangladesh, Sri Lanka and Melanesia currently have the highest global oral cancer incidence rates (Shrivastava et al. 2014).

Regardless of the easy accessibility of the oral cavity for direct examination, these malignancies are often detected at late stages. Alarmingly, patients who survive the primary cancer in the oral cavity are reported to have up to a 20-fold increased risk of developing a second primary oral cancer. This increased risk lasts for 5–10 years. Despite advances in surgery, radiation and chemotherapy, the five-year survival rates in many countries remain at 50%, one of the lowest of the major cancers (Shibahara 2017).

The Indian subcontinent, Sri Lanka, India, Bangladesh and Pakistan alone account for one-third of the global oral cancer burden (Khan 2012; Coelho 2012). In many regions of India, oral cancer is the second most common malignancy diagnosed in men, accounting for up to 20% of cancers, and the fourth most common in women. In India, 90–95% of newly diagnosed malignancies are OSCC. Nearly 70 000 new cases and more than 48 000 oral cancer-related deaths happen every year (Khan 2012; Coelho 2012; Sharma et al. 2018). Oral cancer represents the most common cancer type among males with a crude rate of 20.6/100 000 and the eighth most common cancer type among females with a crude incidence of 5.2/100 000 in Sri Lanka. Moreover, 83% of oral cancers are OSCC. There has been approximately a 40% increase in oral cancer patients over the past seven years. Age-standardised incidence rates were reported as 19.1/100 000 for males and 4.3/100 000 for females (National Cancer Control Programme, Sri Lanka 2019).

7.6 Oral Microbiome as a Biomarker in Oral Cancer

Contemporary advancements in next-generation sequencing (NGS), especially in 'omics' technologies, have provided an extraordinary opportunity to study microbial communities in any ecosystem (Kilian et al. 2016; Perera et al. 2018). Metagenomics studies provide the taxonomic profile of a microbial community under different conditions. Nevertheless, it is not possible to find out whether they are alive or dead. Metatranscriptomics provides us with the genes that are expressed by the community as a whole (Al-Hebshi et al. 2019).

Most of the research on the oral microbiome has focused on the oral bacteriome which is the main component of the oral microbiome. Nevertheless, there is emerging interest in the potential role of fungi (oral mycobiome) and viruses (oral virome) in oral carcinogenesis (Perera et al. 2016; Al-Hebshi et al. 2019).

During the past decade, the epidemiological association between oral bacteria and OSCC has been extensively assessed by metagenomic studies (Perera et al. 2016; Al-Hebshi et al. 2019). In healthy conditions, resident bacteria maintain a homeostasis or equilibrium with the host by symbiosis (Caselli et al. 2020). However, in disease conditions, this symbiosis turns into dysbiosis. Hence, an oral cancer-associated 'specific bacteriome' was observed in the majority of the metagenomic studies comparing oral cancer patients and healthy controls. Nevertheless, there is no consensus on the specific bacterial composition or patterns associated with oral cancer (Perera et al. 2018). Moreover, the variations observed in microbiome profiles associated with oral cancer may reflect the proinflammatory status with functional redundancy (Perera et al. 2018).

Therefore, in reality what becomes a cause for concern is that different species may be enriched in different samples but still would serve the same functions. Thus, more consistent and more useful findings are likely to be achieved with functional analysis with a metatranscriptomic approach rather than with compositional analysis (Al-Hebshi et al. 2019). Evidence is emerging for the potential role of the microbiome in oral carcinogenesis (Perera et al. 2016). In vitro studies have provided evidence for carcinogenic properties of two main periodontal pathogens, *Fusobacterium nucleatum* and *Porphyromonas gingivalis* (Perera et al. 2016). It has been found that the microbial dysbiosis and proinflammatory bacteriome within the tumour microenvironment probably contribute to tumour progression by sustaining chronic inflammation (Perera et al. 2018).

The oral microbiota is metabolically versatile and can adapt easily to environmental and biological changes in the tumour microenvironment (Perera et al. 2018). Shifts in composition and/or function of the oral microbiota might offer new useful diagnostic biomarkers to explore cancer risk, and prognostic markers to assess treatment response (Chattopadhyay et al. 2019). Moreover, genetically manipulated bacteria can be used in targeted therapies, especially in immune therapies, and deliver anticancer drugs (Liu et al. 2014).

7.7 Aetiological Factors of Oral Cancer

Most of the aetiological carcinogens/mutagens (inducing or capable of causing genetic mutations) have been well established by strong epidemiological and laboratory evidence. They are categorised as substances carcinogenic to humans (Group 1) by the International Agency for Research on Cancer (IARC) (IARC 2022a). The aetiological factors for oral potentially malignant disorders (OPMD) and oral cancer act individually or synergistically to cause oral cancer. For example, betel chewing with or without tobacco, areca nut chewing, smoking and alcohol consumption which are lifestyle-related risk habits together as well as individually could cause OPMD and oral cancers (Petti et al. 2013). The amount of each of those substances consumed and duration of exposure to each of those habits are directly proportional to the risk of developing oral cancer (Petti et al. 2013: Gupta and Johnson 2014). Nevertheless, risk can be minimised or controlled by habit intervention as all these aetiological agents are associated with substance abuse and lifestyle-related risk habits (Petti et al. 2013; Gupta and Johnson 2014).

7.7.1 Tobacco smoking

The smoked tobacco category consists of cigarettes, cigars, beedies and pipes. Of these, cigarettes represent the most popular form of smoked tobacco across the globe. Tobacco smoke contains more than 7000 chemical compounds, of which several are proven carcinogens (IARC 2022a). Nicotine is a highly addictive dinitrogen alkaloid compound present in the tobacco plant (*Nicotiana tabacum*). Well-known carcinogens in tobacco smoke can be broadly classified into polycyclic aromatic hydrocarbons (PAH), nicotine-derived nitrosamine ketone (NNK), together with a range of tobacco-specific toxins, including volatile aldehyde and phenolic amines (IARC 2022a,b).

7.7.2 Smokeless Tobacco

Smokeless tobacco is available in many forms, with names specific to the country or region of origin. However, the products are usually classified as loose leaf or twists for chewing, flakes, shredded, solid compressed products in the form of chunks and sticks, viscous pastes and dry or moist ground tobacco (snuff) for oral or nasal use. Smokeless tobacco is mainly consumed as one of the ingredients in betel quid/paan. Moist snuff (shammah) is used in different forms such as tea bag-like pouches, dissolvable tobacco lozenges, tobacco toothpicks and tobacco-smoke water for gargling. Furthermore, smokeless tobacco products are flavoured with sugar, salted and/or aromatised with substances like essences, spices and perfumes. A substantial number of people in South-East Asia use smokeless tobacco together with areca nut.

Smokeless tobacco products contain more than 3000 chemicals and at least 28 of these are carcinogens (IARC 2022a,b; Asthana et al. 2019; Islam et al. 2019). Smokeless tobacco usage exposes the person to tobacco-specific nitrosamines, volatile *N*-nitrosamines, *N*-nitrosamine acids and volatile aldehydes such as formaldehyde and acetaldehyde. Moreover, 4-(methylnitrosamino)-1-(3-pyridyl)-1-butanol (NNAL) is considered the most carcinogenic tobacco-specific nitrosamine. Smokeless tobacco also contains heavy metals such as cadmium, lead, arsenic, nickel and radioactive elements. In addition, it generates reactive oxygen species/oxidative stress which may initiate or progress oral carcinogenesis by multiple molecular and cellular pathways.

7.7.3 Areca Nut and Areca Nut-based Products

The areca nut is the seed of the oriental palm *Areca catechu*. It is common in countries such as India, Sri Lanka, Bangladesh, Myanmar, Taiwan and numerous islands in the south-western Pacific, especially Melanesia. Furthermore, the areca nut is popular in parts of Thailand, Indonesia, Malaysia, Cambodia, Vietnam, the Philippines and China. Areca nut trees are native to Sri Lanka, west Malaysia and Melanesia. An estimated 10–20% of the population worldwide consumes areca nut as a masticatory substance. Carbohydrates, fat, protein, fibre, polyphenols (flavonoids and tannins), alkaloids and minerals are the main components of the areca nut (Li et al. 2019).

A range of packaged areca nut products is mostly produced in India and Pakistan. These products are very popular among a new generation of users which means an emerging trend of young and educated groups indulging in areca nut chewing (Mahees et al. 2021). The most common products are gutka, pan-masala, beeda and babul. Gutka is a non-perishable areca nut-based product that is prepared with powdered tobacco, areca nut, slaked lime and condiments.

Arecoline, arecaidine, guvacine and guacoline are well-known alkaloids in areca nut. Nitrosation of these alkaloids produce nitrosamine derivatives. Arecoline-specific nitrosamines such as methyl nitrosamine propionitrile are known to be carcinogenic (Li et al. 2019). Extensive production of nitrosamine by oral biofilm bacteria was observed in the metabolism of areca nut and areca nut-based products by a study conducted among areca nut chewers. Additionally, the production of reactive oxygen species by auto-oxidation of polyphenols has been reported. These reactive oxygen species have the potential to initiate or progress oral carcinogenesis by multiple molecular and cellular pathways (IARC 2022b).

7.7.4 Slaked Lime

Although slaked lime is not in itself a carcinogen, it instigates erosion of the oral mucous membranes, promoting the penetration of carcinogenic compounds. It may operate as a tumour promoter by hydrolysing alkaloids contained in areca nut to cytotoxic and mutagenic compounds. Moreover, extensive production of nitrosamine from areca nut and tobacco substrates may be facilitated by the alkaline pH provided by the slaked lime in betel quid (IARC 2022a,b).

7.7.5 Alcohol Consumption

Alarmingly, consumption of alcohol as well as 'binge drinking' appears to be a major public health problem worldwide. Alcoholic beverages are complex mixtures that contain volatile and non-volatile flavour compounds, but ethanol and water are the main components of almost all alcoholic beverages.

Ethanol giving rise to a genotoxic effect upon metabolism to acetaldehyde is well known. Acetaldehyde is the agent mainly implicated for carcinogenesis. However, at least 18 carcinogenic compounds have been identified in alcoholic beverages: acetaldehyde, acrylamide, aflatoxins, arsenic, benzene, cadmium, ethanol, ethyl carbamate, formaldehyde, furan, glyphosate, lead, 3-MCPD, 4-methylimidazole, *N*-nitrosodimethylamine, pulegone, ochratoxin A and safrole. However, there is no evidence to support that alcohol is a primary aetiological factor for oral cancer. It has a synergistic effect on tobacco and areca nut-related carcinogens.

7.7.6 Human Papilloma Virus

Human papilloma virus (HPV) belongs to a large family of viruses, the *Papillomaviridae*. They are small in diameter (55 nm) and epitheliotropic, with a genome of 7200–8000 base pairs in length. Based on their nucleotide sequences, HPVs are classified into more than 100 different genotypes, about 15 of which are regarded as 'high risk' due to their oncogenic potential. HPV16 and HPV18 are especially linked with malignant transformation (Shaikh et al. 2015).

Oral sex practices are considered the main mode of transmission for this virus. The oral carcinogenesis caused by HPV is a different entity from that caused by tobacco and betel quid chewing. Accordingly, head and neck squamous cell carcinomas (HNSCC) are divided into two main prognostic and therapeutic groups: HPV-positive and HPV-negative tumours. Of these, HPV-positive tumours have a better prognosis (Shaikh et al. 2015).

Human papillomavirus is established as an aetiological agent for a subset of HNSCCs, especially in the oropharynx (C10) and tonsils (C09). Furthermore, there is sufficient evidence for the causality of high-risk HPV 16 in the oral cavity (C00-C06), especially at the base of the tongue. In recent years, HPV has appeared as a prominent aetiological agent for OSCC across the globe in younger patients who were not exposed to other aetiological factors (Shaikh et al. 2015).

7.8 Predisposing Factors for Oral Cancer

Host factors that facilitate pathogenesis are known as predisposing factors. Genetic susceptibility, dietary micronutrient deficiencies, immunosuppression and age are the main predisposing factors that may promote oral carcinogenesis. The advancement of age is also a predisposing factor as it leads to less effective immune surveillance.

7.8.1 Genetic Susceptibility

There is evidence of family history and increased risk of developing HNSCC, suggesting the existence of genetic predisposition. Thus, certain individuals inherit susceptible genes with the inability to metabolise carcinogens or procarcinogens or an impaired ability to repair the DNA damage. SNPs are considered the major form of genetic variation. SNPs are areas of genes with altered DNA sequences, which also demonstrate geographic and population specificity.

In the past two decades, several studies have been conducted to identify candidate genes that determine susceptibility to oral carcinogenesis. These show that SNPs of cytochrome P4501A1 (CYP1A1), cytochrome P450 2E1 (CYP2E1), CYP1A1, GSTM1 ±, NAT2, ADH and ALDH genes appeared to increase susceptibility to carcinogenesis. These genes encode specific enzymes responsible for xenobiotic (alcohol, tobacco, areca nut) metabolism. These specific enzymes are responsible for the inactivation or detoxification of carcinogens such as polycyclic aromatic hydrocarbons (PAHs), acetaldehyde and aromatic amines. Therefore, polymorphism of these genes plays an important role in alcohol, tobacco and areca nut-induced head and neck cancers.

Polymorphisms in *CYP1A1* (*m2/m2*) and *GSTM1* genes and ADH and ALDH genes, which encode alcohol dehydrogenase *and* aldehyde dehydrogenase enzymes, are important in alcohol metabolism which increases susceptibility to oral cancer. In contrast, genetic polymorphisms in cytochrome P450 2E1 (CYP2E1) is mainly associated with tobacco-related oral cancer.

Polymorphisms of MTHFR-C677T- and XRCC1 Arg194Trp DNA repair gene alter folate levels and DNA methylation that may lead to carcinogenesis and changes in the base excision repair pathway respectively. It appears that the p73G4C14-to-A4T14 homozygous variant genotype might be a risk factor for cancer development via deregulation of programmed cell death.

7.8.2 Dietary Micronutrient Deficiencies

Dietary micronutrient deficiencies have shown a significant association with all head and neck cancers in epidemiological and laboratory studies. Frequent consumption of fresh vegetables, especially carrots, tomatoes, green peppers and leafy vegetables, and fruits including melon, papaya, orange and mango has health benefits. They are rich in antioxidants. Provitamin A carotenoids, beta-carotene, vitamins C and E, and selenium seem to be especially protective against most epithelial cancers and their precursor lesions. Antioxidants are exogenous or endogenous molecules comprising man-made or natural substances (dietary micronutrients) which could prevent or delay some types of cell damage. Diets high in vegetables and fruits, which are rich sources of antioxidants, have proven superior to antioxidant supplements. Examples of antioxidants include vitamins C and E, selenium, carotenoids, such as beta-carotene, lycopene, lutein and zeaxanthin. Antioxidants could mitigate any form of oxidative/nitrosative stress or its consequences. Free radicals (highly unstable molecules) resulting from environmental exposures and smoking give rise to oxidative stress which is a process resulting in cell damage. Nitrosative stress is defined as overproduction of nitric oxides and antioxidants may act directly by scavenging free radicals and increasing antioxidative defences (Rodríguez-Molinero et al. 2021).

7.8.3 Immunosuppression

Immunosuppressed patients, including organ transplant patients, demonstrate a higher susceptibility to oral cancer than normal patients. Interestingly, recent laboratory studies reveal that the immune response is critical in mediating the phenotypic consequences of oncogene addiction in oncogene inactivation. The immunosurveillance mechanism depends on $CD4^+$ and $CD8^+$ T cells, interferon (IFN)-gamma and the IFN-gamma receptor to control neoplastic cells. $CD4^+$ T cells have been suggested to play an important role in the remodelling of the tumour microenvironment. Adaptive and innate immune cells are likely to be involved in the mechanism of tumour regression. In addition, new pathways of elimination, especially by immune cells of the innate immune system have been recently reported. Carcinogenesis itself creates an immunosuppressive status which diminishes immunosurveillance, especially in the elimination stage of immune editing. Thus, the pre-existing immune-suppressive status of the host can promote the oral carcinogenesis process, while further retarding immunosurveillance.

7.8.4 Age

Oral squamous cell carcinomas usually occur in older men, aged 50 years and above, with a history of tobacco (smoked/smokeless), alcohol consumption and betel quid chewing for more than 10 years (Johnson et al. 2018). Therefore, an increased incidence of oral cancer is evident in older age predominantly attributed to consumption of tobacco and tobacco-related products, alcohol and areca nut over a considerable period. Furthermore, immune surveillance and cell repair may be reduced with advanced age. Nevertheless, oral cancers are reported among younger age groups as well.

7.8.5 Socioeconomic Factors

Socioeconomic factors primarily assessed by the level of education, occupation and income have been widely recognised as major determinants of health. Oral cancer risk is high among socially disadvantaged groups (Conway et al. 2008). This increased risk is predominantly attributed to lifestyle-related risk habits that are more common among low socioeconomic groups compared to their better-off counterparts, thus indicating synergy of low socioeconomic status demonstrated by low levels of education, lower income and low levels of occupation such as manual workers indulging in risk habits.

7.9 Risk Factors for Oral Cancer

Besides aetiological and predisposing factors, several environmental factors, as well as infection and the inflammatory response of the host, can increase the risk for oral cancer. These are collectively known as risk factors. The rate of DNA mutation is greatly boosted by an array of population and geographic area-specific risk factors. Their association with increased risk of oral carcinogenesis has been proven by epidemiological studies. However, more laboratory studies are warranted to establish causality, especially in the initiation of oral carcinogenesis.

7.9.1 Exposure to Excessive Solar Radiation and UV Light

Prolonged exposure to solar ultraviolet (UV) radiation is considered one of the most significant environmental DNA-damaging agents to which humans are exposed. Sunlight, specifically UVB and UVA, triggers various types of DNA damage. Thus, excessive exposure to sunlight appears as a risk factor for OSCC, especially on the lips. Thus, it is considered an occupational hazard for people who engage in outdoor activities, such as farmers and fishermen.

Depending on the limited evidence from epidemiological studies conducted in Sweden, Greece, Finland and India, solar radiation is categorised by the IARC as a probable cause of lip cancer (IARC 2022a,b). Mechanisms by which oral carcinogenesis occurs via directly or indirectly induced UV radiation are not clear at present. However, DNA damage of keratinocytes in oral epithelium due to the oxidation of pyrimidine dimers and oxidised bases may contribute to UV-induced carcinogenesis. Under normal conditions, DNA repair pathways protect cells against sunlight-induced oxidised DNA damage. It seems that there are predisposing conditions such as xeroderma pigmentosum (XP) as a result of a defect in the DNA repair system. Further laboratory and large cohort human studies are needed to understand the relative roles of the various forms of sunlight-induced DNA damage in oral carcinogenesis.

7.9.2 Sulfur Dioxide, Pesticides, Aerosols from Strong Inorganic Acids

Aerosols and vapours containing sulfuric acid are present in the environment due to the release of sulfur compounds from both natural and anthropogenic sources. Volcanic eruptions, biogenic gas emissions and oceans are the primary natural sources of sulfur emissions.

Chemical manufacturing (sulfuric acid, nitric acid, synthetic ethanol, vinyl chloride), building and construction, manufacture of lead-acid batteries, manufacture of phosphate fertilisers, pickling and other acid treatments of metals, manufacture of petroleum and coal products, oil and gas extraction, printing and publishing, manufacture of paper and allied products, and tanneries are industries which generate strong acid aerosols.

Occupational exposure to sulfuric acid (H_2SO_4) aerosols is reported to be associated with carcinogenesis, exclusively in the larynx and lungs. Moreover, an increased incidence of cancer of the paranasal sinuses among factory workers due to H_2SO_4 has been reported (IARC 1997). Based on this evidence, sulfuric acid has been classified as carcinogenic to humans. The carcinogenic activity of sulfuric acid is most likely to cause genotoxicity in low-pH environments, which are known to increase the rates of depurination of DNA and deamination of cytidine. This indicates a potential role of occupational exposures to H_2SO_4 in OSCC.

Thus, epidemiological studies are needed to understand the independent association of environmental exposure to aerosols and vapours containing carcinogens, after controlling for confounding factors (tobacco use, alcohol consumption, betel quid chewing). Laboratory studies are needed to understand the carcinogenic mechanisms of acid aerosol-associated carcinogens.

7.9.3 Indoor Air Pollution

It has been reported that nearly three billion people use solid fuel as their source of household energy, in certain parts of the world. Coal makes up the main part of solid fuel and the rest consists of various forms of biomass. Wood, crop residues and animal dung are classic examples of various forms of biomass. The burning of these fuels can cause household air pollution (HAP). Furthermore, HAP is known to cause an increase in household air levels of sulfur dioxide, carbon monoxide, fluorine and known carcinogens such as polycyclic aromatic hydrocarbons (PAHs), benzene, arsenic, 1,3-butadiene and formaldehyde. They can cause DNA mutations which may lead to oral carcinogenesis (Raj et al. 2017).

7.9.4 Infection, Inflammation and Periodontitis

Nearly 15% of the oral cancers cannot be explained by aetiological factors according to current knowledge (Perera et al. 2016). This indicates a need to search for other possible risk factors for OSCC.

The association between chronic inflammation and a range of epithelial malignancies has been known since the observation of Virchow who, in 1863, hypothesised that cancer arises in sites of inflammation. Inflammation is the body's response to noxious stimuli such as infectious, physical or chemical agents. The body's immune defence mechanism plays a role in the inhibition or promotion of cancer and its progression. Acute bacterial infections can inhibit tumour growth often with complete remission. Tumour regression is usually attributable to direct tumour cell killing by apoptosis and/or necrosis, depending on the applied bacteria and indirect immune stimulation via natural killer (NK) cells and cytotoxic T cells. In contrast, chronic inflammation triggers oral carcinogenesis via inflammatory mediators such as growth factors, chemokines and cytokines. Reactive oxygen species (ROS) and nitrogen species (RNS) activate transcriptional factors (NF-KB, STAT-3, HIF 1-alpha) and bring about cellular proliferation, genomic instability, angiogenesis, resistance to apoptosis, invasion and metastasis.

Most malignancies are associated with an inflammatory microenvironment being converted into a protumourigenic microenvironment. PAMPs or DAMPS expressed on pathogens or tissue injury are recognised by a specialised pattern expressed on the host, known as pattern recognition receptors (PRR), including NOD-like receptors and Toll-like receptors, which trigger receptors on myeloid cells, causing inflammation-induced activation of innate immune cells and inflammation-induced cancer by the production of cytokine-mediated NF-kappa-B activation. There is sound evidence that chronic microbial inflammation initiates or triggers carcinogenesis. Hence, chronic periodontitis (CP), which is a polymicrobial inflammatory disease, is linked with an increased risk of oral carcinogenesis according to epidemiological studies. There is promising laboratory evidence on the possible roles of inflammatory bacteriomes dominated by periodontal pathogens, especially *Porphyromonas gingivalis* and *Fusobacterium nucleatum*. Moreover, there is voluminous epidemiological research, mostly case-control studies exploring association between periodontitis and oral cancers. Those studies reported significant associations between oral cancers and periodontitis.

7.10 Mechanism of Carcinogenesis of Known Oral Carcinogens

Carcinogens are responsible for causing sister chromatid exchanges, point mutations and DNA adducts which may cause activation of oncogenes and inactivation of tumour suppressor genes. At the same time, these mutations can inhibit the activity of DNA repair genes.

7.10.1 Polycyclic Aromatic Hydrocarbons

Polycyclic aromatic hydrocarbons undergo metabolic activation to diol-epoxides, which bind covalently to DNA to form PAH-DNA adducts. PAH-DNA adduct formation is essential for carcinogenicity. Thus, epidemiological studies have suggested that HAP may be associated with oral cancer and nasopharyngeal cancer. The possible effect of PAH on the mucosal and endothelial lining of upper aerodigestive tract carcinogenesis has been suggested by epidemiological studies. Moreover, a positive correlation between the level of PAH exposure and the number of PAH-DNA adducts has been found in epidemiological studies.

The carcinogenic potential of certain PAH-DNA adducts has been identified in animal models. These studies revealed that PAHs undergo metabolic activation to diol-epoxides, which bind covalently to DNA. The DNA binding of activated PAHs is considered to be essential for the carcinogenic effect. However, a refined repair system has evolved to eliminate carcinogenic PAH-DNA adducts from the genome by nucleotide excision repair. In any case, if the adducts are left unrepaired, they may cause permanent mutations.

7.10.2 Nicotine-derived Nitrosamine Ketone (NNK) and N′-nitrosonornicotine (NNN)

Metabolically activated NNK and NNN induce deleterious mutations in oncogenes and tumour suppressor genes by forming DNA adducts, which could be considered the initiation of oral carcinogenesis.

7.10.3 Reactive Oxygen and Nitrogen Species

Oxidative/nitrosative stress produced by free radicals/reactive oxygen and nitrogen species (RONS) may initiate or progress oral carcinogenesis by multiple molecular and cellular events. They cause DNA damage, genome instability and alteration in cell signalling which convert normal cells into malignant cells in the tumour microenvironment.

7.10.4 Acetaldehyde

Acetaldehyde associated with alcohol/alcoholic beverage consumption is designated as a group 1 carcinogen by the IARC. Acetaldehyde can cause sister chromatid exchanges and point mutations and interfere with the DNA repair system. Additionally, acetaldehyde forms DNA adducts to initiate carcinogenesis.

7.10.5 HPV Oncoproteins

According to current knowledge, two viral oncoproteins of high-risk HPV (E6 and E7) are responsible for oncogenesis by preventing tumour suppression. E6 inactivates the *p53* tumour suppressor gene inhibiting p53-dependent cell cycle arrest and apoptosis. Furthermore, E6 oncoproteins also enhance telomerase activity, favouring the immortalisation of affected keratinocytes. Meanwhile, E7 promotes cellular proliferation by downregulating the cyclin-dependent kinase (CDK) inhibitors p21 and p27, and by inactivating Rb (retinoblastoma) protein which is a tumour suppressor protein.

7.11 Oral Bacteria and Immunological Tolerance

Bacteria living in the healthy adult human body are thought to outnumber the human cells by at least 10-fold. This was the estimation widely accepted for many years but revisits to this estimation claim that the bacterial cell to human cell ratio is much closer to 1 (Sender et al. 2016). However, there is no conclusive evidence for actual ratios. Furthermore, according to the popular notion, the collective genome of these bacteria (metagenome) surpasses the human genome by orders of magnitude (>150-fold in terms of gene content). Thus, humans could be considered as a 'supra organism' or 'holobiont' as the metagenome can influence immunological and metabolic activities. Nevertheless, current revisits to human and bacterial cell ratios may pose some challenges to these assumptions yet the massive influence of the human microbiome in health and disease is unchallenged.

The oral cavity harbours the second most diverse microbial community in the human body, next to the gut (Kilian et al. 2016). With at least 687 bacterial species/phylotypes present, the oral bacteriome is the major component of the oral microbiome. These species belong to 185 genera and 12 phyla, namely Firmicutes, Fusobacteria, Proteobacteria, Actinobacteria, Bacteroidetes, Chlamydiae, Chloroflexi, Spirochaetes, SR1, Synergistetes, Saccharibacteria (TM7) and Gracilibacteria (GN02). Thirty-two percent of these species have not been cultured and 14% have not been named. When it comes to genera levels, *Streptococcus*, *Rothia*, *Leptotrichia*, *Gemella*, *Capnocytophaga*, *Fusobacterium*, *Prevotella*, *Haemophilus*, *Granulicatella*, and *Veillonella* are reported to be common in healthy oral bacteriome.

Colonisation is a harmless process. Hence, there is a unique balance between the immune response of the host and the colonisation of oral microbes. The mucosal dendritic cells are predisposed to a tolerogenic state, resulting in the secretion of anti-inflammatory immunomodulators such as interleukin (IL)-10, transforming growth factor (TGF)-beta and prostaglandin. These effectors act by suppressing the activity of the immune system and generating T regulatory cells (Tregs) in the tissue, thereby propagating a tolerant state.

There is a dearth of information on how mucosal dendritic cells induce a state of tolerance. Nevertheless, certain studies have proposed a role of immune exhaustion, in which antigen-presenting cells (APCs) are no longer activated in response to specific commensal antigens, essentially becoming desensitised in immune tolerance of mucosal dendritic cells. Moreover, the pathogen-associated molecular patterns (PAMPs) of normal mucosa do not trigger an inflammatory response and the expression and character of these PAMPs do not necessarily change during a pathogenic shift because the transition is not always associated with novel antigenic features in some pathogens. The expression of virulence factors such as adhesins and enzymes does remain crucial in pathogenesis which helps the detection of commensal-turned-pathogen for the immune system to take prompt action to eliminate the pathogen.

7.12 Oral Bacterial Synergy and Dysbiosis in Inflammatory Diseases

In inflammatory diseases, the homeostasis of the oral bacteriome, called 'normobiosis', is lost, resulting in an 'ecological shift' or 'dysbiosis', creating an opportunity for commensals to become pathogenic. Communication among constituent species establishes polymicrobial synergy among metabolically compatible or keystone pathogens, even at low abundance. This elevates community virulence and the resulting dysbiotic community targets specific aspects of host immunity. This further disables immune surveillance while promoting an overall inflammatory response. Inflammophilic organisms benefit from proteinaceous substrates derived from inflammatory tissue breakdown. Inflammation and dysbiosis reinforce each other and the escalating environmental changes further select a pathobiotic community.

7.13 Oral Bacterial Synergy and Dysbiosis in Oral Cancer

The associations between oral bacteria and oral cancer were assessed by a substantial number of epidemiological studies. Consequently, based on metagenomic studies, dysbiosis of the oral bacteriome was found to be associated with OSCC (Perera et al. 2016: Sarkar et al. 2021). However, the role of any specific bacterial species or consortium is yet to be confirmed in the OSCC tumour microenvironment. Furthermore, species richness and diversity are lower in OSCC cases compared with normal tissues. In contrast, species diversity and richness are higher in OSCC cases compared with healthy controls.

In OSCC tissues, several bacterial genera, especially *Fusobacterium*, were significantly abundant along with *Campylobacter*, *Parvimonas* and *Prevotella*. However, significant variations were observed in the composition of the bacteriome at species level associated with OSCC from one cohort to another and from one subject to another within the same cohort. These observed compositional variations of the oral bacteriome relating to the occurrence of OSCC have been blamed for variations and inherent limitations in methods of bioinformatics that are used to analyse genome and proteome sequencing data.

Oral bacteriome synergy and dysbiosis among metabolically compatible periodontal pathogens acquiring functional redundancy have been described. Lipopolysaccharide (LPS) biosynthesis pathways were enriched in OSCC tissues when compared with healthy controls. This highlights the impending importance of conducting metatranscriptomic and metabolomic studies rather than performing compositional analysis by metagenomic studies to find out the role of these metabolically compatible members present in the tumour microenvironment. The compatible members lack the information to understand all mechanisms by which periodontal pathogens initiate oral carcinogenesis. The influence of periodontal pathogens in oral carcinogenesis may either be direct or indirect.

7.14 Role of Bacteria in Oral Carcinogenesis

Current epidemiological and laboratory evidence is not sufficient to confirm the causative role/initiation of oral carcinogenesis by a single species or consortium of oral microbes. However, there is laboratory evidence (in vivo/in vitro) on mechanisms by which two major periodontal pathogens, *P. gingivalis* and *F. nucleatum*, promote oral carcinogenesis. These mechanisms are mainly categorised into two: direct and indirect (Perera et al. 2016).

7.14.1 Direct Influence of Bacteria in Oral Carcinogenesis

Several virulence factors of bacterial origin, namely nucleoside diphosphate kinase (NDK), FimA, LPS and carcinogenic metabolites lead to the expression of oncogenic but not tumour suppressor markers. This is consistent with increased cell proliferation and the promotion of other stages of oral carcinogenesis.

7.14.1.1 Inhibition of Apoptosis
Porphyromonas gingivalis was shown to inhibit apoptosis by (i) activating JAK1/STAT3 and PI3K/Akt signalling pathways, (ii) suppressing proapoptic BCL-2-associated death promoter, (iii) blocking caspase-3 and caspase-9 activities, (iv) upregulating microRNA-203, and (v) preventing ATP-dependent P2X7-mediated apoptosis.

7.14.1.2 Promotion of Proliferation
Porphyromonas gingivalis also activates cell proliferation in a variety of ways: (i) accelerating the progression of gingival epithelial cells through the S and G2 phases of the cell cycle via upregulation of cyclins (A, D and E), activation of cyclin-dependent kinases (CDKs) through phosphorylation and diminishing the level of p53 tumour suppressor. Since bacterial LPS has been reported to dysregulate p53, a similar role by *P. gingivalis* LPS is possible; (ii) contributing to a proliferative phenotype in gingival epithelial cells through activation of beta-catenin via the gingipain-dependent proteolytic process.

In addition, cell proliferation is promoted by *F. nucleatum* which can upregulate several activating kinases, the majority of which are involved in cell proliferation and cell survival signalling as well as DNA repair.

7.14.1.3 Production of Carcinogenic Substances
Several other bacteria, namely *Streptococci*, *Neisseria*, *Rothia*, *Porphyromonas gingivalis* and *Candida*, can produce carcinogenic acetaldehydes, particularly in heavy alcohol drinkers.

7.14.1.4 Upreugulation of receptors on squamous carcinoma cells
Both B7-H1 and B7-DC receptors were upregulated on oral squamous carcinoma cells, SCC-25, and BHY, and on human primary gingival epithelial cells by *P. gingivalis* strains (W83 and ATCC 33277).

7.14.2 Indirect Influence of Bacteria in Oral Carcinogenesis

7.14.2.1 Chronic Inflammatory Status and Carcinogenesis
Acute bacterial infections can prevent carcinogenesis by complete remission of tumours. In contrast, chronic bacterial infections can cause chronic inflammation and promote carcinogenesis via two pathways.

In the intrinsic pathway of inflammation-induced cancer, MYC and RAS family oncogenes remodel the tumour microenvironment by activating transcription factors through recruitment of leucocytes, lymphocytes, chemokines, cytokine expression and angiogenic switch induction. Oncoproteins such as MYC, RAS and RET drive proinflammatory cytokines and chemokines (IL-8, IL-6, IL-1-beta, CCL2 and CCL20) by activation of signalling pathways.

In the extrinsic pathway of inflammation, inflammatory cells in the tumour microenvironment or the chronic inflammatory process can lead to the progression of cancer. These pathways are activated by either mono- or polymicrobial infections, increasing the expression of proinflammatory molecules such as IL-6, IL-8, IL-1-beta and TNF-alpha (Multhof et al. 2012).

Several periodontal pathogens have been shown to activate inflammatory pathways associated with several stages of cellular transformation as they can migrate to the tumour microenvironment from periodontal pockets. These bacteria induce NF-kappa-B pathway-mediated responses such as promotion of cell survival, activation of oncogenic pathways, reduction of proapoptotic protein expression, increase in cell migration/invasion and activation of epithelial-mesenchymal transition (EMT)-associated proteins, and enhance metastasis (Perera et al. 2016).

7.14.2.2 Immune Suppression and Inhibiting Immune Surveillance

The immune surveillance mechanisms in cancer control comprise three phases. First, in the elimination phase, tumour growth is controlled by the destruction of nascent cancer cells by T-cell activation via antigen presentation. Second, in the equilibrium phase, genetic instability of cells gives rise to tumour heterogeneity and as a result, tumour growth maintains a steady state, either by growth enhancement or by inhibition. Third, in the escape phase, tumour cells escape or suppress the immune system, thereby leading to tumour progression. Periodontal pathogen *P. gingivalis* disrupts immune surveillance by generating myeloid-derived dendritic suppressor cells (MDDSCs) from monocytes. MDDSCs inhibit CTLs and induce FOXP3$^+$ Tregs through an antiapoptotic pathway.

7.15 Role of Viruses in Oral Carcinogenesis

Viruses are considered the most infective agents in humans, and they can cause acute, latent or persistent infections not only in eukaryotes but also in archaea and bacteria as well. The viral members are thus abundant in different parts of the body, including the oral cavity. Nevertheless, very few studies have described viral communities and their roles in the oral cavity. Their interactions with each other and other oral microbial inhabitants can influence the host's genetic, metabolic and immunological activities in health and disease.

The oral virome of healthy individuals consists of bacteriophages and eukaryotic viruses. Bacteriophages are mostly from *Siphoviridae*, *Myoviridae* and *Podoviridae* families. Analysis at the family level showed that several dominant viral families, such as *Siphoviridae* and *Myoviridae*, are universally present among all sites with similar distribution patterns (Li et al. 2022). Eukaryotic viruses include a vast array of viruses that permanently infect the host and can exist for decades in asymptomatic individuals. Eukaryotic viruses consist of the human herpes virus, followed by retroviruses, papillomaviruses, poxviruses, circoviruses and anelloviruses (Edlund et al. 2015).

The presence of virulence factor homologues in the oral virome suggests that viruses may serve as reservoirs for pathogenic gene functions and may play an important role in shaping the bacterial ecology in the oral cavity as they have a predatory action on bacteria.

7.15.1 Human Herpes Viruses Associated with Oral Cancer

Human herpes viruses (HHV) such as Epstein–Barr virus (EBV) and herpes simplex virus (HSV-1 and HSV-2) have shown oncogenic potential in oral cancer (Polz-Gruszka et al. 2015). After initial infection, the virus remains latent in neurons, a key feature of alpha herpes viruses. Thus, the asymptomatic host is still capable of spreading the infection to other humans via shedding of the virions.

Reactivation of the virus is attributed to a variety of factors including emotional or physical stress, which subsequently trigger viral replication in epithelial cells. Associations of these viruses with oral cancer have been shown in several epidemiological studies but findings are inconclusive at present to establish a causative role.

7.15.1.1 Epstein–Barr Virus (EBV/HHV-4)

Epstein–Barr virus belongs to the family *Herpesviridae* and the subfamily *Alphaherpesvirinae*. More than 90% of the adult population is infected asymptomatically with EBV. This virus is reported to be associated with various malignancies demonstrating geographic specificity and immunological heterogeneity. EBV appears as a co-factor in the pathogenesis of many types of human cancers, especially nasopharyngeal, brain and salivary gland cancers. A strong correlation between EBV and OSCC has been demonstrated recently.

Epstein–Barr virus is the causative agent of nasopharyngeal cancers, stomach cancers and non-Hodgkin lymphomas. Thus, EBV has been categorised as a group I carcinogen by the IARC. Conditional evidence of a considerable association between EBV and OSCC has been reported.

During the past decade, several studies on EBV have been conducted and the prevalence of EBV in OSCC cases varies from 0% to 82.5% while that in healthy controls is up to 50%. Thus, the prevalence of EBV in OSCC must be interpreted cautiously because a high proportion of individuals shed EBV in saliva, which carries the inevitable risk of contaminating oral tissue biopsies with EBV, resulting in high detection rates.

Several EBV proteins have been identified in OSCC tissues that link with the tumour phenotype. Co-infections of hepatitis B virus (HBV) with HPV and HSV have been observed in studies conducted to determine the prevalence of HHVs in OSCC tissues. Epidemiological evidence is emerging for possible interaction between EBV seropositivity and tobacco use in nasopharyngeal carcinoma (NPC).

This EBV has a double tropism for B lymphocytes and epithelial cells of the upper aerodigestive tract. The viral latent membrane proteins (LMP), especially LMP1 and LMP2, and EBV nuclear antigens (EBNA1) are involved in the modulation of key factors contributing to malignant transformation. These proteins seem to participate in the regulation of important cell signalling pathways through modulating the activity of kinases. LMP1 is an active transmembrane receptor that appears to facilitate malignant transformation by triggering the NF-kappa-B), c- jun N-terminal kinase (JNK) and phosphatidylinositol 3-kinase (P13K)/AKT signalling pathways.

The EBV genome has demonstrated the capacity to integrate with the host genome. Thus, the EBV genome appears to regulate oncogenic activity at the posttranscriptional level by encoding miRNAs. In vitro experiments also demonstrated that the concentration of *p53* gene expression governs cell cycle arrest and apoptosis in EBV-infected B cells. Interactions between *p53* and EBV oncoproteins have been observed in many types of cancers, including head and neck. EBV factors may manipulate the host epigenetic machinery or act in a 'hit and run' manner, meaning that EBV participates in the early stages of tumour development by initiating oncogenic changes within the cell. In vitro experiments demonstrate that cigarette smoke extract promotes EBV DNA replication in EBV-positive Akata, CNE2 and B95-8 cell lines and upregulates the early transcription factors Zta and Rta as well as the lytic-phase late genes *BFRF3* and *gp350*. Thus, tobacco may act as an inducer of recurrent EBV reactivation, which has been shown to promote genome instability and enhance tumour progression of cancer cells.

Apart from employing mechanisms to initiate oncogenesis by the transformation of normal cells into tumours, EBV can further sustain cancer by displaying complex mechanisms of immune escape. They achieve this by interacting with and modulating certain immune-checkpoint inhibitors.

7.15.1.2 Herpes Simplex Virus

Herpes simplex virus type 1 and 2 are highly prevalent human pathogens causing life-long infections. HSV-1 and HSV-2 can avoid immune detection and establish latency in up to 80% and 40% of human adults respectively. They are capable of establishing latencies in trigeminal (HSV-1) or sacral (HSV-2) ganglia due to their unique abilities to enter into cells of the epithelia for viral gene expression and replication, and eventually spread from cell to cell to innervating nerves. Hence, HSV entry into host cells marks the first and perhaps the most critical step in viral pathogenesis.

Herpes simplex virus-1 and HSV-2 antigens and DNA are present in OSCC cases as well as in healthy people. Furthermore, seropositivity has been observed in OSCC patients, OPMD patients and healthy controls. Depending on these results, it has been suggested that the herpes viruses may play a role in OSCC. It has been shown that patients with HNSCC are often co-infected with HHV-1, but the infection is usually asymptomatic. Higher HHV-1 shedding in patients treated for HNSCC is considered to be due to the high level of stress associated with hospital procedures and healing trauma. HSV-1 is also reported to enhance oral carcinogenesis in individuals who are already current smokers and have HPV infections. Thus, co-infections of HSV with EBV and HPV are a reality in OSCC.

In vitro studies demonstrated that the oncogenic transformation takes place as the virus acts as a mutagen. A region of the viral genome has been isolated which raises the mutation frequency in cultured cells. However, it is a cumbersome task to study the association because the transformed malignant cells do not retain the virus. Thus, viral antigens or viral DNA cannot be detected, therefore mutations or phenotypic changes leading to herpes-induced malignancies remain inconclusive.

The question of whether HHV-1 and HHV-2 play an active role in oral carcinogenesis or whether they are just bystanders in the immune-deficient area around a tumour remains unanswered.

7.15.1.3 HHV 8 and Kaposi Sarcoma

Human herpes virus-8 is the aetiological agent for Kaposi sarcoma and uncommon neoplasms such as metacentric Castleman disease (MCD) and primary effusion lymphoma (PEL) typically associated with HIV-infected patients.

Thus, HHV-8 has been categorised as a group I carcinogen by the IARC. This virus is present in the oropharynx and can be recovered from saliva/oral fluid samples. Further, HHV-8 is regularly identified in HIV-positive HNSCC patients.

Molecular pathological evidence reveals mechanisms of carcinogenesis of HHV-8, via molecular mimicry and viral encoded proteins, which are said to activate several cellular signalling cascades whilst evading immune surveillance.

7.15.2 Cytomegalovirus

Cytomegalovirus (CMV) has demonstrated co-infections with EBV in OSCC. Chemoresistance properties of CMV have been identified by cell culture-based in vitro experiments. Promising laboratory evidence has emerged on possible mechanisms by which EBV contributes to oral carcinogenesis.

It is still unclear about the exact oncogenic mechanisms by which CMV induces oral carcinogenesis. The oncogenic process is thought to commence with the integration of CMV DNA into the host keratinocyte genome to commence oral carcinogenesis. CMV oncoproteins have shown the ability to cause chromosomal aberrations/mutations in oncogenes, tumour suppressor genes and DNA repair genes. Consequently, they affect DNA repair mechanism, cell cycle progression and inhibition of apoptotic pathways. Further, overexpression of VEGF is followed by cell motility and migration.

7.16 Role of Fungi in Oral Cancer

Advances in high-throughput sequencing and bioinformatics tools in recent years have paved the way to understanding the complexity of the human microbial world. The study of the mycobiome in health and disease, 'mycobiomics', is a rapidly evolving field. The mycobiome, which is a less abundant (<0.1%) component of the total microbiome, has been termed the 'rare biosphere' and is far more complicated than previously thought.

7.16.1 Oral Mycobiome in Health and Disease

The healthy oral mycobiome mainly consists of *Candida*, followed by *Malassezia*, *Cladosporium*, *Aspergillus*, *Fusarium*, *Cryptococcus*, *Gibbrella* and *Saccharomyces*. The impact of the mycobiome on health is important, as animal models have demonstrated that *Candida* interacts with the oral bacteria to maintain equilibrium/homeostasis. All of these fungi are commensals in the oral cavity under normal conditions. Nevertheless, *Candida* can cause invasive oral infections in immunosuppressive status. Interestingly, there is laboratory evidence on some species of these fungal genera, including *Aspergillus tamarii*, *A. alternata* and *Fusarium solani* to produce compounds with anticancer and anti-inflammatory properties (Bandara et al. 2019).

Fungal infections, especially invasive candidiasis, are much more common in immunosuppressive patients such as HIV, organ transplant, cancer chemotherapy and diabetes as well as antibiotic use. Furthermore, fungi have shown correlations with inflammatory diseases such as inflammatory bowel disease (IBD), cystic fibrosis and hepatitis. There is ever increasing evidence of a significant role for the mycobiome in immune regulation, chronic inflammatory diseases, metabolism and other physiological processes. Interactions between the host and the mycobiome are likely to be carefully balanced, leading to clearance, asymptomatic infection, latency or disease. Virulence factors of the fungi can cause tissue destruction while stimulating the host's immune system to produce immune cells and immune mediators. In disease conditions, these activities will disrupt the homeostatic balance between them and other microbes as well as with the host (Bandara et al. 2019).

7.16.1.1   Oral Mycobiome Dysbiosis Dominated by *Candida albicans* in Oral Cancer

Candida species have been considered the most common commensal fungi that colonise the oral mucosa, with carriage rates ranging from 3% to 70% in healthy individuals. Possible association between candidiasis and precancerous oral neoplasia dates back to 1969. Three decades ago, Krogh's group assessed the nitrosation potential of *Candida* strains isolated from oral leucoplakia lesions and found strains with high potential for nitrosation to be associated with increased levels of dysplasia. The overall malignant transformation rates varied from 2.5% to 28.7%.

A substantial number of studies published between 1994 and 2013 used periodic acid–Schiff (PAS) staining and cultivation techniques to detect/isolate yeasts in mucosal swabs or biopsies of oral dysplasia or OSCC. The presence of yeasts, especially *Candida* species, was significantly greater in dysplasia and OSCC, and such elevation correlated with the severity of dysplasia. Yeasts including *Rhodotorula*, *Saccharomyces* and *Kloeckera* are encountered. *C. albicans* is the most isolated *Candida* species in OSCC. A dysbiotic mycobiome dominated by *C. albicans* associated with OSCC was observed recently by sequencing the internal transcribed spacer (ITS) to characterise the mycobiome within OSCC tissues compared to that in fibroepithelial polyps (Perera et al. 2017).

7.16.1.2 Mechanisms of Oral Carcinogenesis by Fungi

Among oral fungi, *Candida albicans* demonstrates carcinogenic potential. There is a dearth of information to categorise *Candida* as a causative agent of oral cancer. It has been indicated that certain attributes of *C. albicans* may directly or indirectly influence oral and oropharyngeal carcinogenesis. These attributes can be broadly categorized into the production of carcinogenic metabolites and the production of carcinogenic inflammatory mediators, stimulating the host's immune system.

Production of Acetaldehydes Among *Candida* species, *C. albicans*, *C. tropicalis*, *C. parapsilosis* and *C. glabrata* are reported to produce carcinogenic acetaldehydes by oxidation as well as by glucose fermentation from alcohol in heavy drinkers.

Production of Nitrosoamines Endogenous nitrosation is considered a co-factor in oral carcinogenesis. *C. albicans* demonstrates the highest potential but *C. tropicalis*, *C. parapsilosis* and *Torulopsis glabrata* reveal the lowest potential to produce potent carcinogen N-nitrosobenzyl methylamine (NBMA).

Production of Inflammatory Mediators Dysbiosis of the mycobiome dominated by *C. albicans* can lead to excessive production of Th 17 cells and Tregs. This can cause chronic mucosal inflammation. Excessive production of Tregs causes immunosuppression. Consequently, *C. albicans* plays an important role in the development of OSCC via its interaction with epithelial cells, resulting in the production of epithelial cytokines and matrix metalloproteinases (MMPs) and proinvasive phenotypes. Moreover, *C. albicans* possesses the ability to enhance the invasion of genetically altered epithelial cells by reducing keratinocyte cohesion followed by assisting their passage to the basement membrane. It has been revealed that *C. albicans* produces IL-8 secretion from endothelial cells by stimulating the cells to produce TNF-alpha. The transcription factor NF-kappa-B is a key co-ordinator of inflammation and an important tumour promoter. NF-kappa-B activates genes encoding inflammatory cytokines and enzymes such as COX-2. Members of the TLR family are known to be vital in the recognition of *C. albicans* and induction of cytokines. Production of cytokines and enzymes in the prostaglandin synthesis pathway such as COX-2 could be considered as another potential mechanism of *C. albicans* that might influence the early stages of progression of oral cancer (Kang et al. 2016).

Moreover, cancer-related inflammation is involved in the metastasis of malignant cells. This carcinogenic effect is probably connected with both the form of candidal growth (whether yeast or hyphal) and the interaction with other microbial species in a mixed biofilm.

7.17 Association and Causation

Despite voluminous research and publications on the oral microbiome and oral cancers, there are still many knowledge gaps and unanswered questions on causation of oral cancers by the oral microbiome. Considering the multifactorial, multistage complex aetiology of oral cancers controlled by multifactorial events including genetic events, addressing all knowledge gaps on the role of oral microbiome in causation of oral cancers will take time. Nevertheless, the well-proven evidence for oral cancer associated with the microbiome could be a cause, consequence, coincidence or even a complication. For example, poor oral hygiene and a high burden of periodontal disease are commonly reported among oral cancer patients and in advanced stages of oral cancers it becomes difficult to practise oral hygiene measures. On the other hand, oral cancer associated with the microbiome could influence the initiation as well as progression of cancers by increasing the risk of carcinogenesis and cancer progression.

Moreover, association does not mean causation per se, but an associated factor could be or could not be a causal factor. As for an association becoming a causal association in epidemiological studies, the Bradford Hill Criteria should be considered, namely strength of association, consistency, specificity, temporality, biological gradient, plausibility, coherence, experiment and analogy. Further, advances in genetics, molecular biology, toxicology, exposure science and statistics have widened the horizons of analytical capabilities for exploring potential cause-and-effect relationships, as well as providing greater understanding of the complexity behind human disease onset and progression. Therefore, new knowledge is being added to the existing knowledge gaps on the oral microbiome and oral cancer almost on a daily basis.

7.18 Conclusion

In healthy conditions, resident microbes maintain homeostasis or equilibrium with the host by symbiosis. However, in disease conditions, this symbiosis turns into dysbiosis with compositional changes and functional redundancy. Hence, an oral cancer-associated 'specific bacteriome' was observed in all metagenomic studies based on oral cancer patients compared with healthy controls. There was no consensus on specific bacterial composition or patterns associated with oral cancer.

Laboratory evidence is emerging on the potential role of the microbiome in oral carcinogenesis. In vitro studies have provided promising evidence for carcinogenic properties of two main periodontal pathogens: *Fusobacterium nucleatum* and *Porphyromonas gingivalis*. Thus, it has been found that microbial dysbiosis due to an inflammatory bacteriome within the tumour microenvironment probably contributes to tumour progression by sustaining chronic inflammation and changing the immune response. The oral cancer-related microbiome appears as a co-factor in the aetiology of oral carcinogenesis. *Fusobacterium nucleatum* has shown positive correlations with OSCC tissues in almost all epidemiological/clinical studies based on oral cancer patients and some carcinogenic mechanisms of this bacterium were demonstrated in laboratory studies. Thus, *Fusobacterium nucleatum* is more suitable to consider as a risk marker for OSCC. Further research is necessary to understand the changes in inflammatory and immune responses evoked by different types of microbiome in oral carcinogenesis.

References

Al-Hebshi, N.N., Borgnakke, W.S. and Johnson, N.W (2019). The microbiome of oral squamous cell carcinomas: a functional perspective. *Curr. Oral Health Rep.* 6: 145–160.

Al-Marzooq, F., Al Kawas, S., Rahman, B. et al. (2022) Supragingival microbiome alternations as a consequence of smoking different tobacco types and its relation to dental caries. *Sci. Rep.* 12 (1): 2861.

Asthana, S., Labani, S., Kailash, U., Sinha, D.N. and Mehrotra, R. (2019). Association of smokeless tobacco use and oral cancer: a systematic global review and meta-analysis. *Nicotine Tob. Res.* 21 (9): 1162–1171.

Bandara, H., Panduwawala, C.P. and Samaranayake, L.P. (2019). Biodiversity of the human oral mycobiome in health and disease. *Oral Dis.* 25 (2): 363–371.

Berger, D., Rakhamimova, A., Pollack, A. and Loewy, Z. (2018). Oral biofilms: development, control, and analysis. *High Throughput* 7 (3): 24.

Bray, F., Ferlay, J., Soerjomataram, I., Siegel, R.L., Torre, L.A. and Jemal, A. (2018). Global cancer statistics 2018: GLOBOCAN estimates of incidence and mortality worldwide for 36 cancers in 185 countries. *CA Cancer J. Clin.* 68 (6): 394–424. Erratum in: *CA Cancer J. Clin.* 2020; 70(4): 313.

Caselli, E., Fabbri, C., D'Accolti, M. et al. (2020). Defining the oral microbiome by whole-genome sequencing and resistome analysis: the complexity of the healthy picture. *BMC Microbiol.* 20 (1): 120.

Chakraborty, P., Karmakar, T., Arora, N. and Mukherjee, G. (2018). Immune and genomic signatures in oral (head and neck) cancer. *Heliyon* 4 (10): e00880.

Chattopadhyay, I., Verma, M. and Panda, M. (2019). Role of oral microbiome signatures in diagnosis and prognosis of oral cancer. *Technol. Cancer Res. Treat.* 18: 1533033819867354.

Coelho, G.D.P., Ayres, L.F.A., Barreto, D.S., Henriques, B.D., Prado, M. and Passos, C.M.D. (2021). Acquisition of microbiota according to the type of birth: an integrative review. *Rev. Lat. Am. Enfermagem.* 29: e3446.

Coelho, K.R. (2012). Challenges of the oral cancer burden in India. *J. Cancer Epidemiol.* 2012: 701932.

Conway, D.I., Petticrew, M., Marlborough, H., Berthiller, J., Hashibe, M. and Macpherson, L.M. (2008). Socioeconomic inequalities and oral cancer risk: a systematic review and meta-analysis of case-control studies. *Int. J. Cancer.* 122 (12): 2811–2819.

Deo, P.N. and Deshmukh, R. (2019). Oral microbiome: unveiling the fundamentals. *J. Oral Maxillofac. Pathol.* 23 (1): 122–128.

Dominguez-Bello, M.G., Costello, E.K., Contreras, M. et al. (2010). Delivery mode shapes the acquisition and structure of the initial microbiota across multiple body habitats in newborns. *Proc. Natl Acad. Sci. USA* 107 (26): 11971–11975.

Dumache, R., Rogobete, A.F., Andreescu, N. and Puiu, M. (2015). Genetic and epigenetic biomarkers of molecular alterations in oral carcinogenesis. *Clin. Lab.* 61 (10): 1373–1381.

Edlund, A., Santiago-Rodriguez, T.M., Boehm, T.K. and Pride, D.T. (2015). Bacteriophage and their potential roles in the human oral cavity. *J. Oral Microbiol.* 7: 27423.

Fan, X., Peters, B.A., Jacobs, E.J. et al. (2018). Drinking alcohol is associated with variation in the human oral microbiome in a large study of American adults. *Microbiome* 6 (1): 59.

Farah, C.S., Shearston, K., Nguyen, A.P. and Kujan, O. (2019). Oral carcinogenesis and malignant transformation. In: *Premalignant Conditions of the Oral Cavity. Head and Neck Cancer Clinics* (eds P. Brennan, T. Aldridge and R. Dwivedi). Singapore: Springer.

Gillings, M.R., Paulsen, I.T. and Tetu, S.G. (2015). Ecology and evolution of the human microbiota: fire, farming and antibiotics. *Genes* 6 (3): 841–857.

Gomez-Arango, L.F., Barrett, H.L., McIntyre, H.D., Callaway, L.K., Morrison, M. and Nitert, M.D. (2017). Contributions of the maternal oral and gut microbiome to placental microbial colonization in overweight and obese pregnant women. *Sci. Rep.* 7 (1): 2860.

Groussin, M., Mazel, F., Sanders, J.G. et al. (2017). Unraveling the processes shaping mammalian gut microbiomes over evolutionary time. *Nat. Commun.* 8:14319.

Groussin, M., Mazel, F. and Alm, E.J. (2020). Co-evolution and co-speciation of host-gut bacteria systems. *Cell Host Microbe* 28 (1): 12–22.

Gupta, B. and Johnson, N.W. (2014). Systematic review and meta-analysis of association of smokeless tobacco and of betel quid without tobacco with incidence of oral cancer in South Asia and the Pacific. *PLoS One* 9 (11): e113385.

Heller, D., Helmerhorst, E.J., Gower, A.C., Siqueira, W.L., Paster, B.J. and Oppenheim, F.G. (2016). Microbial diversity in the early in vivo-formed dental biofilm. *Appl. Environ. Microbiol.* 82 (6): 1881–1888.

International Agency for Research on Cancer (IARC) (1997). *Summaries and Evaluations: Occupational Exposures to Mists and Vapours from Sulfuric Acid and Other Strong Inorganic Acids.* Lyon: World Health Organization.

International Agency for Research on Cancer (IARC) (2022a). *IARC Monographs on the Identification of Carcinogenic Hazards to Humans.* https://monographs.iarc.who.int/agents-classified-by-the-iarc/

International Agency for Cancer Research (IARC) (2022b). *IARC Monographs on the Evaluation of Carcinogenic Hazards to Humans*, Volume 85. Lyon: World Health Organization.

Islam, S., Muthumala, M., Matsuoka, H. et al. (2019). How each component of betel quid is involved in oral carcinogenesis: mutual interactions and synergistic effects with other carcinogens – a review article. *Curr. Oncol. Rep.* 21 (6): 53.

Jia, Y.J., Liao, Y., He, Y.Q. et al. (2021). Association between oral microbiota and cigarette smoking in the Chinese population. *Front. Cell Infect. Microbiol.* 11: 658203.

Johnson, N.W., Amarasinghe, A., Qualliotine, J.R. and Farkhry, C. (2018). Epidemiology. In: *Oral, Head and Neck Oncology and Reconstructive Surgery* (eds R. Bell, R. Fernandes and P. Andersen). St Louis, MO: Elsevier.

Kaan, A.M.M., Kahharova, D. and Zaura, E (2021). Acquisition and establishment of the oral microbiota. *Periodontology 2000* 86 (1): 123–141.

Kang, J., He, Y., Hetzl D. et al. (2016). Candid assessment of the link between oral candida containing biofilms and oral cancer. *Adv. Microbiol.* 6 (02): 115.

Khan, Z. (2012). An overview of oral cancer in Indian subcontinent and recommendations to decrease its incidence. WebmedCentral CANCER 3 (8):WMC003626.

Kilian, M., Chapple, I.L., Hannig, M. et al. (2016). The oral microbiome – an update for oral healthcare professionals. *Br. Dent. J.* 21 (10): 657–666.

Li, S., Guo, R., Zhang, Y. et al. (2022). A catalog of 48,425 nonredundant viruses from oral metagenomes expands the horizon of the human oral virome. *iScience* 25 (6): 104418.

Li, W., Tapiainen, T., Brinkac, L. et al. (2021). Vertical transmission of gut microbiome and antimicrobial resistance genes in infants exposed to antibiotics at birth. *J. Infect. Dis.* 224 (7): 1236–1246.

Li, Y.C., Cheng, A.J., Lee, L.Y., Huang, Y.C. and Chang, J.T. (2019). Multifaceted mechanisms of areca nuts in oral carcinogenesis: the molecular pathology from precancerous condition to malignant transformation. *J. Cancer* 10 (17): 4054–4062.

Liu, S., Xu, X., Zeng, X., Li, L., Chen, Q. and Li, J. (2014). Tumor-targeting bacterial therapy: a potential treatment for oral cancer (review). *Oncol. Lett.* 8 (6): 2359–2366.

Mahees, M., Amarasinghe, H.K., Usgodaararachchi, U. et al. (2021). Sociological analysis and exploration of factors associated with commercial preparations of smokeless tobacco use in Sri Lanka. *Asian Pac. J. Cancer Prev.* 22 (6): 1753–1759.

Markéta, H., Pařízek, A. and Koucký, M. (2021). The role of the microbiome in pregnancy. *Ceska Gynekol.* 86 (6): 422–427.

Marsh, P.D. and Bradshaw, D.J. (1995). Dental plaque as a biofilm. *J. Ind. Microbiol.* 15 (3): 169–175.

Mascolo, M., Siano, M., Ilardi, G. et al. (2012). Epigenetic disregulation in oral cancer. *Int. J. Mol. Sci.* 13 (2): 2331–2353.

Mukherjee, C., Moyer, C.O., Steinkamp, H.M. et al. (2021). Acquisition of oral microbiota is driven by environment, not host genetics. *Microbiome* 9 (1): 54.

Multhoff, G., Molls, M. and Radons, J. (2012). Chronic inflammation in cancer development. *Front. Immunol.* 2: 98.

Odell, E., Kujan, O., Warnakulasuriya, S. and Sloan, P. (2021). Oral epithelial dysplasia: recognition, grading and clinical significance. *Oral Dis.* 27 (8): 1947–1976.

O'Toole, G., Kaplan, H.B. and Kolter, R. (2000). Biofilm formation as microbial development. *Annu. Rev. Microbiol.* 54: 49–79.

Perera, M., Al-Hebshi, N.N., Speicher, D.J., Perera, I. and Johnson, N.W. (2016). Emerging role of bacteria in oral carcinogenesis: a review with special reference to perio-pathogenic bacteria. *J. Oral Microbiol.* 8: 32762.

Perera, M., Al-Hebshi, N.N., Perera, I. et al. (2017). A dysbiotic mycobiome dominated by *Candida albicans* is identified within oral squamous-cell carcinomas. *J. Oral Microbiol.* 9 (1): 1385369.

Perera, M., Al-Hebshi, N.N., Perera, I. et al. (2018). Inflammatory bacteriome and oral squamous cell carcinoma. *J. Dent. Res.* 97 (6): 725–732.

Petti, S., Masood, M. and Scully, C. (2013). The magnitude of tobacco smoking-betel quid chewing-alcohol drinking interaction effect on oral cancer in South-East Asia. A meta-analysis of observational studies. *PLoS One* 8 (11): e78999.

Polz-Gruszka, D., Stec, A., Dworzański, J. and Polz-Dacewicz, M. (2015). EBV, HSV, CMV and HPV in laryngeal and oropharyngeal carcinoma in Polish patients. *Anticancer Res.* 35 (3): 1657–1661.

Raj, A.T., Patil, S., Sarode, S.C., Sarode, G.S. and Rajkumar, C. (2017). Evaluating the association between household air pollution and oral cancer. *Oral Oncol.* 75: 178–179.

Rodríguez-Molinero, J., Migueláñez-Medrán, B.D.C., Puente-Gutiérrez, C. et al. (2021). Association between oral cancer and diet: an update. *Nutrients* 13 (4): 1299.

Sarkar, P., Malik, S., Laha, S. et al. (2021). Dysbiosis of oral microbiota during oral squamous cell carcinoma development. *Front. Oncol.* 11: 614448.

Sarode, G., Maniyar, N., Sarode, S.C., Jafer, M., Patil, S. and Awan, K.H. (2020). Epidemiologic aspects of oral cancer. *Dis. Mon.* 66 (12): 100988.

Sender, R., Fuchs, S. and Milo, R. (2016). Revised estimates for the number of human and bacteria cells in the body. *PLoS Biol.* 14 (8): e1002533.

Seneviratne, C.J., Zhang, C.F. and Samaranayake, L.P. (2011). Dental plaque biofilm in oral health and disease. *Chin. J. Dent Res.* 14 (2): 87–94.

Shaikh, M.H., McMillan, N.A. and Johnson, N.W. (2015). HPV-associated head and neck cancers in the Asia Pacific: a critical literature review and meta-analysis. *Cancer Epidemiol.* 39 (6): 923–938.

Sharma, S., Satyanarayana, L., Asthana, S., Shivalingesh, K.K., Goutham, B.S. and Ramachandra, S. (2018). Oral cancer statistics in India on the basis of first report of 29 population-based cancer registries. *J. Oral Maxillofac. Pathol.* 22 (1): 18–26.

Shibahara, T. (2017). [Oral cancer – diagnosis and therapy.]. *Clin. Calcium* 27 (10): 1427–1433.

Shrivastava, S.R., Shrivastava, P.S. and Ramasamy, J. (2014). Oral cancer in developing countries: the time to act is upon us. *Iran J. Cancer Prev.* 7 (1): 58–59.

Sulyanto, R.M., Thompson, Z.A., Beall, C.J., Leys, E.J. and Griffen, A.L. (2019). The predominant oral microbiota is acquired early in an organized pattern. *Sci. Rep.* 9 (1): 10550.

Uehara, O., Hiraki, D., Kuramitsu, Y. et al. (2021). Alteration of oral flora in betel quid chewers in Sri Lanka. *J. Microbiol. Immunol. Infect.* 54 (6): 1159–1166.

Verma, D., Garg, P.K. and Dubey, A.K. (2018). Insights into the human oral microbiome. *Arch. Microbiol.* 200 (4): 525–540.

Weyrich, L.S. (2021). The evolutionary history of the human oral microbiota and its implications for modern health. *Periodontology 2000* 85 (1): 90–100.

Xiao, J., Fiscella, K.A. and Gill, S.R. (2020). Oral microbiome: possible harbinger for children's health. *Int. J. Oral Sci.* 12 (1): 12.

Xu, H., Tian, B., Shi, W., Tian, J., Wang, W. and Qin, M. (2022). Maturation of the oral microbiota during primary teeth eruption: a longitudinal, preliminary study. *J. Oral Microbiol.* 14 (1): 2051352.

8

Oral Microbiome and Periodontitis

Rathna Devi Vaithilingam and Chia Wei Cheah

Department of Restorative Dentistry, University of Malaya, Kuala Lumpur, Malaysia

8.1 Introduction

Periodontitis is a chronic inflammatory disease of the periodontal tissues. It is a multifactorial disease with the microbial dental biofilm or dental plaque as its initiator (Kinane 1999). Periodontitis is preceded by gingivitis which is chronic inflammation of the gingival tissues and comprises clinical signs such as gingival bleeding, swelling and the formation of false pockets (Figure 8.1). It is the term used when the disease becomes destructive and the damage to the host tissues becomes irreversible. Destruction of the periodontium is attributed to microbial dysbiosis as well as the excessive immune response of the host (Kinane et al. 2017). At these sites, apical migration of the epithelial attachment onto the root surfaces following loss of periodontal ligament, connective tissue and alveolar bone takes place. Clinically, periodontitis presents with clinical attachment loss (CAL) and increased probing pocket depths (PPD) (Figure 8.2).

Epidemiological studies indicate that severe periodontitis, which is the sixth most prevalent disease globally, affects 743 million people worldwide with an overall prevalence of 11.2% (Tonetti et al. 2017). This chapter will discuss the dental biofilm as the aetiology of periodontitis, the bacterial composition within the dental biofilm and their roles in driving inflammatory response. The currently available treatment modalities and alternatives are also briefly discussed.

8.2 Dental Biofilm

The dental biofilm is an adherent bacterial biofilm that forms on all intraoral hard and soft tissues. The experimental gingivitis study by Loe and co-workers (1965) and other studies on immunologic data as well as the efficacy of antibiotics in the treatment of periodontitis have provided overwhelming evidence to support the view that the dental biofilm is the primary aetiological factor in periodontal disease (Ebersole and Taubman 1994; van Winkelhoff et al. 1996).

8.2.1 Structure and Function of the Dental Biofilm

A structurally and functionally organised microbial dental biofilm is produced through an orderly sequence of events (Socransky and Haffajee 2002; Marsh 2005; Berezow and Darveau 2011). These events include the following (Figure 8.3).

1) The formation of an acquired pellicle which consists of salivary glycoproteins such as proline rich proteins, statherin and fibronectin (Bernimoulin 2003).
2) Reversible adhesion followed by more permanent attachment between the acquired pellicle and the microbial cell surface of the primary colonisers such as Gram-positive coccoid bacterial cells, usually streptococci, especially the *Streptococcus sanguinis* group. Streptococci are able to bind to each other (auto-aggregation) (Jenkinson and Lamont 1997) and also to other Gram-positive bacteria (co-aggregation) such as *Actinomycetes*, *Haemophilus* and *Veillonella* (Kolenbrander 1993).

Immunology for Dentistry, First Edition. Edited by Mohammad Tariqur Rahman, Wim Teughels and Richard J. Lamont.
© 2023 John Wiley & Sons Ltd. Published 2023 by John Wiley & Sons Ltd.

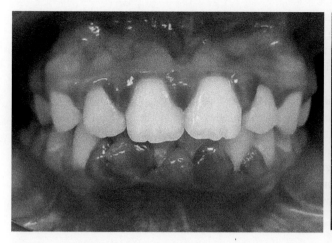

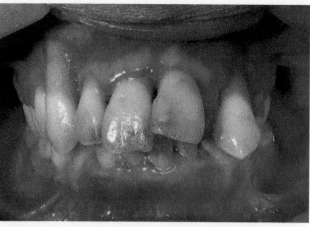

Figure 8.1 Gingivitis. Intraoral photo of a 13-year-old girl with poor oral hygiene.

Figure 8.2 Periodontitis. Intraoral photo of a 50-year-old man showing severe attachment loss.

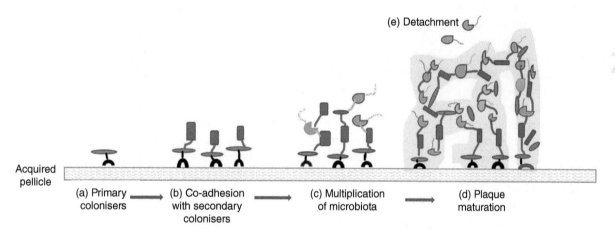

Figure 8.3 Dental biofilm formation. The process involves an orderly sequence of events.

3) Co-adhesion between the secondary colonisers such as *Fusobacterium* and receptors on the attached primary colonisers.

4) Multiplication of the attached microbiota leading to increased biomass and synthesis of exopolymers which forms the matrix of the biofilm, leading to plaque maturation whereby the biofilm takes on a distinctive architecture.

5) And finally, detachment of the attached cells which then colonise at distant sites. As the population grows and becomes more complex, a shift from mainly Gram-positive bacteria to Gram-negative occurs. Late colonisers of the oral cavity such as *Porphyromonas gingivalis*, *Aggregatibacter actinomycetemcomitans* and *Tannarella forsythia* adhere almost exclusively with the long rod-shaped bacterium, *Fusobacterium* (Kolenbrander 1993).

The unique structure of biofilms includes regions where there is inclusion of water channels to allow metabolites to circulate, cell growth at different rates and there is the presence of nutrient gradients (Berezow and Darveau 2011). This complex structural organisation allows the biofilm to exhibit functional heterogeneity with metabolic and phenotypic flexibility (Marsh et al. 2015). The distribution and metabolic activity of the microbiota in the dental biofilm are also dependent on several environmental factors such as the temperature, redox potential, pH, nutrients, host defences, microbial interactions, host genetics, health and lifestyle (Marsh and Devine 2011).

Dental biofilms thus comprise polymicrobial communities where the microbiota lives in a community, which provides several advantages to the colonising species, allowing them to grow (Marsh 2005). These advantages include protection from competing micro-organisms, facilitating the processing and uptake of nutrients, removal of potentially harmful metabolic products and the development of an appropriate physicochemical environment by properly reducing the oxidation reduction potential (Marsh et al. 2015).

The dental biofilm also reduces the susceptibility of the microbiota to antimicrobial agents (Gilbert et al. 2002). Bacterial cells within biofilms can produce enzymes such as beta-lactamase against antibiotics (Allison 2003) or catalases and superoxide dismutases against oxidising ions released by phagocytes (Socransky and Haffajee 2002). These enzymes are released into the matrix, producing an almost impregnable line of defence. Additionally, antibodies are also unable to get through the biofilm matrix (Fux et al. 2005). The bacteria and microcolonies in the biofilm are also able to communicate with one another through quorum sensing and this has an influence on the plaque community structure by encouraging the growth of beneficial species and discouraging the growth of competitors (Socransky and Haffajee 2002; Li et al. 2002; Suntharalingam and Cvitkovitch 2005).

8.2.2 Changes in Dental Biofilm from Health to Disease

The changes in the dental biofilm from oral health to disease relate to shifts in its microbial community. The search for these changes has passed through many phases. During the initial phase, spirochaetes, streptococci, amoeba and fusiform bacteria were implicated in the aetiology of periodontitis (Socransky and Haffajee 1992). In the nineteenth century, the non-specific plaque hypothesis was introduced which believed that accumulation of virtually any microbial species at the gingival margin would lead to gingivitis and then to periodontitis (Miller 1890). Later, the specific plaque hypothesis was introduced whereby mixed infections were studied and microbial complexes were suggested as aetiological agents of periodontitis, for example mixed infections of fusospirochaetes and mixed infections of black pigmented *Bacteroides*. Loesche (1976) added support for the specific plaque hypothesis when it was suggested that plaque control was essential in the treatment of periodontal patients. In 1986, Theilade suggested that not all micro-organisms in plaque may be equally capable of causing destructive periodontitis and thus the concept of non-specificity in destructive periodontal disease re-emerged (Theilade 1986).

The 'ecological plaque hypothesis' was proposed after combining the key concepts of the earlier hypotheses. According to this hypothesis, environmental conditions determine the composition of microbial communities. For instance, ecological stress can result in breakdown of homeostasis, leading to a shift in the balance of the microflora in favour of disease-related pathogens (Marsh 1994).

Following this, periodontal disease was attributed to polymicrobial synergy and dysbiosis, leading to host-mediated disruption of microbial homeostasis, particularly subgingival bacterial communities (Hajishengallis et al. 2012). Presence of certain microbial pathogens at low abundance can lead to a change in normal microbiota (in terms of quantity and composition) as described in the keystone pathogen hypothesis (Hajishengallis et al. 2012). The changes in subgingival microbial communities will then induce gingival inflammation, together with immune cell infiltration, leading to subsequent periodontal tissue destruction (Cekici et al. 2014; Darveau 2010). Furthermore, this model highlighted that the host immune response is initially subverted by *P.gingivalis* as a 'keystone pathogen' with the aid of accessory pathogens (Hajishengallis 2015), leading to breakdown of homeostasis with destructive inflammation in those susceptible individuals.

8.3 Microbial Diagnostic Methods

Knowledge of the complexity of oral microbial communities present in the oral cavity has evolved over the years from initial identifications using microscopy in the 1670s by Antoni van Leeuwenhoek (Listgarten and Helldén 1978) which was later upgraded with the use of dark-field and phase-contrast microscopy. Culture methods were subsequently used and have been considered the gold standard against which other microbiological identification methods have been compared.

Following this, immunoassays that employ antibodies that recognise specific bacterial antigens to detect target micro-organisms were used. Methods using commercially available immunoassays include immunofluorescence microscopy, enzyme-linked immunosorbent assay (ELISA), membrane assays, latex agglutination assays and flow cytometry.

With advancement in technologies, researchers have now moved towards culture-independent techniques, especially for mixed bacterial communities. These techniques target the bacterial DNA for bacteria identification. In clinical microbiology, molecular genetic techniques are increasingly being used to detect and/or differentiate uncultivable, anaerobic or fastidious micro-organisms. These culture-independent molecular diagnostic techniques include DNA probe technology, restriction endonuclease activity, polymerase chain reaction (PCR) and the currently more sophisticated techniques using high-throughput sequencing molecular methods.

8.3.1 Human Microbiome Project

The findings from these diagnostic techniques have enabled identification of the diverse microbial communities that exist in the oral cavity. This has culminated in the development of the Human Oral Microbiome Database (www.homd.org). From this database, over 400 microbial species have been found in the periodontium using 16S rRNA amplification, cloning and Sanger sequencing (Sanger et al. 1977; Dewhirst et al. 2010; Mira et al. 2017).

8.4 Microbes in Health and Periodontitis

Our understanding of the microbiota present in periodontal health and disease has evolved over the years. In 1998, using the DNA:DNA checkerboard hybridisation technique, Socransky and co-workers were able to analyse plaque samples from 185 subjects using whole genomic probes for 40 bacterial species (Socransky et al. 1998). They defined bacterial complexes into colour-coded groupings which were associated with either periodontal health or disease. The complexes associated with periodontal health were presented as yellow, green, purple and blue complexes, which were the initial/primary colonisers (Figure 8.4). The orange complex species came in as later colonisers, which were also the bridging link between the primary colonisers and the red complex that comprised the most periodontally pathogenic complex.

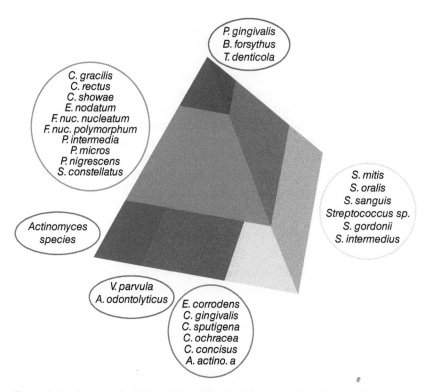

Figure 8.4 Association of the subgingival microbial species with periodontal health and disease. The DNA:DNA checkerboard hybridisation technique was used to analyse samples which were then categorised into colour-coded complexes. *Source:* Reproduced from Socransky et al. 2022/With permission of Munksgaard.

Certain bacteria such as *Aggregatibacter actinomycetemcomitans* serotype b and *Selenomonas noxia* were outliers with little relation to each other and the six major complexes.

Supragingival plaque, which is mainly composed of Gram-positive bacteria, is attached to the tooth surface and is dominated by *Actinomyces* species in most plaque samples in both health and disease (Socransky and Haffajee 2002). Subgingival plaque is more complex with both a tooth-associated and epithelial cell-associated biofilm separated by loosely bound or planktonic cells (Ximénez-Fyvie et al. 2000). The subgingival plaque attached to the tooth surface is an extension of the supragingival plaque. However, the plaque attached to the epithelial surface of the pocket contains mainly spirochaetes and Gram-negative bacterial species such as *Porphyromonas gingivalis* (*P. gingivalis*), *Treponema denticola* and *Tannarella forsythia* (Socransky and Haffajee 2002).

The current research on microbiology that was based on high-throughput technology such as 16S rRNA gene sequencing has enabled the study of the microbiome as a community, which is the case in the context of periodontitis. A diverse bacterial community has been associated with the healthy oral condition. Six major phyla have been identified: Firmicutes, Actinobacteria, Proteobacteria, Fusobacteria, Bacteroidetes and Spirochaetes constituting 96% of the total oral bacteria. The oral microbial community is resistant to perturbances (Zaura et al. 2015).

During the initial phase of periodontal disease, there is an increase in diversity due to a nutritionally richer environment (Camelo-Castillo et al. 2015). Eventually, when disease is established with increased tissue destruction, the bacterial community becomes associated with predominantly disease-associated species (Van Dyke et al. 2020). Hajishengallis and co-workers (2012) have identified *P. gingivalis* as a keystone pathogen orchestrating oral dysbiosis in the pathogenesis of periodontitis. This bacterium has been linked to many other diseases as it can communicate with accessory pathogens and elevate the virulence of the whole community (Hajishengallis and Lamont 2016). It has also been associated with oral cancer together with *Fusobacterium nucleatum* and *Prevotella intermedia*.

Studies have also reported a transition of bacteria in the community from being commensals to having a pathogenic behaviour under disease conditions (Duran-Pinedo et al. 2014; Jorth et al. 2014). This microbial shift can be observed during the gingivitis stage. Negative correlations have been noted from predominantly aerobic and facultatively anaerobic Gram-positive cocci and rods with clinical parameters such as bleeding on probing. This includes members of the genera *Actinomyces*, *Rothia* and *Streptococcus* (classic early colonisers of the tooth surface). At the same time, the Gram-negative taxa of the genera *Campylobacter*, *Fusobacterium*, *Lautropia*, *Leptotrichia*, *Porphyromonas*, *Selenomonas* and *Tannerella* (mostly obligate anaerobes) increased in relative abundance as gingivitis developed and were positively correlated with bleeding on probing (Diaz et al. 2006).

For periodontitis, microbial communities from members of the genera *Prevotella*, *Fusobacterium*, *Treponema*, *Selenomonas* and *Porphyromonas* have been reported to be more abundant while *Actinomyces* and *Streptococcus* were less abundant in subgingival samples of subjects with periodontitis compared with healthy subjects (Griffen et al. 2012). Subjects with severe periodontitis (863 phylotypes) were also found to be more diverse than healthy subjects (686 phylotypes) in a Taiwanese population (Tsai et al. 2018). Bacteroidetes was the most significant phylum in all diseased subjects and its abundance decreased in healthy subjects. The genera most significantly enriched in the group with severe periodontitis were *Porphyromonas*, *Tannarella*, *Treponema*, *Aggregatibacter*, *Peptostreptococcus* and *Filifactor* while the healthy group were enriched with the genera *Lautropia*, *Parvimonas*, *Actinomyces*, *Capnocytophaga*, *Paludibacter*, *Streptococcus*, *Haemophilus* and *Corynebacterium*.

8.4.1 Factors Affecting Microbial Composition

The microbial composition can be modulated by several factors including age and lifestyle factors.

Significant differences in the microbial composition have been reported when comparing those aged 18–45 years old with those above 65 years old. There was a lower relative abundance of *Porphyromonas endodontalis* and *Alloprevotella tannerae* (phylum: Bacteroidetes), *Filifactors alocis* (phylum: Firmicutes), *Treponema* sp. (phylum: Spirochaetes), *Lautropia mirabilis* (phylum: Proteobacteria) and *Pseudopropionibacterium sp._HMT_194* (phylum: Actinobacteria) in the older age group. This has been attributed to changes in the inflammatory state or adaptive immunity in the oral cavity of the elderly (Schwartz et al. 2021). Among centenarians, differences have also been reported between dentate and edentulous subjects (Sekundo et al. 2022).

A diet rich in protein has also been reported to support the growth of proteolytic and amino acid-degrading periodontopathogens as the alkaline products raise the average pH to neutral or slightly alkaline values (Nyvad and Takahashi 2020).

Lifestyle factors such as smoking changes the environment of the oral cavity and thus influences the overall composition of the oral microbial community by altering certain metabolic pathways. The genera *Actinomyces*, *Atopobium*, *Prevotella*,

Moryella, *Oribacterium*, *Megasphaera*, *Veillonella*, *Bulleidia* and *Campylobacter* have been associated with cigarette smoking (Jia et al. 2021). Additionally, histopathological examination has shown signs of epithelial dysplasia such as bulbous rete ridges, loss of polarity and an increase in parabasal cells with potential malignant transformation (Jalayer Naderi et al. 2015).

Chronic alcohol drinkers have been associated with damaged oral epithelial/mucosal tissue and impairment of immune function (Feng and Wang 2013), with an increased risk for microbial infection and changes to the oral microbiome. In a study done on a Chinese population of alcohol drinkers, genera *Prevotella* and *Moryella* and species *Prevotella melaninogenica* and *P. tannerae* were significantly enriched, while genera *Lautropia*, *Haemophilus* and *Porphyromonas* and species *Haemophilus parainfluenzae* were significantly depleted (Liao et al. 2022).

8.5 Microbial Interaction with the Host

Periodontal pathogens can infect periodontal sites by attaching to epithelial cells, existing micro-organisms or the tooth surface and by competing effectively with the resident large microbial population (Slots and Ting 1999). The tissue-destructive potential of these pathogens may include the production of toxins and enzymes or the induction of immunopathological reactions (Slots and Ting 1999).

Neutrophils play a major role in periodontal tissue homeostasis by being in the first line of defence during a bacterial challenge (Page and Schroeder 1976), recruitment of T cells, storage for antimicrobial peptides and enzymes, as well as their proinflammatory, anti-inflammatory or immunoregulatory properties (Scapini and Cassatella 2014; Hajishengallis and Korostoff 2017).

The major fimbriae present on the cell surface of *P. gingivalis* are important in the bacterial adhesion and co-aggregation required for its colonisation (Bao et al. 2014). *P. gingivalis* produces proteases that can block the production of immunoglobulins, degrade IL-8, MCP-1 and complement components C3a and C3b. Collectively, these proteases block its opsonisation, reducing its phagocytosis and thus ensuring survival of the bacteria (Slaney and Curtis 2008). Additionally, the HRGpA gingipain from the surface molecules of *P. gingivalis* can allow the bacteria to escape the action of the complement system (Hajishengallis 2015). Gingipains produced by *P. gingivalis* are also able to alter the co-aggregation of *A. actinomycetemcomitans*, thereby influencing the complexity of the microbial community. The nucleases produced by *P. intermedia* are also able to evade phagocytosis by degrading neutrophil extracellular traps (NETs) released by neutrophils (Doke et al. 2017).

Under normal conditions, there is a constant influx of neutrophils into the gingival sulcus, thereby creating a fine balance between the microbial community and the host immune response (Graves et al. 2019). Periodontal pathogens residing in the deeply anaerobic environment of the periodontal pockets may compromise the important antimicrobial mechanisms of neutrophils and other protective host cells (Slots and Ting 1999). This increase in disease-associated bacteria leads to microbial dysbiosis and tip the balance towards an overactivated immune response (Hajishengallis et al. 2012). The dental biofilm has also been reported to provide an environment for the bacteria present to be more resistant to neutrophil phagocytic activity and more able to replicate (Carvalho et al. 2009). Microbial virulence factors and toxic derivatives could interfere with humoral or cellular antibacterial defence mechanisms, eliciting alveolar bone resorption (Hajishengallis 2014). Moderate immune responses induced by oral microbiota may be beneficial for alveolar bone homeostasis, whereas the expression of large numbers of proinflammatory cytokines induced by excessive immune responses promotes alveolar bone loss (Cheng et al. 2021).

The major inflammatory cells involved in the pathogenesis of periodontitis are summarised in Table 8.1.

Other than regulating the oral immune system, oral bacteria also play crucial roles in oral mucosal integrity. The oral mucosa is considered a mirror of an individual's systemic health (Şenel 2021). Disruption of the epithelial cell-to-cell adhesion, known as a 'leaky gum' condition, is associated with the initiation and progression of periodontal disease (Ye et al. 2000). Bacteria are known to destroy and cause downregulation of this tight junction (Takahashi et al. 2019) by undergoing protein posttranslational modifications (PTMs) (Reiche and Huber 2020). This has been hypothesised as one of the mechanisms linking the involvement of oral microbiota in the pathogenesis of systemic conditions. To survive in the dynamic oral environment, oral bacteria depend on PTMs to quickly respond to external stimuli and regulate their physiological processes. The common protein modifications of oral bacterial species include phosphorylation, acetylation, glycosylation, citrullination, succinylation and glutathionylation (Wu et al. 2019; Zeng et al. 2020). A compromise or dysfunction of the tight junctions in epithelial layers has been implicated in chronic inflammatory conditions (Bhat et al. 2018).

Table 8.1 Inflammatory cells involved in the pathogenesis of periodontitis.

Host immune cells	Functions
Neutrophils	First immune cells in inflammatory response, emigration from bloodstream controlled by intercellular adhesion molecule-1 (ICAM-1) and E-selectin expression. Enhancement of periodontal tissue breakdown. Main source of host proteolytic enzymes, including neutrophil elastase, matrix metalloproteinases, cathepsins and serine proteases
Mast cells	Enhancement of periodontitis
Macrophages	Recruitment of lymphocytes and other immune cells
	M1 (proinflammatory): alveolar bone resorption, osteoclastogenesis, collagen degradation
	M2 (anti-inflammatory): local tissue repair, wound healing
T helper cells	Activation of other immune cells such as neutrophils and B cells
Treg cells	Suppression of immune response and promotion of pathogen survival
B cells	Associated with advanced stages of periodontitis. Dual function: protective – by improving bacterial clearance and destructive – by increasing inflammation, bone resorption and matrix dissolution
Interleukin-8	Polymorphonuclear leucocyte chemoattractant, direct actions on osteoclast differentiation and activity by signalling through the specific receptor, chemokine (C-X-C motif) receptor 1
Nuclear factor kappa-B pathway	Kappa-B receptor activator (RANKL) and osteoprotegerin are key regulators of bone remodelling and are directly involved in the differentiation, activation and survival of osteoclasts and precursors of osteoclasts

P. gingivalis and *F. nucleatum* have also been shown to impair gingival keratinocyte proliferation in an in vitro study (Bhattacharya et al. 2014) which led to a compromised epithelial barrier.

Accumulating evidence suggests that cellular senescence, stem cell exhaustion and immuno-ageing are hallmarks of biological ageing implicated in the impairment of periodontal homeostasis and pathophysiology of periodontitis (Baima et al. 2022).

8.6 Effect of Periodontal Therapy on the Microbiota

The inflammation and tissue breakdown that occur in periodontitis sustain a dysbiotic microbial community in the dental biofilm by providing nutrients that help in its proliferation. Resolution of inflammation and restoration of symbiosis are achieved by regular and thorough disruption of the biofilm (Kilian et al. 2016). This is achieved by a good oral hygiene regime and mechanical plaque removal by professionals.

Studies have reported a key role of supragingival plaque control in recolonisation of subgingival bacteria after non-surgical periodontal therapy (NSPT) whereby major changes in supragingival plaque may bring changes to the composition of subgingival plaque (Magnusson et al. 1984; Xajigeorgiou et al. 2006). It is also believed that following supragingival plaque control, a decrease in gingival inflammation and gingival crevicular fluid flow occurs. Therefore, the microbes would no longer access the nutrients present as the inflammation is treated and the source of collagen peptides on which the Gram-negative anaerobes feed is no longer present (Daly and Highfield 1996; Ramberg et al. 1996). Although oral health intervention by itself may be able to improve clinical parameters, this may not show significant reduction in microbial counts (Asad et al. 2017).

The importance of mechanical plaque removal in periodontal therapy is demonstrated when significant improvements in clinical as well as microbiological profiles are shown after NSPT (Badersten et al. 1981; Kaldahl et al. 1993; Morrison et al. 1980). A decline in the levels of *P. gingivalis*, *A. actinomycetemcomitans* and *P. intermedia* at three months post NSPT was reported, but these pathogens were not totally eliminated (Beikler et al. 2004; Derdilopoulou et al. 2007; Doungudomdacha et al. 2001; Sakamoto et al. 2004). Similarly, in another study, the reduction in frequency and intensity of certain periodontal pathogens including *P. gingivalis* and *T. forsythia* was maintained even nine months after treatment (Colombo et al. 2005; Cugini et al. 2000). Similar findings of a reduction in the presence and bacterial load of disease-causing bacteria but not total elimination of these bacteria were also reported following surgical periodontal therapy (Checchi and Pascolo 2018).

While these mechanical procedures can prevent the formation of a disease-triggering dysbiotic biofilm, they do not directly affect the latent dysregulated inflammatory cascade in susceptible hosts. Based on these findings, adjunctive therapies such as antiseptics, antibiotics, probiotics, photodynamic therapy and ozone therapy have been considered in the periodontal management of severe periodontitis cases.

8.6.1 Antiseptics

The recent European Federation of Periodontology (EFP) consensus guidelines have suggested that for the control of gingival inflammation in periodontitis patients in supportive periodontal care, antiseptic mouth rinse formulations that can be used adjunctively are products containing chlorhexidine (CHX), essential oils and cetylpyridinium chloride, while antiseptics that are recommended to be used in dentifrices are chlorhexidine, triclosan-co-polymer and stannous fluoride-sodium hexametaphosphate (Sanz et al. 2020).

Chlorhexidine has been routinely prescribed in dental settings, due to its antimicrobial effect against bacteria, viruses and fungi. It is used as a short-term adjunct to mechanical periodontal therapy. The EFP guidelines have recommended that 'adjunctive antiseptics may be considered, specifically chlorhexidine mouth rinses for a limited period of time, in periodontitis therapy, as adjuncts to mechanical debridement, in specific cases' (Sanz et al. 2020).

Chlorhexidine must be used with caution as recent studies using next-generation sequencing found that the oral microbiome demonstrated reduced diversity, thus becoming more dysbiotic, following a week's use of chlorhexidine mouthwash. This was reported in a study by Bescos et al. (2020) on healthy individuals who were instructed to rinse with CHX mouthwash for one minute over seven days; an increase in the acidic condition with a major shift and lower diversity of the salivary microbiome was found. The authors also reported lower nitrite availability with an increase in systolic blood pressure due to depletion in bacterial nitrate-reducing activity such as by *Veillonella*. The reduced microbial biodiversity may cause an increased risk for oral disease. In addition, it has also been suggested that the use of chlorhexidine in hypertensive subjects should be properly reviewed due to the possibility of an increased mortality rate (Deschepper et al. 2018).

8.6.2 Antibiotics

A wide range of antibiotics have been prescribed as adjuncts to mechanical periodontal therapy. Antibiotics for periodontitis have traditionally been delivered either locally or systemically.

Herrera and colleagues (2020) demonstrated statistically significant improvements in clinical periodontal parameters at 6–9 months post therapy compared to controls in their systematic review and meta-analyses on the use of locally delivered antibiotics as adjuncts to mechanical periodontal therapy. They reported that groups using doxycycline- or tetracycline-based products such as Atridox®, Actisite® and Ligosan® showed the largest benefits.

Another systematic review and meta-analysis which assessed the use of systemically delivered antibiotics as adjunctive therapy following scaling and root debridement (SRD) reported statistically significant full-mouth periodontal pocket reduction and clinical attachment level gain compared to controls at six months post therapy which was maintained up to one year (Teughels et al. 2020). The level of evidence was highest for the combination of metronidazole and amoxicillin, followed by metronidazole alone and azithromycin. The findings for the metronidazole and amoxicillin combination did not distinguish between chronic periodontitis and aggressive periodontitis patients. The reason given for the similarity in the effects against both forms of periodontitis was that both conditions have similar microbiota as well as host response mechanisms to the microbiota (Mombelli et al. 2002; Duarte et al. 2015; Teughels et al. 2020).

Currently, the use of adjunctive systemic antibiotics has very low-certainty evidence for long-term follow-up in the non-surgical treatment of periodontitis (Khattri et al. 2020). The 6th European Workshop recommended that the use of systemic antimicrobials as adjuncts in periodontitis therapy should be restricted to patients with severe and progressing forms of periodontitis (Sanz and Teughels 2008). Over the years, we are now seeing the emergence of antibiotic-resistant strains (Sukumar et al. 2020). One study showed that the effect of antibiotics on oral bacteria lasted only one month but the disturbance to the gut microbiome lasted up to one year (Zaura et al. 2015). A recent review concluded that complex interactions exist amongst the members of the vastly diverse microbial community and therapeutic concepts that target bacterial species or strains are unrealistic (Mombelli 2018). Therefore, the decision to use systemic antibiotics as adjuncts to periodontal therapy must be taken judiciously.

8.6.3 Probiotics

Probiotics are 'live micro-organisms which, when administered in adequate amounts, confer a health benefit on the host' (FAO/WHO). Probiotics can disrupt the established dysbiosis present in the deep niches of periodontal pockets and thus re-establish the symbiotic relationship present in periodontal health. In a recent systematic review, probiotics were shown to improve periodontal clinical parameters and reduce the load of *P. gingivalis*, *T. forsythia* and *F. nucleatum* and also pro-inflammatory markers (Gheisary et al. 2022). Probiotics such as *Lactobacillus* (Mennigen et al. 2009) (recently known as *Limosilactobacillus*) and *Bifidobacterium* (Hojo et al. 2007) have been shown to positively regulate the epithelial barrier function by direct and indirect mechanisms and maintaining the integrity of the epithelial tight junction (Takahashi et al. 2019).

A recent systematic review assessing the effect of different strains of probiotics as adjuncts to SRD reported that *Lactobacillus* spp. showed statistically significant differences in intergroup comparisons for bleeding on probing (Vives-Soler and Chimenos-Küstner 2020). Vivekananda and colleagues (2010) suggested *L. reuteri*'s antimicrobial effect in short-term measurements in a split-mouth study comparing probiotics lozenges either alone or in combination with SRD. Significant improvements in clinical parameters (pocket depth and percentage of bleeding reduction) and reduced counts of *A. actinomycetencomitans*, *P. gingivalis* and *P. intermedia* was seen at sites treated with SRD and probiotics (Vivekananda et al. 2010). Additionally, in the probiotics group, sites without mechanical debridement also showed reduction in bleeding.

Probiotics have also been used as part of periodontal maintenance therapy. Probiotics lozenges were prescribed to a group of successfully treated patients who were initially diagnosed with periodontitis Stage 3 to 4, Grade C. The patients were followed up every three months for one year. The reduction in percentage of gingival bleeding was significant up to the one-year follow-up period (Grusovin et al. 2020).

Further studies need to be done on the effect of different strains of probiotics using larger cohorts of subjects.

8.6.4 Photodynamic Therapy

Antimicrobial photodynamic therapy (aPDT) is based on the principle that photosensitiser dye molecules brought into the pocket can be activated by laser light or light of a suitable wavelength to produce free oxygen radicals, which react with bacteria and their products and cause bacterial cell death (Wilson 1994). Using aPDT, levels of *F. nucleatum*, *E. nodatum*, *P. gingivalis*, *T. forsythia*, *T. denticola* and *E. corrodens* in subjects with periodontitis were found to be significantly reduced (Joseph et al. 2017).

A systematic review on the use of aPDT as an adjunct to SRD in patients with aggressive periodontitis found that this combination demonstrated significant improvements in clinical parameters as well as the reduction of periodontopathogens (Vohra et al. 2016). However, the findings from a study that investigated the effect of single verses double episodes of aPDT in addition to instrumentation in the management of periodontitis reported no significant difference in the detection frequencies of micro-organism from baseline to three or six months (Müller Campanile et al. 2015).

In their systematic review on the use of aPDT as an adjunct to professional mechanical plaque removal, Trombelli and colleagues (2020) reported that aPDT did not enhance the magnitude of CAL gain or BOP and PD reduction when sites with probing depth ≥4 mm were repeatedly treated in supportive periodontal therapy. However, their findings differed from the findings reported by Xue and Zhao (2017) which reported significant improvements in PD reductions and CAL gain when aPDT was used adjunctively with SRD. The EFP consensus guidelines reported that aPDT did not provide additional benefits and there was also the concern of additional costs involved for the use of laser therapy (Sanz et al. 2020). It is recommended that more randomised clinical trials with well-defined control groups are needed to explore this adjunctive approach.

8.6.5 Other Therapies

There are currently a few other techniques being studied that can be used as adjuncts to periodontal therapy.

Ozonated water and ozonated oils have been used in the field of dentistry. In a recent study, patients with generalised severe periodontitis were treated with the combination of full-mouth ultrasonic SRD and a 10-day administration of hyperbaric ozone therapy (Lombardo et al. 2020). The findings from this study demonstrated effective reduction of bleeding on probing and slower bacterial recolonisation when compared to the control group.

Photobiomodulation, previously known as low-level laser therapy, uses red and near infra-red wavelengths of the electromagnetic spectrum to improve the tissue repair process (Dalvi et al. 2021). The effect of photobiomodulation therapy as an adjunct to SRD compared to conventional treatment alone remains debatable, as concluded from a systematic review (Dalvi et al. 2021).

Quorum sensing signalling is important in the regulation of the dental biofilm. To disrupt biofilm formation, the quorum sensing mechanism needs to be disrupted and this process is also known as quorum quenching (Yada et al. 2015). Studies looking at the effect of quorum sensing inhibitors as adjuncts in periodontal therapy need to be explored further (Bizzarro et al. 2016).

8.7 Conclusion

Dental microbial dysbiosis has been seen as one of the main players in the aetiology and progression of periodontal disease. With the introduction of advanced diagnostic techniques, our understanding of the diverse microbial communities that exists in the healthy and diseased periodontal condition has increased. Knowledge of how these disease-associated pathogens may compromise important antimicrobial mechanisms in the host cells will be instrumental in guiding clinicians in their management of periodontal disease. This will bring about improvements in periodontal health status and also the overall health of patients as the periodontal microbiota and its dysbiosis play an important role in regulating human health and disease.

References

Allison, D.G. (2003). The biofilm matrix. *Biofouling* 19 (2): 139–150.

Asad, M., Abdul Aziz, A.W., Raman, R.P. et al. (2017). Comparison of nonsurgical periodontal therapy with oral hygiene instruction alone for chronic periodontitis. *J. Oral Sci.* 59 (1): 111–120.

Badersten, A., Nilvéus, R. and Egelberg, J. (1981). Effect of nonsurgical periodontal therapy. *J. Clin. Periodontol.* 8 (1): 57–72.

Baima, G., Romandini, M., Citterio, F., Romano, F. and Aimetti, M. (2022). Periodontitis and accelerated biological aging: a geroscience approach. *J. Dent. Res.* 101 (2): 125–132.

Bao, K., Belibasakis, G.N., Thurnheer, T., Aduse-Opoku, J., Curtis, M.A. and Bostanci, N. (2014). Role of Porphyromonas gingivalis gingipains in multi-species biofilm formation. *BMC Microbiol* 14 (1): 258.

Beikler, T., Abdeen, G., Schnitzer, S. et al. (2004). Microbiological shifts in intra-and extraoral habitats following mechanical periodontal therapy. *J. Clin. Periodontol.* 31 (9): 777–783.

Berezow, A.B. and Darveau, R.P. (2011). Microbial shift and periodontitis. *Periodontology 2000* 55 (1): 36–47.

Bernimoulin, J.-P. (2003). Recent concepts in plaque formation. *J. Clin. Periodontol.* 30 (s5): 7–9.

Bescos, R., Ashworth, A., Cutler, C. et al. (2020). Effects of Chlorhexidine mouthwash on the oral microbiome. *Sci. Rep.* 10 (1): 5254.

Bhat, A.A., Uppada, S., Achkar, I.W. et al. (2018). Tight junction proteins and signaling pathways in cancer and inflammation: a functional crosstalk. *Front. Physiol.* 9: 1942.

Bhattacharya, R., Xu, F., Dong, G. et al. (2014). Effect of bacteria on the wound healing behavior of oral epithelial cells. *PLoS One* 9 (2): e89475.

Bizzarro, S., Laine, M.L., Buijs, M.J. et al. (2016). Microbial profiles at baseline and not the use of antibiotics determine the clinical outcome of the treatment of chronic periodontitis. *Sci. Rep.* 6 (1): 20205.

Camelo-Castillo, A J., Mira, A., Pico, A. et al. (2015). Subgingival microbiota in health compared to periodontitis and the influence of smoking. *Front. Microbiol.* 6: 119.

Carvalho, R.P., Mesquita, J.S., Bonomo, A., Elsas, P.X. and Colombo, A.P. (2009). Relationship of neutrophil phagocytosis and oxidative burst with the subgingival microbiota of generalized aggressive periodontitis. *Oral Microbiol. Immunol.* 24 (2): 124–132.

Cekici, A., Kantarci, A., Hasturk, H. and Van Dyke, T.E. (2014). Inflammatory and immune pathways in the pathogenesis of periodontal disease. *Periodontology 2000* 64 (1): 57–80.

Checchi, V. and Pascolo, G. (2018). Microbiological response to periodontal therapy: a retrospective study. *Open Dent. J.* 12: 837–845.

Cheng, X., Zhou, X., Liu, C. and Xu, X. (2021). Oral osteomicrobiology: the role of oral microbiota in alveolar bone homeostasis. *Front. Cell Infect. Microbiol.* 11: 751503.

Colombo, A.P.V., Teles, R.P., Torres, M.C. et al. (2005). Effects of non-surgical mechanical therapy on the subgingival microbiota of Brazilians with untreated chronic periodontitis: 9-month results. *J. Periodontol.* 76 (5): 778–784.

Cugini, M., Haffajee, A., Smith, C., Kent, R. and Socransky, S. (2000). The effect of scaling and root planing on the clinical and microbiological parameters of periodontal diseases: 12-month results. *J. Clin. Periodontol.* 27 (1): 30–36.

Dalvi, S., Benedicenti, S. and Hanna, R. (2021). Effectiveness of photobiomodulation as an adjunct to nonsurgical periodontal therapy in the management of periodontitis – a systematic review of in vivo human studies. *Photochem. Photobiol.* 97 (2): 223–242.

Daly, C. and Highfield, J. (1996). Effect of localized experimental gingivitis on early supragingival plaque accumulation. *J. Clin. Periodontol.* 23 (3): 160–164.

Darveau, R.P. (2010). Periodontitis: a polymicrobial disruption of host homeostasis. *Nat. Rev. Microbiol.* 8 (7): 481–490.

Derdilopoulou, F.V., Nonhoff, J., Neumann, K. and Kielbassa, A.M. (2007). Microbiological findings after periodontal therapy using curettes, Er: YAG laser, sonic, and ultrasonic scalers. *J. Clin. Periodontol.* 34 (7): 588–598.

Deschepper, M., Waegeman, W., Eeckloo, K., Vogelaers, D. and Blot, S. (2018). Effects of chlorhexidine gluconate oral care on hospital mortality: a hospital-wide, observational cohort study. *Intensive Care Med.* 44 (7): 1017–1026.

Dewhirst, F.E., Chen, T., Izard, J. et al. (2010). The human oral microbiome. *J. Bacteriol.* 192 (19): 5002–5017.

Diaz, P.I., Chalmers, N.I., Rickard, A.H. et al. (2006). Molecular characterization of subject-specific oral microflora during initial colonization of enamel. *Appl. Environ. Microbiol.* 72 (4): 2837–2848.

Doke, M., Fukamachi, H., Morisaki, H., Arimoto, T., Kataoka, H. and Kuwata, H. (2017). Nucleases from Prevotella intermedia can degrade neutrophil extracellular traps. *Mol. Oral Microbiol.* 32 (4): 288–300.

Doungudomdacha, S., Rawlinson, A., Walsh, T. and Douglas, C. (2001). Effect of non-surgical periodontal treatment on clinical parameters and the numbers of Porphyromonas gingivalis, Prevotella intermedia and Actinobacillus actinomycetemcomitans at adult periodontitis sites. *J. Clin. Periodontol.* 28 (5): 437–445.

Duarte, P.M., Bastos, M.F., Fermiano, D. et al. (2015). Do subjects with aggressive and chronic periodontitis exhibit a different cytokine/chemokine profile in the gingival crevicular fluid? A systematic review. *J. Periodont. Res.* 50 (1): 18–27.

Duran-Pinedo, A.E., Chen, T., Teles, R. et al. (2014). Community-wide transcriptome of the oral microbiome in subjects with and without periodontitis. *ISME J.* 8 (8): 1659–1672.

Ebersole, J.L. and Taubman, M.A. (1994). The protective nature of host responses in periodontal diseases. *Periodontology 2000* 5: 112–141.

Feng, L. and Wang, L. (2013). Effects of alcohol on the morphological and structural changes in oral mucosa. *Pak. J. Med. Sci.* 29 (4): 1046–1049.

Fux, C.A., Costerton, J.W., Stewart, P.S. and Stoodley, P. (2005). Survival strategies of infectious biofilms. *Trends Microbiol.* 13 (1): 34–40.

Gheisary, Z., Mahmood, R., Harri Shivanantham, A. et al. (2022). The clinical, microbiological, and immunological effects of probiotic supplementation on prevention and treatment of periodontal diseases: a systematic review and meta-analysis. *Nutrients* 14 (5).

Gilbert, P., Maira-Litran, T., McBain, A.J., Rickard, A.H. and Whyte, F.W. (2002). The physiology and collective recalcitrance of microbial biofilm communities. *Adv. Microb. Physiol.* 46: 202–256.

Graves, D.T., Corrêa, J.D. and Silva, T.A. (2019). The oral microbiota is modified by systemic diseases. *J. Dent. Res.* 98 (2): 148–156.

Griffen, A.L., Beall, C.J., Campbell, J.H. et al. (2012). Distinct and complex bacterial profiles in human periodontitis and health revealed by 16S pyrosequencing. *ISME J.* 6 (6): 1176–1185.

Grusovin, M.G., Bossini, S., Calza, S. et al. (2020). Clinical efficacy of Lactobacillus reuteri-containing lozenges in the supportive therapy of generalized periodontitis stage III and IV, grade C: 1-year results of a double-blind randomized placebo-controlled pilot study. *Clin. Oral Invest.* 24 (6): 2015–2024.

Hajishengallis, G. (2014). Immunomicrobial pathogenesis of periodontitis: keystones, pathobionts, and host response. *Trends Immunol.* 35 (1): 3–11.

Hajishengallis, G. (2015). Periodontitis: from microbial immune subversion to systemic inflammation. *Nat. Rev. Immunol.* 15 (1): 30–44.

Hajishengallis, G. and Lamont, R.J. (2016). Dancing with the stars: how choreographed bacterial interactions dictate nososymbiocity and give rise to keystone pathogens, accessory pathogens, and pathobionts. *Trends Microbiol.* 24 (6): 477–489.

Hajishengallis, G. and Korostoff, J. M. (2017). Revisiting the Page and Schroeder model: the good, the bad and the unknowns in the periodontal host response 40 years later. *Periodontology 2000* 75 (1): 116–151.

Hajishengallis, G., Darveau, R.P. and Curtis, M.A. (2012). The keystone-pathogen hypothesis. *Nat. Rev. Microbiol.* 10 (10): 717–725.

Herrera, D., Matesanz, P., Martín, C., Oud, V., Feres, M. and Teughels, W. (2020). Adjunctive effect of locally delivered antimicrobials in periodontitis therapy: a systematic review and meta-analysis. *J. Clin. Periodontol.* 47 (Suppl 22): 239–256.

Hojo, K., Mizoguchi, C., Taketomo, N. et al. (2007). Distribution of salivary Lactobacillus and Bifidobacterium species in periodontal health and disease. *Biosci. Biotechnol. Biochem.* 71 (1): 152–157.

Jalayer Naderi, N., Semyari, H. and Elahinia, Z. (2015). The impact of smoking on gingiva: a histopathological study. *Iran J. Pathol.* 10 (3): 214–220.

Jenkinson, H.F. and Lamont, R.J. (1997). Streptococcal adhesion and colonization. *Crit. Rev. Oral Biol. Med.* 8 (2): 175–200.

Jia, Y.J., Liao, Y., He, Y.Q. et al. (2021). Association between oral microbiota and cigarette smoking in the Chinese population. *Front. Cell Infect. Microbiol.* 11: 658203.

Jorth, P., Turner, K.H., Gumus, P., Nizam, N., Buduneli, N. and Whiteley, M. (2014). Metatranscriptomics of the human oral microbiome during health and disease. *mBio* 5 (2): e01012–01014.

Joseph, B., Janam, P., Narayanan, S. and Anil, S. (2017). Is antimicrobial photodynamic therapy effective as an adjunct to scaling and root planing in patients with chronic periodontitis? A systematic review. *Biomolecules* 7 (4): 79.

Kaldahl, W.B., Kalkwarf, K.L. and Patil, K.D. (1993). A review of longitudinal studies that compared periodontal therapies. *J. Periodontol.* 64 (4): 243–253.

Khattri, S., Kumbargere Nagraj, S., Arora, A. et al. (2020). Adjunctive systemic antimicrobials for the non-surgical treatment of periodontitis. *Cochrane Database Syst. Rev.* 11 (11): Cd012568.

Kilian, M., Chapple, I.L., Hannig, M. et al. (2016). The oral microbiome – an update for oral healthcare professionals. *Br. Dent. J.* 221 (10): 657–666.

Kinane, D.F. (1999). Periodontitis modified by systemic factors. *Ann. Periodontol.* 4 (1): 54–64.

Kinane, D.F., Stathopoulou, P.G. and Papapanou, P.N. (2017). Periodontal diseases. *Nat. Rev. Dis. Primers* 3: 17038.

Kolenbrander, P.E. (1993). Coaggregation of human oral bacteria: potential role in the accretion of dental plaque. *J. Appl. Bacteriol.* 74 (Suppl): 79s–86s.

Li, Y.H., Tang, N., Aspiras, M.B. et al. (2002). A quorum-sensing signaling system essential for genetic competence in Streptococcus mutans is involved in biofilm formation. *J. Bacteriol.* 184 (10): 2699–2708.

Liao, Y., Tong, X.T., Jia, Y.J. et al. (2022). The effects of alcohol drinking on oral microbiota in the Chinese population. *Int. J. Environ. Res. Public Health* 19 (9): 5729.

Listgarten, M.A. and Helldén, L. (1978). Relative distribution of bacteria at clinically healthy and periodontally diseased sites in humans. *J. Clin. Periodontol.* 5 (2): 115–132.

Loe, H., Theilade, E. and Jensen, S.B. (1965). Experimental gingivitis in man. *J. Periodontol.* 36: 177– 187.

Loesche, W.J. (1976). Chemotherapy of dental plaque infections. *Oral Sci. Rev.* 9: 65–107.

Lombardo, G., Pardo, A., Signoretto, C. et al. (2020). Hyperbaric oxygen therapy for the treatment of moderate to severe periodontitis: a clinical pilot study. *Undersea Hyperb. Med.* 47 (4): 571–580.

Magnusson, I., Lindhe, J., Yoneyama, T. and Liljenberg, B. (1984). Recolonization of a subgingival microbiota following scaling in deep pockets. *J. Clin. Periodontol.* 11 (3): 193–207.

Marsh, P.D. (1994). Microbial ecology of dental plaque and its significance in health and disease. *Adv. Dent. Res.* 8 (2): 263–271.

Marsh, P.D. (2005). Dental plaque: biological significance of a biofilm and community life-style. *J. Clin. Periodontol.* 32 (Suppl 6): 7–15.

Marsh, P.D. and Devine, D.A. (2011). How is the development of dental biofilms influenced by the host? *J. Clin. Periodontol.* 38 (s11): 28–35.

Marsh, P.D., Head, D.A. and Devine, D.A. (2015). Dental plaque as a biofilm and a microbial community – implications for treatment. *J. Oral Biosci.* 57 (4): 185–191.

Mennigen, R., Nolte, K., Rijcken, E. et al. (2009). Probiotic mixture VSL#3 protects the epithelial barrier by maintaining tight junction protein expression and preventing apoptosis in a murine model of colitis. *Am. J. Physiol. Gastrointest. Liver Physiol.* 296 (5): G1140–1149.

Miller, W.D. (1890). *The Micro-organisms of the Human Mouth: The Local and General Diseases which are Caused by Them.* Lakewood, NJ: S.S. White Dental Manufacturing Company.

Mira, A., Simon-Soro, A. and Curtis, M.A. (2017). Role of microbial communities in the pathogenesis of periodontal diseases and caries. *J. Clin. Periodontol.* 44 (Suppl 18): S23–s38.

Mombelli, A. (2018). Microbial colonization of the periodontal pocket and its significance for periodontal therapy. *Periodontology 2000* 76 (1): 85–96.

Mombelli, A., Casagni, F. and Madianos, P.N. (2002). Can presence or absence of periodontal pathogens distinguish between subjects with chronic and aggressive periodontitis? A systematic review. *J. Clin. Periodontol.* 29 (Suppl 3): 10–21; discussion 37–18.

Morrison, E., Ramfjord, S. and Hill, R. (1980). Short-term effects of initial, nonsurgical periodontal treatment (hygienic phase). *J. Clin. Periodontol.* 7 (3): 199–211.

Müller Campanile, V.S., Giannopoulou, C., Campanile, G., Cancela, J.A. and Mombelli, A. (2015). Single or repeated antimicrobial photodynamic therapy as adjunct to ultrasonic debridement in residual periodontal pockets: clinical, microbiological, and local biological effects. *Lasers Med. Sci.* 30 (1): 27–34.

Nyvad, B. and Takahashi, N. (2020). Integrated hypothesis of dental caries and periodontal diseases. *J. Oral Microbiol.* 12 (1): 1710953.

Page, R.C. and Schroeder, H.E. (1976). Pathogenesis of inflammatory periodontal disease. A summary of current work. *Lab. Invest.* 34 (3): 235–249.

Ramberg, P., Furuichi, Y., Volpe, A., Gaffar, A. and Lindhe, J. (1996). The effects of antimicrobial mouthrinses on de novo plaque formation at sites with healthy and inflamed gingivae. *J. Clin. Periodontol.* 23 (1): 7–11.

Reiche, J. and Huber, O. (2020). Post-translational modifications of tight junction transmembrane proteins and their direct effect on barrier function. *Biochim. Biophys. Acta Biomembranes* 1862 (9): 183330.

Sakamoto, M., Huang, Y., Ohnishi, M., Umeda, M., Ishikawa, I. and Benno, Y. (2004). Changes in oral microbial profiles after periodontal treatment as determined by molecular analysis of 16S rRNA genes. *J. Med. Microbiol.* 53 (6): 563–571.

Sanger, F., Nicklen, S. and Coulson, A.R. (1977). DNA sequencing with chain-terminating inhibitors. *Proc. Natl Acad. Sci. USA* 74 (12): 5463–5467.

Sanz, M. and Teughels, W. (2008). Innovations in non-surgical periodontal therapy: Consensus Report of the Sixth European Workshop on Periodontology. *J. Clin. Periodontol.* 35 (8 Suppl): 3–7.

Sanz, M., Herrera, D., Kebschull, M. et al. (2020). Treatment of stage I–III periodontitis – The EFP S3 level clinical practice guideline. *J. Clin. Periodontol.* 47 (S22): 4–60.

Scapini, P. and Cassatella, M.A. (2014). Social networking of human neutrophils within the immune system. *Blood* 124 (5): 710–719.

Schwartz, J.L., Peña, N., Kawar, N. et al. (2021). Old age and other factors associated with salivary microbiome variation. *BMC Oral Health* 21 (1): 490.

Sekundo, C., Langowski, E., Wolff, D., Boutin, S. and Frese, C. (2022). Maintaining oral health for a hundred years and more? An analysis of microbial and salivary factors in a cohort of centenarians. *J. Oral Microbiol.* 14 (1): 2059891.

Şenel, S. (2021). An overview of physical, microbiological and immune barriers of oral mucosa. *Int. J. Mol. Sci.* 22 (15): 7821.

Slaney, J.M. and Curtis, M.A. (2008). Mechanisms of evasion of complement by Porphyromonas gingivalis. *Front. Biosci.* 13: 188–196.

Slots, J. and Ting, M. (1999). Actinobacillus actinomycetemcomitans and Porphyromonas gingivalis in human periodontal disease: occurrence and treatment. *Periodontology 2000* 20: 82–121.

Socransky, S.S. and Haffajee, A.D. (1992). The bacterial etiology of destructive periodontal disease: current concepts. *J. Periodontol.* 63 (4 Suppl): 322–331.

Socransky, S.S. and Haffajee, A.D. (2002). Dental biofilms: difficult therapeutic targets. *Periodontology 2000* 28: 12–55.

Socransky, S.S., Haffajee, A.D., Cugini, M.A., Smith, C. and Kent, R.L. Jr (1998). Microbial complexes in subgingival plaque. *J. Clin. Periodontol.* 25 (2): 134–144.

Sukumar, S., Martin, F.E., Hughes, T.E. and Adler, C.J. (2020). Think before you prescribe: how dentistry contributes to antibiotic resistance. *Austral. Dent. J.* 65 (1): 21–29.

Suntharalingam, P. and Cvitkovitch, D.G. (2005). Quorum sensing in streptococcal biofilm formation. *Trends Microbiol.* 13 (1): 3–6.

Takahashi, N., Sulijaya, B., Yamada-Hara, M., Tsuzuno, T., Tabeta, K. and Yamazaki, K. (2019). Gingival epithelial barrier: regulation by beneficial and harmful microbes. *Tissue Barriers* 7 (3): e1651158.

Teughels, W., Feres, M., Oud, V., Martín, C., Matesanz, P. and Herrera, D. (2020). Adjunctive effect of systemic antimicrobials in periodontitis therapy: a systematic review and meta-analysis. *J. Clin. Periodontol.* 47 (S22): 257–281.

Theilade, E. (1986). The non-specific theory in microbial etiology of inflammatory periodontal diseases. *J. Clin. Periodontol.* 13 (10): 905–911.

Tonetti, M.S., Jepsen, S., Jin, L. and Otomo-Corgel, J. (2017). Impact of the global burden of periodontal diseases on health, nutrition and wellbeing of mankind: a call for global action. *J. Clin. Periodontol.* 44 (5): 456–462.

Trombelli, L., Farina, R., Pollard, A. et al. (2020). Efficacy of alternative or additional methods to professional mechanical plaque removal during supportive periodontal therapy: a systematic review and meta-analysis. *J. Clin. Periodontol.* 47 (Suppl 22): 144–154.

Tsai, C.Y., Tang, C.Y., Tan, T.S. et al. (2018). Subgingival microbiota in individuals with severe chronic periodontitis. *J. Microbiol. Immunol. Infect.* 51 (2): 226–234.

Van Dyke, T.E., Bartold, P.M. and Reynolds, E.C. (2020). The nexus between periodontal inflammation and dysbiosis. *Front. Immunol.* 11: 511.

van Winkelhoff, A.J., Rams, T.E. and Slots, J. (1996). Systemic antibiotic therapy in periodontics. *Periodontology 2000* 10: 45–78.

Vivekananda, M.R., Vandana, K.L. and Bhat, K.G. (2010). Effect of the probiotic Lactobacilli reuteri (Prodentis) in the management of periodontal disease: a preliminary randomized clinical trial. *J. Oral Microbiol.* 2.

Vives-Soler, A. and Chimenos-Küstner, E. (2020). Effect of probiotics as a complement to non-surgical periodontal therapy in chronic periodontitis: a systematic review. *Med. Oral Patol. Oral Cir. Bucal.* 25 (2): e161–e167.

Vohra, F., Akram, Z., Safii, S.H. et al. (2016). Role of antimicrobial photodynamic therapy in the treatment of aggressive periodontitis: a systematic review. *Photodiagn. Photodyn. Ther.* 13: 139–147.

Wilson, M. (1994). Bactericidal effect of laser light and its potential use in the treatment of plaque-related diseases. *Int. Dent. J.* 44 (2): 181–189.

Wu, L., Gong, T., Zhou, X. et al. (2019). Global analysis of lysine succinylome in the periodontal pathogen Porphyromonas gingivalis. *Mol. Oral Microbiol.* 34 (2): 74–83.

Xajigeorgiou, C., Sakellari, D., Slini, T., Baka, A. and Konstantinidis, A. (2006). Clinical and microbiological effects of different antimicrobials on generalized aggressive periodontitis. *J. Clin. Periodontol.* 33 (4): 254–264.

Ximénez-Fyvie, L.A., Haffajee, A.D. and Socransky, S.S. (2000). Comparison of the microbiota of supra- and subgingival plaque in health and periodontitis. *J. Clin. Periodontol.* 27 (9): 648–657.

Xue, D. and Zhao, Y. (2017). Clinical effectiveness of adjunctive antimicrobial photodynamic therapy for residual pockets during supportive periodontal therapy: a systematic review and meta-analysis. *Photodiagn. Photodyn. Ther.* 17: 127–133.

Yada, S., Kamalesh, B., Sonwane, S., Guptha, I. and Swetha, R.K. (2015). Quorum sensing inhibition, relevance to periodontics. *J. Int. Oral Health* 7 (1): 67–69.

Ye, P., Chapple, C.C., Kumar, R.K. and Hunter, N. (2000). Expression patterns of E-cadherin, involucrin, and connexin gap junction proteins in the lining epithelia of inflamed gingiva. *J. Pathol.* 192 (1): 58–66.

Zaura, E., Brandt, B.W., Teixeira de Mattos, M.J. et al. (2015). Same exposure but two radically different responses to antibiotics: resilience of the salivary microbiome versus long-term microbial shifts in feces. *mBio* 6 (6): e01693–01615.

Zeng, J., Wu, L., Chen, Q. et al. (2020). Comprehensive profiling of protein lysine acetylation and its overlap with lysine succinylation in the Porphyromonas gingivalis fimbriated strain ATCC 33277. *Mol. Oral Microbiol.* 35 (6): 240–250.

9

Periodontitis and Systemic Diseases

Rathna Devi Vaithilingam and Nor Adinar Baharuddin

Department of Restorative Dentistry, University of Malaya, Kuala Lumpur, Malaysia

9.1 Introduction

Periodontal disease is a chronic inflammatory disease of the periodontium, comprising two main categories: gingivitis, affecting the gingival tissues alone, and periodontitis, which results in irreversible periodontal attachment loss, alveolar bone destruction and ultimately tooth loss if left untreated (Philstrom et al. 2005). The clinical features of periodontal disease (Figure 9.1) include signs and symptoms such as alterations of the colour, volume and texture of the gingiva, bleeding upon probing (BOP), increased periodontal pocket depth (PPD) due to reduction of resistance to probing of soft marginal gingival tissues, clinical attachment loss (CAL), gingival recession, alveolar bone loss, root furcation exposure, increased tooth mobility and drifting.

The periodontitis–systemic disease link has been gaining importance over the past few decades. This is based on increasing evidence associating periodontitis with systemic diseases such as type 2 diabetes mellitus (T2DM), cardiovascular disease (CVD), obesity, adverse pregnancy outcomes, respiratory diseases and more recently rheumatoid arthritis.

9.2 Prevalence of Periodontitis

Periodontitis is the sixth most prevalent oral condition worldwide, with a prevalence of 30–35%, and represents a major contributor to the global burden of disease (WHO 2007; Marcenes et al. 2013). Severe periodontitis is estimated to affect 11.2% of the global adult population (Kassebaum et al. 2014) and is a major cause of tooth loss, nutritional compromise, altered speech, low self-esteem and poorer overall quality of life.

In the USA, the National Health and Nutrition Examination Survey (NHANES 2009–2012) estimated that 46% of adults aged 30 and older suffer from periodontitis, with 8.9% of them having severe periodontitis (Eke et al. 2015). In the United Kingdom, 9% of the population 16 years and older have severe periodontitis (White et al. 2012). It has also been reported that Asians in developing nations are more susceptible to periodontitis than their Caucasian counterparts (Corbet and Leung 2011). However, the prevalence in these countries needs to be interpreted carefully due to the different methodologies used in its determination. In Malaysia, the prevalence of periodontitis increased from 1990 (23%) to 2000 (25.2%) and doubled in 2010 (48.5%) (Tuti et al. 2013). Out of this, 18.2% were categorised as severe periodontitis (NOHSA 2010). These findings could reflect persistent ineffective oral hygiene practices, lack of periodontal health awareness and inadequate exposure to treatment provided within the Malaysian population.

9.3 Pathogenesis of Periodontitis

Periodontitis is a multifactorial disease with the dental biofilm as the initiator while the host immune response against resident bacteria present in the dental biofilm (plaque) on the tooth surface causes the ensuing inflammation (Philstrom et al. 2005). The biofilm, through modification of the environment and the host inflammatory response coupled with the

Immunology for Dentistry, First Edition. Edited by Mohammad Tariqur Rahman, Wim Teughels and Richard J. Lamont.

Figure 9.1 A case of periodontitis showing signs of inflammation such as red, swollen and oedematous gingiva and interdental papilla. There are also localised areas of gingival recession. Generalised dental plaque accumulation is also observed along the gingival margins.

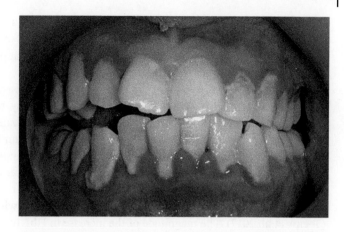

individual's unique susceptibility profile, might become dysbiotic (Hajishengallis et al. 2011; Tonetti et al. 2017). Hence it initiates a disease process that causes inflammatory destruction of the supporting structures of the dentition (cementum, periodontal ligament, alveolar bone) and eventually significant tooth loss if not properly treated (Darveau 2010; Hajishengallis et al. 2011; Tonetti et al. 2017).

9.4 Systemic Spread of Bacteria from the Inflamed Periodontium

During the progression of periodontal disease, ongoing inflammation caused by the disease results in swollen gingiva due to an increase in inflammatory infiltrates. This leads to the formation of a periodontal pocket and the anaerobic environment present at the base of the pocket becomes conducive for the formation of an anaerobic biofilm/plaque. The pocket epithelium becomes ulcerated and allows the migration of periodontitis-associated bacteria into the systemic circulation. The circulating bacteria then gain access to organs at distant sites where they exert their effects. This notion is supported by the presence of the DNA of these circulating bacteria in atheromatous plaques in patients with acute myocardial infarcts (Ohki et al. 2012) as well as in the synovial fluid of inflamed joints in rheumatoid arthritis (RA) subjects (Moen et al. 2006).

9.5 Systemic Spread of Inflammatory Mediators

Being a chronic inflammatory disease, periodontitis involves complex inflammatory and immune responses. Matrix metalloproteinases (MMPs) and reactive oxygen species cause phagocytosis of matrix components and increased destruction of periodontal tissues. The periodontal lesion is a rich source of proinflammatory mediators such as interleukin (IL)-1, transforming growth factor (TGF)-beta, prostaglandin E2 and interferon (IFN)-gamma that migrate into the systemic circulation and increase the systemic load of inflammation. In turn, this contributes to the pathogenesis of other systemic diseases such as diabetes, obesity, rheumatoid arthritis and coronary heart disease. The increased C-reactive protein (CRP) levels seen in periodontitis patients prove that periodontitis is a source of inflammatory mediators which can enter the circulation and be taken to distant organs to cause their effects (Paraskevas et al. 2008).

9.6 Periodontitis and Diabetes

Both diabetes and periodontitis are chronic inflammatory diseases and share similar risk factors such as older age, smoking, obesity, genetic predisposition, male gender and low socioeconomic status (Kocher et al. 2018). A bidirectional relationship has been reported between periodontitis and diabetes; it has been demonstrated that diabetes is a major risk factor for periodontitis and patients with periodontitis have been found to have a higher chance of developing diabetes (Taylor 2001). Additionally, periodontitis has also been confirmed as one of the complications of diabetes. The pathological and clinical link between these two conditions has been established to the extent that periodontitis is regarded as a useful risk indicator for the early screening of diabetes.

Diabetes is one of the most common endocrine disorders and is characterised by hyperglycaemia. The various forms of diabetes are type 1 diabetes mellitus (T1DM), type 2 diabetes mellitus (T2DM) and gestational diabetes. T1DM is caused by autoimmune destruction of the beta cells of the pancreas that produces insulin, while T2DM is mainly caused by a combination of insulin resistance and relative insulin deficiency.

Long-term effects of hyperglycaemia may lead to macrovascular (coronary artery disease, peripheral arterial disease, stroke) and microvascular (diabetic nephropathy, neuropathy, retinopathy) complications.

Based on a five-year longitudinal study of health in Pomerania, non-diabetic subjects with severe periodontitis at baseline had a five times greater increase in glycated haemoglobin (HbA1c) levels compared to those who were periodontally healthy at baseline (Demmer et al. 2010). Similarly, non-diabetic individuals with severe periodontitis demonstrated a significantly higher risk of developing diabetes (adjusted hazard ratio of 1.19–1.33) compared to their periodontally healthy counterparts (Graziani et al. 2018). Furthermore, the number of suspected new diabetics was reported to be higher (18.1%) among those with severe periodontitis compared to those with mild/moderate periodontitis (9.9%) and controls (8.5%) (Teeuw et al. 2017). The magnitude of the increase in HbA1c attributed to periodontitis in T2DM has been reported to be 0.29% (95% confidence interval [CI] 0.20–0.37%) (Graziani et al. 2018).

Periodontitis in both T1DM and T2DM has also been associated with significantly worse diabetes-related complications, especially cardio-renal complications. Diabetic individuals with severe periodontitis have a 3.2 times higher risk of cardio-renal mortality than those with mild or moderate periodontitis. Overall mortality was also significantly associated with periodontitis and diabetes (hazard ratio 3.5–4.5) (Graziani et al. 2018).

9.6.1 Diabetes – A Risk Factor for Periodontitis

Diabetes mellitus is an established risk factor for periodontitis as it contributes to increased prevalence, severity and progression of periodontitis (Borgnakke et al. 2013). According to the widely known Gila River Pima Indian studies, increased prevalence and incidence of periodontal disease were observed among those who had been diagnosed with T2DM compared to their healthy counterparts (Nelson et al. 1990). Individuals with diabetes were found to be approximately twice as likely to have more severe periodontal attachment loss than those without diabetes, after controlling for other variables (Chávarry et al. 2009).

In certain subpopulations, prediabetes has also been suggested as contributing to progressive periodontal disease and tooth loss. However, further studies need to be conducted to support such findings (Kocher et al. 2019). Poorly controlled T2DM has also been shown to increase the risk for progression of periodontitis and tooth loss. In other words, despite being diagnosed with T2DM, having a well-controlled glycaemic index reduces the risk of progression of periodontitis (Demmer et al. 2012).

9.6.2 Effects on Oral Microbiota in Diabetes With or Without Periodontitis

There is a progressive shift in the concept of linking periodontal pathogens and insulin resistance. Earlier studies on the influence of the microbiota on insulin resistance were largely inconclusive. Subsequent studies concluded that the subgingival microbiota was similar in subjects with T1DM or T2DM and healthy controls (Taylor et al. 2013) and the severity of diabetic status did not cause periodontal microbial dysbiosis. According to more recent studies, however, the subgingival microbiota is thought to be involved in inflammation and insulin resistance which in turn is influenced by hyperglycaemia with a concomitant increase in the severity of periodontitis (Demmer et al. 2017; Kocher et al. 2019).

9.6.3 Common Inflammatory Responses in Diabetes and Periodontitis

Several cytokines that are involved in different phases of inflammation were shown to be commonly affected by diabetic conditions and periodontitis. Increased levels of IL-1-beta, IL-6 and receptor activator of nuclear factor-kappa B ligand (RANKL)/osteoprotegerin (OPG) ratios were reported in persons with diabetes and periodontitis compared to periodontitis alone (Taylor et al. 2013). The relationship between these cytokines and glycaemic control appears to be dose dependent. In addition, an increase in levels of tumour necrosis factor (TNF)-alpha, IL-6, and IL-1-beta is shown in the gingival crevicular fluid (GCF) of individuals with diabetes and obesity (Polak and Shapiro 2018; Preshaw et al. 2012).

The hyperglycaemic state in diabetics is also associated with other proinflammatory components such as substance P and iNOS as well as increased expression of innate immunity receptors, such as TLR2 and TLR4 (Polak and Shapiro, 2018), commonly observed in inflamed periodontal tissues. This corroborates the fact that the increased severity and progression of periodontal disease seen in diabetic patients is due to the inflammatory host response to the microbial dental biofilm and not the microbiota per se.

A hyperinflammatory response in diabetic conditions has been attributed to defective neutrophil responses, a hyperinflammatory monocytic phenotype, neutrophil priming due to increased activity of protein kinase C and vascular permeability, and impaired chemotaxis (Lalla and Papapanou 2011). Although a defective neutrophil function in diabetes and periodontitis has been common, the evidence for the role of altered monocyte and T-cell function in individuals with diabetes with periodontitis seems to be limited (Taylor et al. 2013). The hyperglycaemic status and increased levels of advanced glycation endproducts (AGEs) in the gingival tissue may induce and alter PDL fibroblast function and thus cause increased secretion of TNF-alpha, IL-6 and IL-1-beta, activation of TLRs, apoptosis, expression of adhesion molecules and nuclear factor-kappa B ligand (NF-kappa B), thus contributing to the progression and increased severity of periodontitis (Polak and Shapiro 2018).

The receptor for advanced glycation endproducts (RAGE) is a multiligand signalling receptor and a member of the immunoglobulin superfamily of cell surface molecules including AGEs (Lalla and Papapanou 2011). The AGE–RAGE activation plays a role in the development and progression of complications associated with diabetes, such as cardiovascular disease and kidney disease (Yan et al. 2009). In diabetic persons with periodontitis, periodontal infection potentiates an increased level of AGEs and RAGE in the serum and gingival tissues (Lalla and Papapanou 2011).

9.6.4 Cross-talk of Pathogenesis Between Diabetes and Periodontitis

Inflammatory triggers arising from the initial dental biofilm may result in penetration of the biofilm bacteria or their degradation products, such as endotoxins, into the soft tissues of the periodontium and subsequently into the systemic circulation (Kocher et al. 2018).

The dental biofilm-initiated inflammatory response also results in an exaggerated systemic inflammatory response with an acute-phase protein burst and secretion of IL-1-beta, IL-6, prostaglandin E2 (PGE2), TNF-alpha, RANKL and matrix metalloproteinase (MMP)-8, MMP-9 and MMP-13, T cell regulatory cytokines (e.g. IL-12, IL-18) and chemokines which facilitate insulin resistance (Preshaw et al. 2012). TNF-alpha, IL-6 and CRP, the main inducers of acute-phase proteins, have been demonstrated to impair intracellular insulin signalling and thus further contribute to insulin resistance.

Susceptibility also plays a role in the heterogeneity of host response to disease, and this is influenced by genetic, epigenetic and environmental factors (Preshaw et al. 2012). As the inflammation progresses, insulin resistance and markers of systemic inflammation increase gradually in prediabetes ranges of glucose concentrations (Kocher et al. 2018). As the systemic load of inflammation increases, insulin resistance, hyperglycaemia and the diabetic state progress.

9.6.5 The Effect of Therapy on Bidirectional Disease

As inflammation promotes insulin resistance and dysregulates glycaemia, the hypothesis that treatment of periodontal infections and the associated inflammation could result in improved glycaemic control seems to be biologically plausible (Lalla and Papapanou 2011).

At 3–4 months after non-surgical periodontal therapy, a reduction of serum HbA1c levels ranging from 0.27% to 0.48% was detected in patients with diabetes and periodontitis (Madianos and Koromantzos 2018; Sanz et al. 2018). The reported reduction in HbA1c levels after non-surgical periodontal therapy is in agreement with the 0.29% (95% CI 0.20–0.37%) magnitude of increase in HbA1c attributed to periodontitis in T2DM (Graziani et al. 2018; Sanz et al. 2018). However, in patients with poorly controlled diabetes, tissue healing and wound repair are compromised. In these patients, a similar response to periodontal therapy is absent (Lalla and Papapanou 2011).

Furthermore, adjunctive antibiotic therapy does not affect HbA1c reduction beyond scaling and root surface debridement alone among people with T2DM (Sanz et al. 2018). It is estimated that there is a 35% reduction in complications for every 1% decrease in HbA1c levels. It has also been suggested that a 0.2% reduction in HbA1c is associated with a 10% reduction in mortality (Lakschevitz et al. 2011). Thus, the treatment of periodontal disease has been proven as an alternative or adjunct therapy to improve glycaemic control.

Type 2 diabetes has a well-established effect on inflamed periodontal tissues by exacerbating its proinflammatory response. These effects are mediated by hyperglycaemia and AGEs present in these tissues. Studies have also shown that biological mechanisms from circulating proinflammatory mediators mediate the effect of periodontitis on diabetes control.

There is evidence to show that periodontal therapy influences a reduction in HbA1c levels. Further studies are required to explore the biological effects of periodontal inflammation in type 2 diabetes to better understand the link.

9.7 Periodontitis and Cardiovascular Disease

Cardiovascular disease (CVD) is a major cause of death globally that includes ischaemic heart disease, stroke, coronary heart disease (CHD) and hypertension (leading to heart failure). Empirical and clinical evidence arguably support the causal link between severe periodontitis and CVD (Tonetti et al. 2013). Severe periodontitis is independently and significantly associated with cardiovascular mortality in different populations (Linden et al. 2012; Sharma et al. 2016).

9.7.1 Epidemiological Association Between Periodontitis and CVD

Mattila and co-workers (1989) were the first to report an association between poor oral health and acute myocardial infarction (AMI) in two separate case–control studies (100 AMI patients and 102 controls). Dental health indices were significantly worse in those with AMI compared to controls after adjusting the possible confounding factors such as age, social class, smoking, serum lipid concentration and presence of diabetes. On the other hand, periodontitis patients demonstrated thickened carotid arteries independent of cardiovascular risk factors, significantly greater thickness of the carotid intima media and elevated arterial calcification scores (Beck et al. 2001).

According to the National Health and Nutrition Examination Survey (NHANES) I (DeStefano et al. 1993), a mild association (relative risk [RR] = 1.25) between periodontitis and an increased risk for CHD was demonstrated after adjustment for confounding variables. A stronger association (RR = 1.72) was observed for younger men (25–49 years). In contrast, using the same NHANES I data a causal association between periodontitis and CHD risk has also been denied (Hujoel et al. 2000). A large-scale longitudinal study using standardised case definition and similar adjustments for confounding factors might be useful to resolve the dispute.

Nevertheless, periodontitis was modestly associated with atherosclerosis, MI and CVD (Scannapieco et al. 2003; Janket et al. 2003). Similarly, a higher risk (RR 1.19; 95% CI 1.08–1.32) of potential CVD was observed in those with periodontal disease, compared to those without (Janket et al. 2003). For example, periodontal disease has been associated with a 19% increase in the risk of future CVD. However, the risk increment between those with or without periodontal disease in the general population is modest (20%), considering that 40% of the population suffers from periodontal disease.

Furthermore, an increased risk of a first cerebrovascular event was reported in those with clinically diagnosed periodontitis or more severe periodontitis compared to those without periodontitis or less severe periodontitis (Dietrich et al. 2013). Nevertheless, opposing views exist to conclude a significant association between periodontitis and secondary cardiovascular events (Dorn et al. 2010; Reichert et al. 2016; Sen et al. 2013). However, relative risk estimates vary between studies, depending on population characteristics and periodontitis case definitions. Clinically speaking, this modest increase has a profound public health impact.

9.7.2 Potential Causal Link Between Periodontitis and CVD

Various mechanisms could explain the potential link between periodontitis and CVD: (i) direct invasion of oral bacteria; (ii) indirectly by bacterial toxins that induce bacterial mediators to enter the bloodstream and contribute to systemic vascular challenge; (iii) common predisposing mechanisms; and (iv) molecular mimicry.

9.7.2.1 Direct Mechanism

Oral bacterial species can enter the circulation and cause bactaeremia, so there has been concern about whether periodontopathogens could invade gingival as well as cardiac tissues. It was hypothesised that periodontal pathogens that can invade atherosclerotic plaques might play a role in the pathogenesis of CHD. However, it was unclear if periodontal pathogens act as causal agents of atherosclerosis or simply invade an already damaged artery. The presence of periodontal pathogens in endothelial cells may lead to injury and/or activation of endothelial cells which can induce an increase in procoagulant activity, secretion of vasoactive and inflammatory mediators and expression of adhesion molecules (Haraszthy et al. 2000).

Oral organisms including periodontal pathogens were found in atherothrombosclerotic plaque and cardiac tissues (Haraszthy et al. 2000; Ford et al. 2005). A positive correlation was observed between the presence of periodontal pathogens in atherothrombotic tissues, with other biological sample sources, in the same patients (Armingohar et al. 2014; Mahendra et al. 2013). At least two studies have demonstrated the presence of *Porphyromonas gingivalis* and *Aggregatibacter actinomycetemcomitans* in atherothrombotic tissue when culturing the atheroma samples (Kozarov et al. 2005).

A higher risk of bacteraemia is associated with gingival inflammation (Tomas et al. 2012). Additionally, a randomised clinical trial (RCT) demonstrated that non-surgical periodontal therapy induced bactaeremia in both gingivitis and periodontitis patients. Though the magnitude and frequency were greater among periodontitis patients (Balejo et al. 2017), this evidence is sufficient to suggest that bactaeremia could result from daily life activities and oral interventions.

9.7.2.2 Indirect Mechanism

During host–bacteria interaction in periodontitis, various proinflammatory cytokines are released and may enter the systemic circulation, consequently affecting other organs. The acute-phase response activated by the periodontal pathogens may result in increased white blood cell counts, fibrinogen, CRP and other inflammatory markers (Ebersole et al. 1997).

C-reactive protein is a crucial marker for increased risk of CVD. In the development and pathogenesis of CVD, CRP is implicated by its proinflammatory effects, ability to bind low-density lipoprotein (LDL) in atherosclerotic plaques and mediate lipid uptake by macrophages (Zhang et al. 1999; Zwaka et al. 2001), activation of complement and increasing macrophage production of tissue factor that promote thrombosis (Lagrand et al. 1999). However, the causal significance of CRP in CVD is largely unknown.

Cross-sectional and prospective studies reported a positive association between increased CRP levels and periodontitis (Craig et al. 2003; Noack et al. 2001; Slade et al. 2000; Wu et al. 2000). Wu and co-workers reported a significant relation between indicators of poor periodontal status and increased CRP and fibrinogen. Slade and co-workers reported similar findings in that people with severe periodontal disease (>10% of sites with periodontal pockets >4 mm) had a doubling in the prevalence of elevated CRP compared with periodontally healthy people (Slade et al. 2000). This observation (raised CRP levels in severe periodontitis) remained in multivariate analyses ($P < 0.01$), with established risk factors for elevated CRP (diabetes, arthritis, emphysema, smoking and anti-inflammatory medications) and sociodemographic factors controlled for. In addition, CRP may be elevated in a dose response due to the pathogenic burden of periodontopathic bacteria (Noack et al. 2001; Wakai et al. 1999). Studies have shown a significant reduction in CRP levels, together with improvements in surrogate measurements of cardiovascular health following periodontal therapy (Demmer et al. 2013; Koppolu et al. 2013).

9.7.2.3 Common Predisposing Mechanisms

Another potential mechanism that could contribute to the association between periodontitis and CVD is a common hyperinflammatory response (Beck et al. 1999). Variations in the genes that regulate IL-1 response have been associated with both periodontal disease and CVD. A pattern of IL-1 polymorphism characterised by IL-1A (+4845) and IL-1B (+3954) markers is associated with periodontitis. Another IL-1 genetic pattern characterised by IL-1B (–511) and IL-1RN (+2018) markers is associated with atherosclerosis, but not periodontitis (Kornman et al. 1999).

Clinical studies have suggested that periodontitis may be associated with hyperlipidaemia (Cutler et al. 1999; Losche et al. 2000). Cutler and co-workers (1999) reported that periodontitis was significantly associated with elevated serum triglycerides and cholesterol levels, as well as serum antibodies to *P. gingivalis*. In addition, Losche and co-workers (2000) reported that total cholesterol, LDL cholesterol and triglycerides were significantly higher in those with periodontitis compared to healthy controls. In contrast, Wu and co-workers (2000) examined the relationship between periodontitis and cardiovascular risk factors using data from the Third National Health and Nutrition Examination Survey (1988–1994). While a weak association between total cholesterol levels was reported, the association between periodontitis and high-density lipoprotein (HDL) has been inconsistent. Despite the association shown between hyperlipidaemia and periodontitis in systemically healthy subjects, it was not clear if periodontitis causes the increase in lipid levels or if periodontitis and CVD merely share hyperlipidaemia as a common risk factor. There is a need for longitudinal human studies to confirm whether periodontal disease causes hyperlipidaemia.

9.7.2.4 Molecular Mimicry

Heat shock protein (HSP) is produced in many human tissues, including the endothelium lining the vessel wall. Certain stressors, including high blood pressure, infection, hypercholesterolaemia, and exposure to lipopolysaccharide (LPS), result in the production of HSP60 (Chun et al. 2005), considered important in the pathogenesis of atherosclerosis (Mori

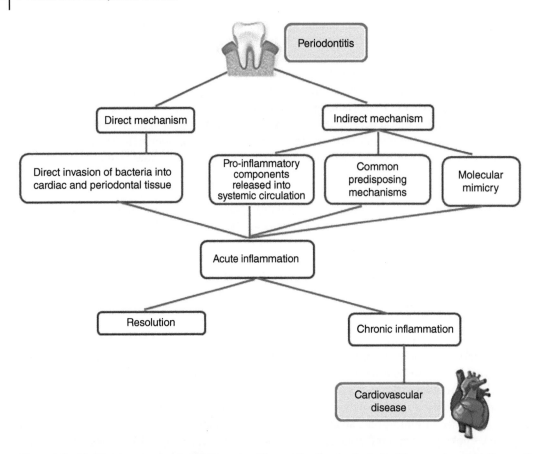

Figure 9.2 The link between periodontitis and cardiovascular disease. Periodontitis causes acute inflammation through either direct or indirect mechanisms. Acute inflammation will then progress to cardiovascular disease.

et al. 2000; Xu et al. 1992). Among bacterial HSP, the molecular chaperone complex GroEL is well investigated in autoimmune reactions because of the sequence similarity with human HSP60. Antibodies to HSP from periodontal pathogens (*P. gingivalis, Tannerella forsythia, A. actinomycetemcomitans* and *Fusobacterium nucleatum*) can cross-react with human HSPs. These antibodies have been shown to activate cytokine production, as well as monocyte and endothelial cell activation. The presence of anticardiolipin antibodies has been significantly associated with periodontitis, which reversed following periodontal therapy. There is some evidence that periodontal pathogens can elicit antibodies that cross-react with cardiolipin (Schenkein and Loos 2013). The antibody titres to HSP60 and bacterial GroEL were significantly higher in peri-odontitis patients and these antibodies were also detected in the gingival tissue and atherosclerotic plaques.

The anti-HSP reactions may be involved in the pathogenesis of periodontitis as well as CVD. The precise mechanism of cross-reaction between bacterial and mammalian HSP remains unclear. However, the elevated levels of antibodies play important roles in periodontal immune and inflammatory responses and may correlate with the pathogenesis and severity of periodontal and cardiovascular diseases. Further understanding of the roles of HSP might lead to a new theranostic strategy of precision medicine for systemic health-related periodontitis.

Figure 9.2 summarises the possible link between periodontitis and CVD.

9.7.3 Impact of Periodontal Therapy on CVD

Periodontal therapy has been shown to affect surrogate markers of CVD, with moderate evidence for reduction of low-grade inflammation as assessed by serum levels of CRP and IL-6, and improvements in measures of endothelial function. There is limited evidence suggesting that periodontal treatment reduces arterial blood pressure and stiffness, subclinical ACVD (as assessed by mean carotid intima-media thickness), and insufficient evidence of an effect on ACVD biomarkers of coagulation, endothelial cell activation and oxidative stress (Sanz et al. 2020).

Studies have consistently suggested that oral health interventions including self-performed oral hygiene habits (de Oliveira et al. 2010; Park et al. 2019), dental prophylaxis (Lee et al. 2015), increased self-reported dental visits (Sen et al. 2018) and periodontal treatment (Holmlund et al. 2017; Lee et al. 2015; Park et al. 2019) contribute to a reduction in the incidence of CVD events.

To date, there are no prospective randomised controlled periodontal intervention studies on primary prevention of cardiovascular diseases (including first ischaemic events or cardiovascular death) (Tonetti et al. 2013). The feasibility of conducting adequately powered RCTs in primary prevention at a population level was questioned due to ethical, methodological and financial considerations.

9.7.4 Summary of Periodontitis and CVD

It is crucial that we recognise the possible links between periodontitis and CVD. Biological arguments could explain this recognised relationship, and even elucidate a possible causal association between both diseases. Epidemiological evidence supports the notion that periodontitis contributes to an increased risk for future atherosclerotic CVD. This impact of periodontitis on CVD can be explained by commonly induced systemic inflammation, and subsequently contribute to the development of atherothrombogenesis. The association between these two conditions is related to shared common risk factors and common underlying physiology and pathophysiology.

There is no exact mechanism that can suggest a complete explanation for the association between periodontitis and CVD. However, the importance of preventing and treating infections, especially chronic infections such as periodontitis, should become vital in terms of the advice and treatment given to patients with CVD. Intervention trials were not sufficiently adequate to draw further conclusions at that time. However, periodontitis patients should be advised that they are at higher risk for CVD and should manage their CVD risk factors. Those diagnosed with periodontitis and CVD should be informed that they may be at higher risk for subsequent CVD complications, and thus should adhere to regular dental treatment (Sanz et al. 2020).

9.8 Periodontitis and Obesity

Obesity is a condition in which abnormal or excessive fat is deposited in the body, resulting from an imbalance between intake and usage of food measured in equivalence of calories. Obesity increases the risk for non-communicable diseases (NCD) such as T2DM, CVD, fatty liver disease, obstructive sleep apnoea, osteoarthritis and destructive periodontal disease (Blüher 2019). Although obesity has been primarily attributed to a sedentary lifestyle – a combination of reduced physical activity and a diet high in fat – it has now become concentrated among the poor (Mariapun et al. 2018). Studies have suggested that periodontitis could be linked to obesity due to their similar pathophysiological pathways.

Worldwide, the prevalence of obesity in the adult population doubled from the 1990s to 2014. Approximately 200 million adults were obese in 1995 and the number increased to 300 million in 2000 (WHO 2008). In 2014, approximately 1.9 billion adults were overweight worldwide. Of these, 600 million were obese, bringing the estimated world's prevalence of obesity to 13%. Females showed a higher prevalence of obesity (15%) compared to males (11%) (WHO 2015). In the South-East Asian region, the prevalence of obesity was estimated at 3% (WHO 2008). Variations in the trends and prevalence of obesity when compared between the countries across the region may depend on the designs of epidemiological studies as well as the ethnic or cultural differences practised by communities.

Interestingly, economic development has shifted the distribution of obesity from the socioeconomically more advantaged to the less advantaged. Mariapun and co-workers (2018) evaluated the socioeconomic trends in overweight, obesity and abdominal obesity among Malaysians across a period of significant economic growth, using the NHMS data sets for the years 1996, 2006 and 2011. They reported that women in peninsular Malaysia demonstrated patterns that were similar to those of developed countries, where the distributions for overweight, obesity and abdominal obesity became concentrated among the poor. Interestingly, for women in east Malaysia, distributions became concentrated among neither the rich nor poor, while distributions for men were still concentrated among the rich.

9.8.1 Common Prevalence of Obesity and Periodontitis

The relationship between obesity and periodontitis was first reported in experimental animals (Perlstein and Bissada 1977). A five-year longitudinal study involving Japanese workers demonstrated a positive relationship between body mass index (BMI) and periodontal disease (Morita et al. 2011). Subsequent human studies demonstrated that obesity increases the risk for periodontitis (Al-Zahrani et al. 2003; Khader et al. 2009; Khan et al. 2015). According to a systematic review based on 26 cross-sectional studies, six case–control studies and one cohort study, a positive association between obesity and periodontitis was confirmed (Suvan et al. 2011). According to a different meta-analysis (Moura-Grec et al. 2014) summarising 25 independent researchers, the risk of periodontitis was associated with obesity (or had a tendency for this). A significant association was concluded between obesity and periodontitis and with mean BMI and periodontal disease.

9.8.2 Possible Mechanisms Linking Obesity and Periodontitis

The association between obesity and periodontitis could be due to these conditions sharing the same pathophysiological pathways. The mechanisms linking the two conditions are: (i) the multidirectional relationship between obesity and diabetes mellitus; and (ii) the direct relationship between obesity and periodontitis.

9.8.2.1 Multidirectional Relationship Between Obesity and Periodontitis

Proinflammatory cytokines may play a crucial role in the relationship between periodontitis, obesity and chronic diseases. Genco proposed that the association may be multidirectional (Genco et al. 2005) involving chronic diseases, genetic and environmental factors (Figure 9.3). The inflamed condition of the periodontal tissues induces the production of proinflammatory cytokines such as IL-1, IL-6 and TNF-alpha. In addition, the release of TNF-alpha by adipose tissue was triggered by LPS (periodontal Gram-negative bacteria) which promote hepatic dyslipidaemia and decrease insulin sensitivity (Saito et al. 2001; Nishimura et al. 2003). An increase in hepatic triglycerides is dependent on the amount of free fatty acids, which were derived from visceral adipose tissue, and was correlated with insulin resistance (Kopelman 2000).

Type 2 DM and decreased insulin sensitivity are associated with the production of AGEs, which subsequently trigger the further release of inflammatory cytokines and predispose them towards inflammatory diseases such as periodontitis (Genco et al. 2005). These observations suggested a possible interaction among obesity, periodontitis and DM as chronic diseases.

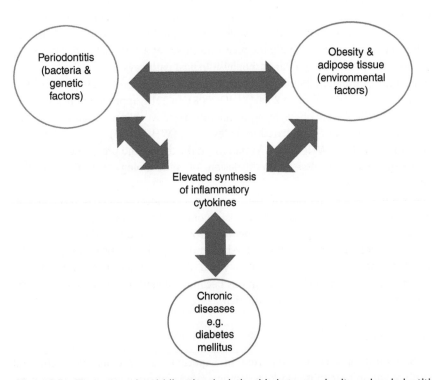

Figure 9.3 The proposed multidirectional relationship between obesity and periodontitis with chronic diseases. *Source:* Adapted and modified from Genco et al. (2005).

9.8.2.2 Direct Relationship

Obesity can be directly associated with periodontitis, independent of the deteriorated glucose level in DM. An earlier animal study showed that obese hypertensive rats had the potential to develop periodontitis, compared to normal rats. Histologically, these obese rats' periodontal blood vessels were presented with intimal thickening, causing diminished blood circulation (Perlstein and Bissada 1977). Conversely, a study in rats with periodontitis showed a proliferation of the junctional epithelium and an increase in bone resorption after these rats were fed a high-cholesterol diet (Tomofuji et al. 2005). High-cholesterol food intake is associated directly with fat accumulation, and therefore elevated serum cholesterol levels may play a part in the association between obesity and periodontitis.

Visceral fat accumulation is also associated with an increased level of fat in the liver. An increase in the waist-to-hip ratio (WHR), independent of BMI, among Japanese obese females showed an increased condition of hepatic steatosis or fatty liver. A significant association between periodontitis and serum aspartate aminotransferase, alanine aminotransferase, cholinesterase levels and the aspartate aminotransferase-to-alanine aminotransferase ratio, which can lead to hepatic steatosis, was observed (Saito et al. 2006). This result indicates a possible relationship between periodontitis and fatty liver disease, an adverse effect of upper body obesity.

Adipose tissue secretes adipocytokines (including TNF-alpha, IL-6, leptin, adiponectin, plasminogen activator inhibitor-1 [PAI-1] and angiotensinogen) that may have a direct effect on the periodontal tissue (Saito and Shimazaki 2007). At elevated levels, the adipocytokines contribute to low-grade chronic inflammation, which in turn alters the host immune response threshold. Subsequently, this shift in balance makes obese individuals more susceptible to incoming microbial plaque insult compared to their normal-weight counterparts. Since the adipocytokine secretions are proportionate to the amount of adipose tissue present (Montague and O'Rahilly 2000), it is reasonable to suggest that obesity may have the potential to modulate the immune system and increase susceptibility to periodontitis (Nishida et al. 2005).

T lymphocytes also secrete proinflammatory cytokines which may also mediate the pathogenesis of periodontitis. Following the immuno-inflammatory response, the balance between T-helper (Th) 1, Th2, Th17 and T regulatory type cytokines released against periodontal pathogens will determine the pattern of periodontal lesions. Stable lesions in periodontitis showed a predominance of Th1 cells, with IL-12, IFN-gamma and TNF-alpha involved in the Th1 immune response pathway. On the other hand, the predominance of the Th2 subset of cells is associated with periodontitis progression (Gemmell et al. 2007). IL-4, IL-5 and IL-13 participated in the Th2 immune response and thus induced humoral immunity (Mosmann and Sad 1996). The Th17 subset of T-helper cells that secrete IL-17 cytokine has been shown to play a role in the pathogenesis of periodontitis (Johnson et al. 2004; Takahashi et al. 2005; Vernal et al. 2005).

9.8.3 Effect of Obesity on Periodontal Therapy

Non-surgical periodontal therapy has been proven effective in treating periodontal disease (Heitz-Mayfield et al. 2002; Van der Weijden et al. 2002; Kwon and Levin 2014), though the outcomes might vary depending on disease severity and the patient's health complications such as obesity (Akram et al. 2016). Non-surgical periodontal therapy has been shown to improve clinical parameters and cytokine levels, as well as producing a reduction in inflammation and periodontal pathogens. A body of research on the effect of obesity on periodontal treatment response has reported conflicting results. Some reported short-term favourable responses to periodontal treatment by showing improvement in both clinical parameters and inflammatory cytokine measurements (Zuza et al. 2011; Al-Zahrani and Alghamdi 2012; Altay et al. 2013). Others reported a negative response to periodontal treatment after two months with an increased BMI and obesity (Suvan et al. 2014).

Mean serum resistin was higher in obese subjects with periodontitis followed by non-obese periodontitis and non-obese healthy subjects (Patel and Raju 2014). Two months after non-surgical periodontal therapy, a greater reduction in resistin was observed in normal-weight subjects with periodontitis than in obese periodontitis subjects (Suresh et al. 2018). In contrast, other studies showed no significant difference in terms of serum levels of resistin at baseline and three months after non-surgical periodontal therapy (Akram et al. 2017; Goncalves et al. 2015). Obesity conditions could enhance the risk of patients exhibiting periodontitis by having high numbers of pathogenic subgingival species. Mean counts of *P. gingivalis* and *T. forsythia* were higher in obese subjects with periodontitis (Suresh et al. 2017; Haffajee and Socransky 2009).

Regardless of obesity status, non-surgical periodontal therapy has a significant impact on visible plaque index (VPI) and gingival bleeding index (GBI) in periodontitis subjects. However, the impact of non-surgical periodontal therapy on serum resistin and periodontal pathogens was non-significant in those with periodontitis (Tahir et al. 2020).

9.9   Periodontitis and Rheumatoid Arthritis

Rheumatoid arthritis (RA), an autoimmune disease with a global prevalence of 1%, is a chronic inflammatory disorder leading to synovial inflammation and destruction of cartilage and bone. Associations between periodontitis and RA have been reported whereby periodontitis is more severe in patients with established RA. Both these diseases result in bone destruction, via the periodontal apparatus in periodontitis and the cartilage and underlying bone in RA. The plausible link between both conditions is based on shared pathogenic similarities regarding risk factors, immunogenetics and tissue destruction pathways.

9.9.1   Epidemiological Evidence on the Association Between RA and PD

From an epidemiological standpoint, an increasing number of studies conclude that there is a considerable positive association between RA and periodontitis. While the relationship is unlikely to be causal, most of these studies have reported that PD is more severe and common in patients with established RA (Bartold et al. 2005).

A cross-sectional study from India reported that the odds for periodontitis were 4.28 times higher in non-smoking RA patients compared to healthy controls (Potikuri et al. 2012). A study from Thailand with 196 RA cases found a high prevalence of moderate to severe periodontitis in patients with RA at 42% and 57% respectively (Khantisopon et al. 2014). In a systematic review and meta-analysis of eight publications, when comparing RA subjects to healthy controls, the odds ratio (OR) for PD was 4.68 (Tang et al. 2017). These authors also reported an OR for PD of 1.28 when comparing RA and non-RA subjects. They concluded that RA is significantly associated with the overall risk of periodontitis.

9.9.2   Plausible Causal Links Between RA and PD

Over the years, several hypotheses have been proposed on how periodontitis interacts or links with RA (Figure 9.4).

According to the earliest hypotheses, periodontitis precedes the development of RA and RA is initiated by humoral response to periodontal pathogens (Rosenstein et al. 2004). Central to this hypothesis is the production of peptidyl arginine deiminase (PAD) enzymes by *P. gingivalis*, known as *P. gingivalis* peptidyl arginine deiminase (PPAD), that can induce autoantibodies via citrullination, allowing for a link between periodontitis and the development of RA (Rosenstein et al. 2004).

Subsequently, a 'two-hit' model hypothesis suggested that a systemic disease like RA can potentially exacerbate or initiate periodontitis and vice versa (Golub et al. 2006). According to this model, the first hit of chronic inflammation via chronic periodontitis is at the periodontal microbial biofilm, followed by a second hit to induce systemic inflammation in RA, leading to an exacerbated inflammatory response (Golub et al. 2006).

Bright and colleagues (2015) proposed a dual-hit hypothesis for the pathogenesis of RA being driven by either citrullination or carbamylation, or both, in inflamed periodontal tissues of a genetically susceptible individual. In this model, chronic inflammation seen in periodontitis (first hit) will result in the extra-articular formation of antibodies directed against the citrullinated and carbamylated peptides, leading to the initial break in immune tolerance. These autoimmune responses will then be translated into inflammatory joint disease in susceptible individuals (second hit). This hypothesis has suggested a plausible mechanistic link associating PD with the pathogenesis of RA via citrullination and carbamylation.

9.9.2.1   Linking Periodontal Pathogens and RA

The microbiological link between PD and RA was first hypothesised in 2004 whereby *P. gingivalis* was implicated in the pathogenic connection through the process of citrullination (Rosenstein et al. 2004). *P. gingivalis*, a common periodontal pathogen, has been reported to be the sole PAD-expressing bacterium (McGraw et al. 1999). PPAD is capable of initiating the citrullination of mammalian proteins as well as the auto-citrullination of bacterial proteins (Rodriguez et al. 2009). However, further investigation will be needed to confirm if the association between PPAD and RA is either related to PPAD causing a change in the immune tolerance or is due to PPAD causing an increase in virulence of *P. gingivalis* and subsequently an increase in the severity of the periodontal inflammation which ultimately leads to the increase in RA severity (Bartold and Lopez-Oliva 2020).

In addition to *P. gingivalis*, other periodontitis-associated bacteria such as *Capnocytophaga* sp., *Desulfobulbus* sp., *Bulleidia* sp., *Dialister pneumosintes*, *Prevotella intermedia*, *Tannarella forsythia*, *Prevotella melaninogenica*, *Filifactor*

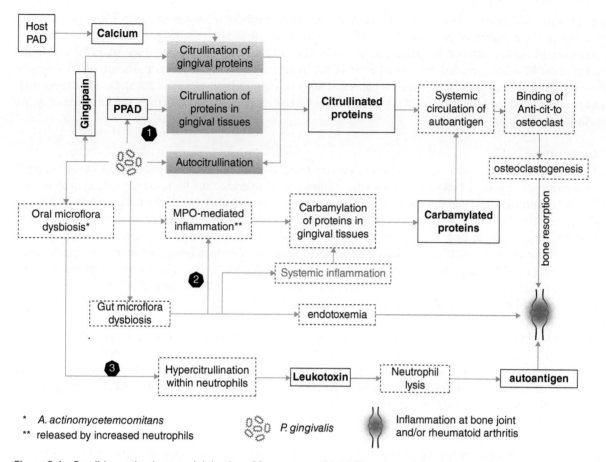

Figure 9.4 Possible mechanisms explaining how PD aggravates RA. (1) The role of *P. gingivalis* in contributing to the formation of autoantigens either directly through protein citrullination or indirectly through inflammation-mediated carbamylation. (2) *P. gingivalis* as a keystone pathogen causing alterations to the gut microflora and potentially leading to endotoxaemia and the persistence of low-grade systemic inflammation which may exacerbate the inflammatory response within the joint. (3) Extracellular release of autoantigens following neutrophil apoptosis as a result of *A. actinomycetemcomitans*-induced hypercitrullination. *Source:* Reproduced with permission from Lee et al. (2019)/International Academy of Periodontology.

alocis, *Prevotella* sp. and *Leptotrichia* sp. have been implicated with RA (Eezammuddeen et al. 2020; Bartold and Lopez-Oliva 2020). This was confirmed by either the presence of their DNA in the synovium or antibodies to these bacteria in the serum of these RA patients (Bartold and Lopez-Oliva 2020). These findings have again emphasised the possibility of the inflamed periodontal tissues being an extra-auricular site for the translocation of bacteria or antibodies to the synovium where they can exacerbate the inflammatory process in the joints of susceptible subjects.

9.9.2.2 Host and Periodontal Pathogen-mediated Citrullination

Citrullination is an enzymatic deimination process where arginine is converted to citrulline by PAD, resulting in a post-translational modification of the tertiary structure, antigenicity and function of proteins (Schellekens et al. 1998, 2000). Such modification may elicit an immune response against self proteins, hence an autoimmune reaction, as citrulline is not a standard amino acid of proteins (Gyorgy et al. 2006). A citrullinated peptide acts as an antigenic determinant that could break the immunological tolerance and evoke an autoimmune response by binding onto antigen-presenting cells. As a result, pathogenic T and B cells will be activated, leading to the formation of RA-specific anticitrullinated protein (anti-CitP) (Schellekens et al. 1998). This anti-CitP will then form immune complexes with citrullinated peptides, resulting in the production of inflammatory mediators and ultimately causing joint destruction in RA (Koziel et al. 2014).

Citrullination, which is a normal physiological process, also takes part in pathological inflammatory conditions as part of the innate response to bacterial infection and cell death mechanism (Wegner et al. 2010). Apart from inflamed synovial joints in RA, citrullinated proteins have also been detected in inflamed periodontal tissues of patients with periodontitis (Nesse et al. 2012). The citrullinated proteins PAD-2 and PAD-4 were also found in inflamed periodontal tissues in periodontitis patients without any signs of RA (Harvey et al. 2012). The fact that the autoimmune response in RA due to the production of anti-CitP often preceded the clinical onset of RA by several years suggests that the origin of RA might be linked to mucosal sites distant to the joints, such as gums and lungs (Rantapaa-Dahlqvist et al. 2003). Based on these findings, it was postulated that periodontitis could provide a conducive environment for citrullination and initiation of ACPA targeting citrullinated peptides in joints.

9.9.2.3 Carbamylation

Carbamylation is a posttranslational modification of proteins involving cyanate that converts lysine residues to homocitrulline via a non-enzymatic reaction. This process breaks the immunological tolerance and leads to the production of autoantibodies known as anti-carbamylated protein (anti-CarP), which has been associated with the pathogenesis of RA (Shi et al. 2014). In a healthy individual, cyanate is present in equilibrium with urea and its concentration is too low to allow excessive carbamylation to occur under the steady physiological state (Bax et al. 2014). However, carbamylation may be enhanced during inflammatory conditions mediated by myeloperoxidase (MPO) which is released from neutrophils during inflammation to aid in the formation of neutrophil extracellular traps (NETs). NETs play an important role in trapping and removing Gram-negative bacteria. As a result, high levels of MPO associated with NETs in sites of inflammation will cause an increased concentration of cyanate by converting thiocyanate to a cyanate which will then lead to extensive carbamylation of proteins (Wang et al. 2007).

Carbamylation has been shown to occur in inflamed periodontal tissues with the presence of a high abundance of MPO associated with NETs (Bright et al. 2015). Therefore, inflamed periodontal tissues may serve as a potential site of MPO-driven protein carbamylation producing anti-CarP. An increased expression of citrullinated and carbamylated proteins occurring with the presence of inflammation was observed in both PD and PD-RA specimens with no statistically significant difference in the level of proteins between them, suggesting that inflamed gingiva could be a local source of citrullinated and carbamylated proteins (Lee et al. 2019).

Additionally, in a case–control study, the serum levels of carbamylated protein and NETs in patients with RA and periodontitis were found to be significantly higher than in the control group (Kaneko and Kobayashi 2018). All these findings suggest that periodontitis could be responsible for prompting the breakdown of immune tolerance to carbamylated proteins leading to RA in susceptible individuals, providing another possible mechanistic link between RA and PD via carbamylation.

9.9.3 Common Tissue Destruction Pathway in RA and PD

The common tissue destruction pathway was suggested based on the common underlying dysregulation of the inflammatory pathway between RA and PD involving a RANKL–OPG–TNF-related apoptosis-inducing ligand (TRAIL) axis (Bartold et al. 2005). The RANKL binds to its receptor RANK on osteoclast precursor cells and promotes the maturation of osteoclasts, which in turn causes bone resorption. OPG acts as a natural inhibitor of RANKL. Therefore, no bone destruction will transpire when OPG binds to RANK (Wang and El-Deiry 2003).

However, Arg-gingipain of *P. gingivalis* has been shown to increase the RANKL/OPG ratio in gingival fibroblast and periodontal ligament cells favouring binding between RANKL and RANK and subsequently enhancing osteoclastogenesis (Belibasakis et al. 2007). Recent studies have shown that individuals with either RA or PD or both have increased serum levels of RANKL (Kindstedt et al. 2018, Panezai et al. 2018). This suggests that dysregulation of inflammatory cascades in patients with RA and PD leads to sustained overproduction of osteoclastogenic mediators and enzymes such as RANKL.

Furthermore, TRAIL and its role in tissue destruction pathway have been gaining prominence. Out of the five types of receptors for TRAIL, two are death receptors with death domains and three are decoy receptors without death domains. Therefore, programmed cell death (apoptosis) can be activated if TRAIL binds to the death receptors whilst it is inhibited when TRAIL binds the decoy receptors (Lucas et al. 2010). Hence, in both RA and PD, the presence of large numbers of chronic inflammatory cells in the diseased tissues may be due to either a reduced expression of TRAIL death receptors or an increased expression of TRAIL decoy receptors (Agnihotri and Gaur 2014; Lucas et al. 2010).

Notably, a decrease in OPG expression leads to vascular damage whereas an increase in RANKL and TRAIL levels may result in the activation of osteoclasts and consequently bone resorption. However, future studies need to investigate the levels of RANKL, OPG and TRAIL simultaneously in both RA and PD lesions to validate this hypothesis.

9.9.4 The Effect of Periodontal Therapy on RA

Non-surgical periodontal therapy was beneficial in checking RA disease activity and treatment outcome (Bartold and Lopez-Oliva 2020). In general, non-surgical periodontal therapy comprising scaling and root surface debridement resulted in a reduction of Disease Activity Score 28 joints (DAS28) scores (Ribeiro et al. 2005; Erciyas et al. 2013), CRP levels (Erciyas et al. 2013) and erythrocyte sedimentation rate (ESR) (Ribeiro et al. 2005; Ortiz et al. 2009).

Non-surgical periodontal therapy on 60 subjects with low, moderate and highly active RA with chronic periodontitis revealed improved DAS28 scores regardless of RA disease activity (Erciyas et al. 2013). Similarly, Kaur et al (2014) also reported that there was a positive trend in the reduction of DAS28 scores following periodontal therapy.

Clear alteration of these biomarkers after non-surgical periodontal therapy and during the active phase of RA implies that a decrease in inflammation at the periodontal level could lead to changes in systemic inflammatory markers, therefore exerting a positive influence upon RA. Based on these findings, it has been suggested that more thorough and larger controlled trials are needed to convincingly substantiate the effect of non-surgical periodontal therapy on the improvement of RA disease activity (Bartold and Lopez-Oliva 2020).

9.9.5 Summary of Periodontitis and RA

There is currently strong evidence to show that there is a relationship between RA and periodontitis. However, the exact mechanism linking the two diseases remains elusive. RA and PD are diseases with similar host-mediated pathogenesis that can cause significant social burdens related to increased patient discomfort and treatment costs. The knowledge gained on the RA–PD link will enable both the physician and/or rheumatologist and periodontist to provide optimum care in terms of intervention and this will lead to better outcomes and improved quality of life.

9.10 Clinical Significance of the Periodontal–Systemic Disease Link

Evidence connecting periodontitis with several NCDs through a systemic link has been gaining strength over recent decades as more studies have been conducted to prove the association. In some cases, this relationship is bidirectional such as periodontitis with diabetes, obesity or rheumatoid arthritis. Knowledge about the importance of this link and the ensuing damage to tissues if left untreated emphasises the urgent need for periodontal therapy to be provided to patients in the high-risk group. It is also imperative for dentists to work as team players with their medical counterparts in promoting this awareness among medical professionals as well as patients so that early screening and detection of both diseases can be done. Ultimately, early referrals and treatment of both diseases will enable these patients to have an improved quality of life.

References

Agnihotri, R. and Gaur, S.(2014). Rheumatoid arthritis in the elderly and its relationship with periodontitis: a review. *Geriatr. Gerontol. Int.* 14: 8–22.

Akram, Z., Safiii, S.H., Vaithilingam, R.D. et al. (2016). Efficacy of non-surgical periodontal therapy in the management of chronic periodontitis among obese and non-obese patients: a systematic review and meta-analysis. *Clin. Oral Invest.* 20: 903–914.

Akram, Z., Baharuddin, N.A., Vaithilingam, R.D. et al. (2017). Effect of nonsurgical periodontal treatment on clinical periodontal variables and salivary resistin levels in obese Asians. *J. Oral Sci.* 59: 93–102.

Altay, U., Gurgan, C.A. and Agbaht, K. (2013). Changes in inflammatory and metabolic parameters after periodontal treatment in patients with and without obesity. *J. Periodontol.* 8: 13–23.

Al-Zahrani, M.S. and Alghamdi, H.S. (2012). Effect of periodontal treatment on serum C-reactive protein level in obese and normal-weight women affected with chronic periodontitis. *Saudi Med. J.* 33: 309–314.

Al-Zahrani, M.S., Bissada, N.F. and Borawski, E.A. (2003). Obesity and periodontal disease in young, middle-aged, and older adults. *J. Periodontol.* 74: 610–615.

Armingohar, Z., Jørgensen, J.J., Kristoffersen, A.K., Abesha-Belay, E. and Olsen, I. (2014). Bacteria and bacterial DNA in atherosclerotic plaque and aneurysmal wall biopsies from patients with and without periodontitis. *J. Oral Microbiol.* 15: 6.

Balejo, R.D.P., Cortelli, J.R., Costa, F.O. et al. (2017). Effects of chlorhexidine pre- procedural rinse on bacteremia in periodontal patients: A randomized clinical trial. *J. Appl. Oral Sci.* 25: 586–595.

Bartold, P., Marshall, R. and Haynes, D. (2005). Periodontitis and rheumatoid arthritis: a review. *J. Periodontol.* 76 (11-s): 2066–2074.

Bartold, P.M. and Lopez-Oliva, I. (2020). Rheumatoid arthritis and periodontitis: an update 2012–2017. *Periodontology 2000* 83 (1): 189–212.

Bax, M., Huizinga, T.W.J. and Toes, R.E.M. (2014). The pathogenic potential of autoreactive antibodies in rheumatoid arthritis. *Semin. Immunopathol.* 36: 313–325.

Beck, J., Elter, J., Heiss, G., Couper, D., Mauriello, S. and Offenbacher, S. (2001) Relationship of periodontal disease to carotid artery intima-media wall thickness: the Atherosclerosis Risk in Communities (ARIC) Study. *Arterioscler. Thromb. Vasc. Biol.* 21: 1816–1822.

Beck, J.D., Pankow, J., Tyroler, H.A. and Offenbacher, S. (1999). Dental infections and atherosclerosis. *Am. Heart J.* 138 (5 Pt 2): S528–S533.

Belibasakis, G.N., Bostanci, N., Hashim, A. et al. (2007). Regulation of RANKL and OPG gene expression in human gingival fibroblasts and periodontal ligament cells by Porphyromonas gingivalis: a putative role of the Arg-gingipains. *Microb. Pathogen.* 43: 46–53.

Blüher, M. (2019). Obesity: global epidemiology and pathogenesis. *Nat. Rev. Endocrinol.* 15: 288–298.

Borgnakke, W.S., Ylostalo, P.V., Taylor, G.W. and Genco, R.J. (2013). Effect of periodontal disease on diabetes: systematic review of epidemiologic observational evidence. *J. Clin. Periodontol.* 40 (Suppl. 14): 135–152.

Bright, R., Proudman, S., Rosenstein, E. and Bartold, P. (2015). Is there a link between carbamylation and citrullination in periodontal disease and rheumatoid arthritis? *Med. Hypothes.* 84 (6): 570–576.

Chávarry, N.G., Vettore, M.V., Sansone, C. and Sheiham, A. (2009). The relationship between diabetes mellitus and destructive periodontal disease: a meta-analysis. *Oral Health Prev. Dent.* 7 (2): 107–127.

Chun, Y.H., Chun, K.J., Olguin, D.A. and Wang, H. (2005). Biological foundation for periodontitis as a potential risk factor for athersclerosis. *J. Periodontal Res.* 40 (1): 87–95.

Corbet, E.F. and Leung, W.K. (2011). Epidemiology of periodontitis in the Asia and Oceania regions. *Periodontology 2000* 56 (1): 25–64.

Craig, R.G., Yip, J.K., So, M.K. et al. (2003). Relationship of destructive periodontal disease to the acute-phase response. *J. Periodontol.* 74 (7): 1007–1016.

Cutler, C., Shinedling, E., Nunn, M. et al. (1999). Association between periodontitis and hyperlipidemia: cause or effect? *J. Periodontol.* 70 (12): 1429–1434.

Darveau, R.P. (2010). Periodontitis: a polymicrobial disruption of host homeostasis. *Nat. Rev. Microbiol.* 8 (7): 481–490.

Demmer, R.T., Desvarieux, M., Holtfreter, B. et al. (2010). Periodontal status and A1C change: longitudinal results from the study of health in Pomerania (SHIP). *Diabetes Care* 33: 1037–1043.

Demmer, R.T., Holtfreter, B., Desvarieux, M. et al. (2012). The influence of type 1 and type 2 diabetes on periodontal disease progression: prospective results from the Study of Health in Pomerania (SHIP). *Diabetes Care* 35 (10): 2036–2042.

Demmer, R.T., Trinquart, L., Zuk, A. et al. (2013). The influence of anti-infective periodontal treatment on C-reactive protein: a systematic review and meta-analysis of randomized controlled trials. *PLoS One* 8: e77441.

Demmer, R.T., Breskin, A., Rosenbaum, M. et al. (2017). The subgingival microbiome, systemic inflammation and insulin resistance: the Oral Infections, Glucose Intolerance and Insulin Resistance Study. *J. Clin. Periodontol.* 44 (3): 255–265.

de Oliveira, C., Watt, R. and Hamer, M. (2010). Toothbrushing, inflammation, and risk of cardiovascular disease: results from Scottish Health Survey. *BMJ* 340: c2451.

DeStefano, J., Anda, R.F., Kahn, H.S., Williamson, D.F. and Russell, C.M. (1993). Dental disease and risk of coronary heart disease and mortality. *BMJ* 306: 688–691.

Dietrich, T., Sharma, P., Walter, C., Weston, P. and Beck, J. (2013). The epidemiological evidence behind the association between periodontitis and incident atherosclerotic cardiovascular disease. *J. Clin. Periodontol.* 40: S70–84.

Dorn, J.M., Genco, R.J., Grossi, S.G. et al. (2010). Periodontal disease and recurrent cardiovascular events in survivors of myocardial infarction (MI): the Western New York Acute MI Study. *J. Periodontol.* 81: 502–511.

Ebersole, J.L., Machen, R.L., Steffen, M.J. and Willmann, D.E. (1997) Systemic acute-phase reactants, C-reactive protein and haptoglobin, in adult periodontitis. *Clin. Exp. Immunol.* 107 (2): 347–352.

Eezammuddeen, N.N., Vaithilingam, R.D., Hassan, N.H.M. et al. (2020). Association between rheumatoid arthritis and periodontitis: recent progress. *Curr. Oral Health Rep.* 7: 139–153.

Eke, P.I., Dye, B.A., Wei, L. et al. (2015). Update on prevalence of periodontitis in adults in the United States: NHANES 2009 to 2012. *J. Periodontol.* 86 (5): 611–622.

Erciyas, K., Sezer, U., Üstün, K. et al. (2013). Effects of periodontal therapy on disease activity and systemic inflammation in rheumatoid arthritis patients. *Oral Dis.* 19 (4): 394–400.

Ford, P.J., Gemmell, E., Hamlet, S.M. et al. (2005) Cross-reactivity of GroEL antibodies with human heat shock protein 60 and quantification of pathogens in atherosclerosis. *Oral Microbiol. Immunol.* 20: 296–302.

Gemmell, E., Yamazaki, K. and Seymour, G.J. (2007). The role of T cells in periodontal disease: homeostasis and autoimmunity. *Periodontology 2000* 47: 14–40.

Genco, R.J., Grossi, S.G., Ho, A., Nishimura, F. and Murayama, Y. (2005). A proposed model linking inflammation to obesity, diabetes and periodontal infections. *J. Periodontol.* 76: 2075–2084.

Golub, L.M., Payne, J.B., Reinhardt, R.A. and Nieman, G. (2006). Can systemic diseases co-induce (not just exacerbate) periodontitis? A hypothetical 'two-hit' model. *J. Dent. Res.* 85 (2): 102–105.

Goncalves, T.E.D., Feres, M., Zimmermann, G.S. et al. (2015). Effects of scaling and root planning on clinical response and serum levels of adipocytokines in patients with obesity and chronic periodontitis. *J. Periodontol.* 86: 53–61.

Graziani, F., Gennai, S., Solini, A. and Petrini, M. (2018). A systematic review and meta-analysis of epidemiologic observational evidence on the effect of periodontitis on diabetes. An update of the EFP-AAP review. *J. Clin. Periodontol.* 45 (2): 167–187.

Gyorgy, B., Toth, E., Tarcsa, E., Falus, A. and Buzas, E. I. (2006). Citrullination: a posttranslational modification in health and disease. *Int. J. Biochem. Cell Biol.* 38 (10): 1662–1677.

Haffajee, A.D. and Socransky, S.S. (2009). Relation of body mass index, periodontitis and Tannerella forsythia. *J. Clin. Periodontol.* 36: 89–99.

Hajishengallis, G., Liang, S., Payne, M.A. et al. (2011). Low-abundance biofilm species orchestrates inflammatory periodontal disease through the commensal microbiota and complement. *Cell Host Microbe* 10 (5): 497–506.

Haraszthy, V.I., Zambon, J.J., Trevisan, M., Zeid, M. and Genco, R.J. (2000). Identification of periodontal pathogens in atheromatous plaques. *J. Periodontol.* 71: 1554–1560.

Harvey, G.P., Fitzsimmons, T.R., Dhamarpatni, A.A., Marchant, C., Haynes, D.R., and Bartold, P.M. (2012). Expression of peptidylarginine deiminase-2 and -4, citrullinated proteins and anti-citrullinated protein antibodies in human gingiva. *J. Periodont. Res.* 48 (2): 252–261.

Heitz-Mayfield, L., Trombelli, L., Heitz, F., Needleman, I. and Moles, D. (2002). A systematic review of the effect of surgical debridement vs. non-surgical debridement for the treatment of chronic periodontitis. *J. Clin. Periodontol.* 29 (s3): 92–102.

Holmlund, A., Lampa, E. and Lind, L. (2017). Oral health and cardiovascular disease risk in a cohort of periodontitis patients *Atherosclerosis* 262: 101–106.

Hujoel P.P., Drangsholt, M., Spiekerman, C. et al. (2000). Periodontal disease and coronary heart disease risk. *JAMA* 284 (11): 1406–1410.

Janket, S.J., Baird, A.E., Chuang, S.K. and Jones, J.A. (2003). Meta-analysis of periodontal disease and risk of coronary heart disease and stroke. *Oral Surg. Oral Med. Oral Pathol. Oral Radiol. Endod.* 95: 559–569.

Johnson, R.B., Wood, N. and Serio, F.G. (2004). Interleukin-11 and IL-17 and the pathogenesis of periodontal disease. *J. Periodontol.* 75 (1): 37–43.

Kaneko, C. and Kobayashi, T. (2018). Circulating levels of carbamylated protein and neutrophil extracellular traps are associated with periodontitis severity in patients with rheumatoid arthritis: a pilot case-control study. *PLoS One* 13 (2): e0192365.

Kassebaum, N.J., Bernabe, E., Dahiya, M., Bhandari, B., Murray, C.J. and Marcenes, W. (2014). Global burden of severe periodontitis in 1990– 2010: a systematic review and meta-regression. *J. Dent. Res.* 93: 1045–1053.

Kaur, S., Bright, R., Proudman, S.M. and Bartold, P.M. (2014). Does periodontal treatment influence clinical and biochemical measures for rheumatoid arthritis? A systematic review and meta-analysis. *Semin. Arthritis Rheum.* 44: 113–122.

Khader, Y., Bawadi, H., Haroun, T., Alomari, M. and Tayyem, R. (2009). The association between periodontal disease and obesity among young adults in Jordan. *J. Clin. Periodontol.* 36: 18–24.

Khan, S., Saub, R., Vaithilingam, R.D. et al. (2015). Prevalence of chronic periodontitis in an obese population: a preliminary study. *BMC Oral Health* 15 (1): 114.

Khantisopon, N., Louthrenoo, W., Kasitanon, N. et al. (2014). Periodontal disease in Thai patients with rheumatoid arthritis. *Int. J. Rheum. Dis.* 17 (5): 511–518.

Kindstedt, E., Johansson, L., Palmqvist, P. et al. (2018). Association between marginal jawbone loss and onset of rheumatoid arthritis and relationship to plasma levels of RANKL. *Arthritis Rheumatol.* 70 (4): 508–515.

Kocher, T., König, J., Borgnakke, W.S., Pink, C. and Meisel, P. (2018). Periodontal complications of hyperglycemia/diabetes mellitus: epidemiologic complexity and clinical challenge. *Periodontology 2000* 78 (1): 59–97.

Kopelman, P.G. (2000). Obesity as a medical problem. *Nature* 404: 635–643.

Koppolu, P., Durvasula, S., Palaparthy, R. et al. (2013). Estimate of CRP and TNF-alpha level be- fore and after periodontal therapy in cardiovascular disease patients. *Pan African Med. J.* 15: 92.

Kornman, K.S., Crane, A., Wang, H.Y. et al. (1997). The interleukin-1 genotype as a severity factor in adult periodontal disease. *J. Clin. Periodontol.* 24: 72–77.

Kozarov, E.V., Dorn, B.R., Shelburne, C.E., Dunn, W.A. Jr and Progulske-Fox, A. (2005). Human atherosclerotic plaque contains viable invasive *Actinobacillus actinomycetemcomitan* and *Porphyromonas gingivalis*. *Arterioscler. Thromb. Vasc. Biol.* 25: e17–18.

Koziel, J., Mydel, P. and Potempa, J. (2014). The link between periodontal disease and rheumatoid arthritis: an updated review. *Curr. Rheumatol. Rep.* 16 (3): 408.

Kwon, T. and Levin, L. (2014). Cause-related therapy: a review and suggested guidelines. *Quintessence Int.* 45 (7): 585–591.

Lagrand, W.K., Visser, C.A., Hermens, W.T. et al. (1999). C-reactive protein as a cardiovascular risk factor: more than an epiphenomenon? *Circulation* 100 (1): 96–102.

Lakschevitz, F., Aboodi, G., Tenenbaum, H. and Glogauer, M. (2011). Diabetes and periodontal diseases: interplay and links. *Curr. Diabetes Rev.* 7: 433–439.

Lalla, E. and Papapanou, P. (2011). Diabetes mellitus and periodontitis: a tale of two common interrelated diseases. *Nat. Rev. Endocrinol.* 7: 738–748.

Lee, Y.H., Lew, P.H., Cheah, C.W. et al. (2019). Potential mechanisms linking periodontitis to rheumatoid arthritis. *J. Int. Acad. Periodontol.* 21 (3): 99–110.

Lee, Y.L., Hu, H.Y., Chou, P. and Chu, D. (2015). Dental prophylaxis decreases the risk of acute myocardial infarction: a nationwide population-based study in Taiwan. *Clin. Int. Aging* 10: 175– 182.

Linden, G.J., Linden, K., Yarnell, J., Evans, A., Kee, F. and Patterson, C.C. (2012). All-cause mortality and periodontitis in 60–70-year-old men: a prospective cohort study. *J. Clin. Periodontol.* 39: 940–946.

Losche, W., Karapetow, F., Pohl, A. and Kocher, T. (2000). Plasma lipid and glucose levels in patients with destructive periodontal disease. *J. Clin. Periodontol.* 27: 537–541.

Lucas, H., Bartold, P., Dharmapatni, A., Holding, C. and Haynes, D. (2010). Inhibition of apoptosis in periodontitis. *J. Dent. Res.* 89: 29–33.

Madianos, P.N. and Koromantzos, P.A. (2018). An update of the evidence on the potential impact of periodontal therapy on diabetes outcomes. *J. Clin. Periodontol.* 45 (2): 188–195.

Mahendra, J., Mahendra, L., Felix, J. and Romanos, G. (2013). Prevalence of periodontopathogenic bacteria in subgingival biofilm and atherosclerotic plaques of patients undergoing coronary revascularization surgery. *J. Indian Soc. Periodontol.* 17: 719724.

Marcenes, W., Kassebaum, N.J., Bernabe, E. et al. (2013). Global burden of oral conditions in 1990–2010: a systematic analysis. *J. Dent. Res.* 92 (7): 592–597.

Mariapun, J., Ng, C. and Hairi, N.N. (2018). The gradual shift of overweight, obesity, and abdominal obesity towards the poor in a multi-ethnic developing country: findings from the Malaysian National Health and Morbidity Surveys. *J. Epidemiol.* 28 (6): 279–286.

Mattila, K.J., Nieminen, M.S., Valtonen, V.V. et al. (1989). Association between dental health and acute myocardial infarction. *BMJ* 298: 779–781.

McGraw, W.T., Potempa, J., Farley, D. and Travis, J. (1999). Purification, characterization, and sequence analysis of a potential virulence factor from Porphyromonas gingivalis, peptidylarginine deiminase. *Infect. Immun.* 67 (7): 3248–3256.

Moen, K., Brun, J.G., Valen, M. et al. (2006). Synovial inflammation in active rheumatoid arthritis and psoriatic arthritis facilitates trapping of a variety of oral bacterial DNAs. *Clin. Exp. Rheumatol.* 24 (6): 656–66.3

Montague, C.T. and O'Rahilly, S. (2000). The perils of portliness: causes and consequences of visceral adiposity. *Diabetes* 49: 883.

Mori, Y., Kitamura, H., Song, Q.H. et al. (2000). A new murine model for athersclerosis with inflammation in the periodontal tissue induced by immunization with heat shock protein. *Hypertens. Res.* 23: 475–481.

Morita, I., Okamoto, Y., Yoshii, S. et al. (2011). Five-year incidence of periodontal disease is related to body mass index. *J. Dent. Res.* 90: 199–202.

Mosmann, T.R. and Sad, S. (1996). The expanding universe of T-cell subsets: Th1, Th2 and more. *Immunol. Today* 17 (3): 138–146.

Moura-Grec, P.G., Marsicano, J.A., Carvalho, C.A. and Sales-Peres, SH. (2014). Obesity and periodontitis: systematic review and meta-analysis. *Cien. Saude Colet.* 19 (6): 1763–1772.

Nelson, R.G., Shlossman, M., Budding, L.M. et al. (1990). Periodontal disease and NIDDM in Pima Indians. *Diabetes Care* 13 (8): 836–840.

Nesse, W., Westra, J., van der Wal, J. E. et al. (2012). The periodontium of periodontitis patients contains citrullinated proteins which may play a role in ACPA (anti-citrullinated protein antibody) formation. *J. Clin. Periodontol.* 39 (7): 599–607.

Nishida, N., Tanaka, M., Hayashi, N. et al. (2005). Determination of smoking and obesity as periodontitis risks using the classification and regression tree method. *J. Periodontol.* 76: 923–928.

Nishimura, F., Iwamoto, Y., Mineshiba, J., Shimizu, A., Soga, Y. and Murayama, Y. (2003). Periodontal disease and diabetes mellitus: the role of tumor necrosis factor-alpha in a 2-way relationship. *J. Periodontol.* 74: 97–102.

Noack, B., Genco, R.J., Trevisan, M., Grossi, S., Zambon, J.J. and De Nardin, E. (2001). Periodontal infections contribute to elevated systemic C-reactive protein level. *J. Periodontol.* 72 (9): 1221–1227.

NOHSA (2010). *National Oral Health Survey in Adults*. Malaysia: Ministry of Health.

Ohki, T., Itabashi, Y., Kohno, T., et al. (2012). Detection of periodontal bacteria in thrombi of patients with acute myocardial infarction by polymerase chain reaction. *Am. Heart J.* 163: 164–167.

Ortiz, P., Bissada, N.F., Palomo, L. et al. (2009). Periodontal therapy reduces the severity of active rheumatoid arthritis in patients treated with or without tumor necrosis factor inhibitors. *J. Periodontol.* 80 (4): 535–540.

Panezai, J., Ghaffar, A., Altamash, M., Engström, P.-E. and Larsson, A. (2018). Periodontal disease influences osteoclastogenic bone markers in subjects with and without rheumatoid arthritis. *PLoS One* 13 (6): e0197235.

Paraskevas, S., Huisinga, J.D. and Loos, B.G. (2008). A systematic review and meta-analyses on C-reactive protein in relation to periodontitis. *J. Clin. Periodontol.* 35: 277–290.

Park, S.Y., Kim, S.H., Kang, S.H. et al. (2019). Improved oral hygiene care attenuates the cardiovascular risk of oral health disease: a population-based study from Korea. *Eur. Heart J.* 40: 1138–1145.

Patel, S.P. and Raju, P.A. (2014). Gingival crevicular fluid and serum levels of resistin in obese and non-obese subjects with and without periodontitis and association with single nucleotide polymorphism at −420. *J. Ind. Soc. Periodont.* 18: 555.

Perlstein, M.I. and Bissada, N.F. (1977). Influence of obesity and hypertension on the severity of periodontitis in rats. *Oral Surg. Oral Med. Oral Pathol.* 43: 707–719.

Philstrom, B.L., Michalowicz, B.S. and Johnson, N.W. (2005). Periodontal diseases. *Lancet* 366: 1809–1820.

Polak, D. and Shapira, L. (2018). An update on the evidence for pathogenic mechanisms that may link periodontitis and diabetes. *J. Clin. Periodontol.* 45 (2): 150–166.

Potikuri, D., Dannana, K.C., Kanchinadam, S. et al. (2012). Periodontal disease is significantly higher in non-smoking treatment-naive rheumatoid arthritis patients: results from a case-control study. *Ann. Rheum. Dis.* 71 (9): 1541–1544.

Preshaw, P.M., Alba, A.L., Herrera, D. et al. (2012). Periodontitis and diabetes: a two-way relationship. *Diabetologia* 55 (1): 1–31.

Rantapaa-Dahlqvist, S., de Jong, B.A., Berglin, E. et al. (2003). Antibodies against cyclic citrullinated peptide and IgA rheumatoid factor predict the development of rheumatoid arthritis. *Arthritis Rheum.* 48 (10): 2741–2749.

Reichert, S., Schulz, S., Benten, A.C. et al. (2016). Periodontal conditions and incidence of new cardiovascular events among patients with coronary vascular disease. *J. Clin. Periodontol.* 43: 918–925.

Ribeiro, J., Leao, A. and Novaes, A.B. (2005). Periodontal infection as a possible severity factor for rheumatoid arthritis. *J. Clin. Periodontol.* 32 (4): 412–416.

Rodriguez, S.B., Stitt, B.L. and Ash, D.E. (2009). Expression of peptidylarginine deiminase from Porphyromonas gingivalis in Escherichia coli: enzyme purification and characterization. *Arch. Biochem. Biophys.* 488 (1): 14–22.

Rosenstein, E.D., Greenwald, R.A., Kushner, L.J. and Weissmann, G. (2004). Hypothesis: the humoral immune response to oral bacteria provides a stimulus for the development of rheumatoid arthritis. *Inflammation* 28 (6): 311–318.

Saito, T. and Shimazaki, Y. (2007). Metabolic disorders related to obesity and periodontal disease. *Periodontology 2000* 43: 254–266.

Saito, T., Shimazaki, Y., Koga, T., Tsuzuki, M. and Ohshima, A. (2001). Relationship between upper body obesity and periodontitis. *J. Dent. Res.* 80 (7): 1631–1636.

Saito, T., Shimazaki, Y., Koga, T., Tsuzuki, M. and Ohshima, A. (2006). Relationship between periodontitis and hepatic condition in Japanese women. *J. Int. Acad. Periodontol.* 8: 89–95.

Sanz, M., Ceriello, A., Buysschaert, M. et al. (2018). Scientific evidence on the links between periodontal diseases and diabetes: consensus report and guidelines of the joint workshop on periodontal diseases and diabetes by the International Diabetes Federation and the European Federation of Periodontology. *J. Clin. Periodontol.* 45 (2): 138–149.

Sanz, M., del Castillo, A.M., Jepsen, S. et al. (2020). Periodontitis and cardiovascular diseases. *Consensus report. Global Heart* 15 (1): 1.

Scannapieco, F.A., Bush, R.B. and Paju, S. (2003). Associations between periodontal disease and risk for atherosclerosis, cardiovascular disease and stroke: a systematic review. *Ann. Periodontol.* 8: 38–53.

Schellekens, G.A., de Jong, B.A., van den Hoogen, F.H., van de Putte, L.B. and van Venrooij, W.J. (1998). Citrulline is an essential constituent of antigenic determinants recognized by rheumatoid arthritis-specific autoantibodies. *J. Clin. Invest.* 101 (1): 273–281.

Schellekens, G.A., Visser, H., de Jong, B.A. et al. (2000). The diagnostic properties of rheumatoid arthritis antibodies recognizing a cyclic citrullinated peptide. *Arthritis Rheum.* 43 (1): 155–163.

Schenkein, H.A. and Loos, B.G. (2013). Inflammatory mechanisms linking periodontal diseases to cardiovascular diseases. *J. Clin. Periodontol.* 40 (Suppl 14): S51–69.

Sen, S., Sumner, R., Hardin, J. et al. (2013). Periodontal disease and recurrent vascular events in stroke/transient ischemic attack patients. *J. Stroke Cerebrovasc. Dis.* 22: 1420–1427.

Sen, S., Giamberardino, L.D., Moss, K. et al. (2018). Periodontal disease, regular dental care use, and incident ischemic stroke. *Stroke* 49: 355– 362.

Sharma, P., Dietrich, T., Ferro, C.J., Cockwell, P. and Chapple, I.L. (2016). Association between periodontitis and mortality in stages 3–5 chronic kidney disease: NHANES III and linked mortality study. *J. Clin. Periodontol.* 43: 104–113.

Shi, J., van de Stadt, L.A., Levarht, E.W. et al. (2014). Anti-carbamylated protein (anti-CarP) antibodies precede the onset of rheumatoid arthritis. *Ann. Rheum. Dis.* 73 (4): 780–783.

Slade, G.D., Offenbacher, S., Beck, J.D., Heiss, G. and Pankow, J.S. (2000). Acute-phase inflammatory response to periodontal disease in the US population. *J. Dent. Res.* 79 (1): 49–57.

Suresh, S., Mahendra, J., Kumar, A., et al. (2017). Comparative analysis of subgingival red complex bacteria in obese and normal weight subjects with and without chronic periodontitis. *J. Indian Soc. Periodontol.* 21: 186–191.

Suresh, S., Mahendra, J., Singh, G., Kumar, A.R.P., Thilagar, S. and Rao, N. (2018). Effect of nonsurgical periodontal therapy on plasma-reactive oxygen metabolite and gingival crevicular fluid resistin and serum resistin levels in obese and normal weight individuals with chronic periodontitis. *J. Indian Soc. Periodontol.* 22: 310–316.

Suvan, J., D'Aiuto, F., Moles, D.R., Petrie, A. and Donos, N. (2011). Association between overweight/obesity and periodontitis in adults. A systematic review. *Obes. Rev.* 12: e381–e404.

Suvan, J., Petrie, A., Moles, D.R. et al. (2014). Body mass index as a predictive factor of periodontal therapy outcomes. *J. Dent. Res.* 93: 49–54.

Tahir, K.M., Malek, A.H., Vaithilingam, R.D. et al. (2020). Impact of non-surgical periodontal therapy on serum Resistin and periodontal pathogen in chronic periodontitis patients with obesity. *BMC Oral Health* 20: article no. 52.

Takahashi, K., Azuma, T., Motohira, H., Kinane, D.F. and Kitetsu, S. (2005). The potential role of interleukin-17 in the immunopathology of periodontal disease. *J. Clin. Periodontol.* 32 (4): 369–374.

Tang, Q., Fu, H., Qin, B. et al. (2017). A possible link between rheumatoid arthritis and periodontitis: a systematic review and meta-analysis. *Int. J. Periodont. Rest. Dent.* 37 (1): 79–86.

Taylor, G.W. (2001). Bidirectional interrelationships between diabetes and periodontal diseases: an epidemiologic perspective. *Ann. Periodontol.* 6: 99–112.

Taylor, J.J., Preshaw, P.M. and Lalla, E. (2013). A review of the evidence for pathogenic mechanisms that may link periodontitis and diabetes. *J. Clin. Periodontol.* 40 (Suppl 14): S113–S134.

Teeuw, W.J., Kosho, M.X., Poland, D.C., Gerdes, V.E. and Loos, B.G. (2017). Periodontitis as a possible early sign of diabetes mellitus. *BMJ Open Diabetes Res. Care* 5 (1): e000326.

Tomas, I., Diz, P., Tobias, A., Scully, C. and Donos, N. (2012). Periodontal health status and bacteraemia from daily oral activities: systematic review/meta-analysis. *J. Clin. Periodontol.* 39: 213–228.

Tomofuji, T., Kusano, H., Azuma, T., Ekuni, D., Yamamoto, T. and Watanabe, T. (2005). Effects of a high-cholesterol diet on cell behaviour in rat periodontitis. *J. Dent. Res.* 84: 752–756.

Tonetti, M.S., Van Dyke, T.E. Working Group 1 of the Joint EFP/AAP Workshop (2013). Periodontitis and atherosclerotic cardiovascular disease. Consensus report of the Joint EFP/AAP Workshop on Periodontitis and Systemic Diseases. *J. Clin. Periodontol.* 40 (Suppl 14): S24–29.

Tonetti, M.S., Jepsen, S., Jin, L. and Otomo-Corgel, J. (2017). Impact of the global burden of periodontal diseases on health, nutrition and wellbeing of mankind: a call for global action. *J. Clin. Periodontol.* 44 (5): 456–462.

Tuti, N.M.D., Khairiyah, A.M., Rasidah, A. et al. (2013). Periodontal status and provision of periodontal services in Malaysia: trends and way forward. *Malay. J. Public Health Med.* 13 (2): 38–47.

Van der Weijden, G. and Timmerman, M. (2002). A systematic review on the clinical efficacy of subgingival debridement in the treatment of chronic periodontitis. *J. Clin. Periodontol.* 29 (s3): 55–71.

Verna, l R., Dutzan, N., Chaparro, A. et al. (2005). Levels of interleukin-17 in gingival crevicular fluid and in supernatants of cellular cultures of gingival tissue from patients with chronic periodontitis. *J. Clin. Periodontol.* 32 (4): 383–389.

Wakai, K., Kawamura, T., Umemura, O. et al. (1999). Associations of medical status and physical fitness with periodontal disease. *J. Clin. Periodontol.* 26 (10): 664–72.

Wang, S. and El-Deiry, W.S. (2003). TRAIL and apoptosis induction by TNF-family death receptors. *Oncogene* 22: 8628–8633.

Wang, Z., Nicholls, S.J., Rodriguez, E.R. et al. (2007). Protein carbamylation links inflammation, smoking, uremia and atherogenesis. *Nat. Med.* 13 (10): 1176–1184.

Wegner, N., Lundberg, K., Kinloch, A. et al. (2010). Autoimmunity to specific citrullinated proteins gives the first clues to the etiology of rheumatoid arthritis. *Immunol. Rev.* 233: 34–54.

White, D.A., Tsakos, G., Pitts, N.B. et al. (2012) Adult Dental Health Survey 2009: common oral health conditions and their impact on the population. *Br. Dent. J.* 213: 567–572.

World Health Organization (WHO) (2007). *The WHO Global Oral Health Data Bank*. Geneva: World Health Organization.

World Health Organization (WHO) (2008). *Global Health Observatory: situation and trends of obesity*. Geneva: World Health Organization.

World Health Organization (WHO) (2015). *Obesity Fact Sheet 311: Obesity and overweight*. Geneva: World Health Organization

Wu, T., Trevisan, M., Genco, R.J., Falkner, K.L., Dorn, J.P. and Sempos, C.T. (2000). Examination of the relation between periodontal health status and cardiovascular risk factors: serum total and high density lipoprotein cholesterol, C-reactive protein, and plasma fibrinogen. *Am. J. Epidemiol.* 151 (3): 273–82.

Xu, Q., Dietrich, H. and Steiner, H.J. (1992). Induction of arthersclerosis in normocholesterolemic rabbits by immunization with heat shock protein 65. *Arterioscler. Thromb.* 12: 789–799.

Yan, S.F., Ramasamy, R. and Schmidt, A.M. (2009). Receptor for AGE (RAGE) and its ligands – cast into leading roles in diabetes and the inflammatory response. *J. Mol. Med.* 87: 235–247.

Zhang, Y.X., Cliff, W.J., Schoefl. G.I. and Higgins, G. (1999). Coronary C-reactive protein distribution: its relation to development of atherosclerosis. *Atherosclerosis* 145 (2): 375–379.

Zuza, E.P., Barroso, E.M., Carrareto, A.L.V. et al. (2011). The role of obesity as a modifying factor in patients undergoing non-surgical periodontal therapy. *J. Periodontol.* 82: 676–682.

Zwaka, T.P., Hombach, V. and Torzewski, J. (2001). C-reactive protein-mediated low density lipoprotein uptake by macrophages: implications for atherosclerosis. *Circulation* 103 (9): 1194–1197.

10

Immunology of Tooth Movement and Root Resorption in Orthodontics

Wan Nurazreena Wan Hassan[1] and Rachel J. Waddington[2]

[1] Department of Paediatric Dentistry and Orthodontics, Faculty of Dentistry, Universiti Malaya, Kuala Lumpur, Malaysia
[2] School of Dentistry, Cardiff University, Cardiff, UK

10.1 Orthodontic Tooth Movement: Definition and Theories

In principle, mechanical loading of orthodontic appliances on teeth transmits the forces applied on the crowns through the roots, and in turn, induces mechanical strain against the periodontal ligament and alveolar bone. The initial phase of tooth movement occurs immediately after force application and lasts for about 24 to 48 hours. This phase is rapid and involves displacement of the tooth in the periodontal ligament (PDL) space within the alveolar socket. There is compression of the PDL where the force is directed, resulting in deformation of the blood vessels and rearrangement of the surrounding tissues. The PDL and blood flow adapt to the compressive force, resulting in metabolic changes in response to hypoxia and decreased nutrients. Hyalinisation of the cell-free zone is observed due to cell death in the PDL of the compressed periodontium. Consequently, the initial stages of orthodontic force application are characterised by an aseptic acute inflammatory response.

Within the periodontium, the capillaries vasodilate to allow the migration of leucocytes and biochemical signals initiate synthesis and secretion of proinflammatory cytokines and chemokines, growth factors and enzymes. Tooth movement is minimal, or absent, during this lag phase which usually lasts about 20–30 days. The necrosed tissue is removed by macrophages and foreign body giant cells, while the alveolar bone proper is resorbed by osteoclasts recruited from the underlying cortical bone. Subsequently, in the post lag phase tooth movement begins about 40 days after the initial force application (Asiry 2018).

Several theories have been proposed for the initation of orthodontic tooth movement.

10.1.1 Pressure–Tension Theory

The foundation of this theory was laid by Sandstedt (1904), Oppenheim (1911) and Schwarz (1932). According to this theory, the tooth moves into the PDL space and creates areas of pressure and tension, through compression and stretching of the PDL tissues (Figure 10.1). The action affects the blood flow of the PDL, whereby the pressure side has reduced blood flow, and subsequently less oxygen and more carbon dioxide, and vice versa on the tension side. Excessive force would result in tissue necrosis (see Figure 10.1) due to the strangulated periodontium. The macrophages would resorb the hyalinised tissue while undermining bone resorption by the osteoclasts occurs alongside the hyalinised tissue. On the tension side, there is an increase in blood flow. Mesenchymal stem cells differentiate into osteoblasts. Mature osteoblasts lay down the osteoid, followed by a mineralisation process to form mature bone (Meikle 2006).

10.1.2 Biological Electric Theory

This theory was introduced by Bassett and Becker in 1962. Alveolar bone is relatively elastic. Orthodontic appliances translate the orthodontic force to flex the alveolar bone. When the alveolar bone bends, it releases electric signals. The ions in

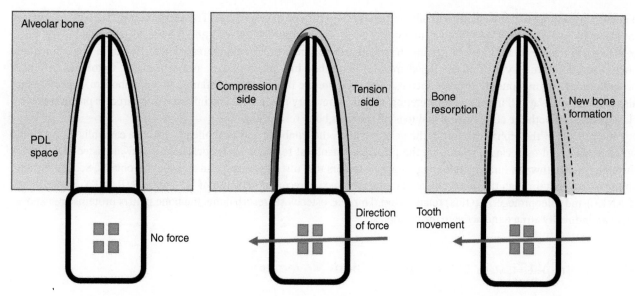

Figure 10.1 Direction of orthodontic force and tooth movement. During a normal physiological state, the periodontium is in equilibrium (left). When orthodontic force is applied (middle), the PDL space on the compressed side may undergo hyalinisation (red line) due to reduced blood flow from excessive force application. Removal of the hyalinised tissue by macrophages subsequently allows for bone remodelling with bone resorption on the compressed side and bone formation on the tension side.

the bone interact with the electric field generated by bone bending. Small charges are produced, known as streaming potential, which is thought to activate osteoclasts and osteoblasts resulting in resorption and deposition for moving teeth (Meikle 2006).

10.1.3 Biomechanical Theory

According to the biomechanical theory, tooth movement is linked to a mechanical distortion of the cell membranes which, in turn, stimulates a cascade of biological responses. This is based on the principle that osteocytes are sensitive to mechanical deformation and act as mechanoreceptors during orthodontic force loading. Mechanical distortion changes the conformation of the cell membrane. The phospholipid bilayer cell membrane activates the production of phospholipase A_2. Subsequently, the arachidonic acid (eicosatetraenoic acid) metabolism via the cyclo-oxygenase (COX) pathway results in the formation of prostaglandins (PGE_2) and thromboxanes. Other metabolites of arachidonic acid such as leukotrienes and hydroxyeicosatetraenoic acids (HETEs) are produced via the lipoxygenase (LOX) pathway.

During orthodontic tooth movement, prostaglandins and leukotrienes facilitate tooth movement via osteoclast formation to induce bone resorption. Thus, mechanical forces are translated into transduction of intracellular signals or secondary messengers via the cell membrane into the cell and nucleus to stimulate DNA synthesis. The secondary messengers implicated in mechanical force transduction include the adenosine 3',5' cyclic monophosphate (cAMP), inositol phosphate and tyrosine kinase. The biomechanical effect of orthodontic forces thus stimulates alveolar bone remodelling for orthodontic tooth movement which involves bone resorption and bone formation processes (Meikle 2006).

10.1.4 Biphasic Theory

According to this theory (Alikhani et al. 2018), tooth movement is divided into two phases: the initial catabolic phase followed by an anabolic phase. During the catabolic phase, osteoclasts resorb bone at both the compression and tension sites and subsequently during the anabolic phase, osteoblasts act to restore the alveolar bone. The tension side is anticipated to have more bone formation because tensile forces stimulate osteoblast activity. The theory supports a prominent role for the PDL as the mechanical trigger for initiation of the catabolic phase rather than bone cells, and notably, implants and ankylosed teeth without PDL do not move orthodontically.

Sustained compressive force during orthodontic loading squeezes the incompressible fluids out of the PDL space, resulting in movement of teeth to further compress the PDL. This immediately causes blood vessel constriction and decreased blood flow, resulting in reduced nutrient and oxygen levels at the compression side. The surrounding PDL cells, in addtion to osteocytes and osteoblasts in the adjacent alveolar bone proper, undergo necrosis and the site becomes hyalinised. Local cells begin to release chemokines, triggering the initial aseptic, acute inflammatory response for inflammation-dependent bone resorption. Monocytes from the bloodstream differentiate into macrophages and osteoclasts. Cytokines that have proinflammatory functions continue to increase and promote the initial aseptic inflammatory catabolism. The cytokines also prevent runaway inflammation by secreting anti-inflammatory mediators. The inflammatory process promotes osteo-clastogenesis on both the compression and tension sides for bone resorption.

The principle of the biphasic theory is the delay between the catabolic and anabolic phases. The catabolic phase would produce abundant osteoclasts, which are the principal osteoblast regulators. Osteoclasts can activate osteoblast activity through three pathways. First, by releasing paracrine factors that directly recruit and activate osteoblasts. Second, by acti-vating osteoblasts through the direct cell-to-cell interactions, i.e. receptor activator of NF-kappa-B (RANK), RANK ligand (RANKL) and osteoprotegerin (OPG) relationship. Third, as osteoclasts resorb bone, the bone matrix proteins are exposed that can indirectly attract and activate the osteoblasts.

10.2   Principal Tissues of Orthodontic Tooth Movement

In many ways, the supporting complex of periodontium represents a unique set of connective tissues that provide for the interdigitation of the Sharpey's fibres of the PDL with the mineralised tissue of the alveolar bone lining the tooth socket and the cementum coating the root dentine (see Figure 10.1). The primary function of the periodontium is to support the attachment of the teeth within their socket, particularly when withstanding the considerable forces brought about by chewing. At the same time, these tissues are capable of responding to occlusal loads for the continued delivery of their primary function. To enable this, the PDL has for many years been identified to have the highest turnover for extracellular matrix components within the human body (Sodek 1977), thus allowing for quick repair and remodelling of the tissues to an array of biomechanical forces encountered on a daily basis. Equally, the responsiveness of the PDL to mechanical forces is now recognised to be central to facilitating orthodontic tooth movement.

When considering supraphysiological forces applied during orthodontic tooth movement, inflammatory cells resident within the periodontal ligament, and their associated signalling factors, take centre stage to accelerate tissue remodelling. Consequently, orthodontic tooth movement relies on the generation of a controlled aseptic inflammatory environment within the PDL. It is noteworthy that ankylosed teeth and dental implants lack PDL and are unable to respond to mechani-cal forces because they have lost the cell populations vital for orchestrating bone remodelling.

10.2.1   Periodontal Ligament and Cells Within

The extracellular matrix of the PDL is mainly composed of type I and III collagen fibrous bundles. These terminally form into Sharpey's fibre insertion points embedding into either the alveolar bone or the cementum. The fibres form into prin-cipal fibre groups which vary slightly concerning their orientation along the length of the root, helping the PDL to with-stand the different axial and lateral compressional, tipping and rotational loads, which vary according to the changing magnitude of the functional loads delivered around the alveolar socket. Paradoxically, mechanical loading is important not only for damage repair but also in maintaining joint function, placing the tooth in an optimal occlusal position to provide efficient biting and chewing. As a consequence of this dynamic remodelling process, Sharpey's inserts at the PDL bone interface are regularly and necessarily resorbed and remodelled.

Fundamental to this process are the cells residing within the PDL (Figure 10.2). Resident fibroblasts, and their precursor mesenchymal cells, make up 50–60% of the cell population. There is a wide phenotypic variation within the fibroblast popu-lation, which respond differently to extracellular signalling factors, including growth factors and cytokines involved in an inflammatory response (Menicanin et al. 2010). The PDL is also known to contain discrete populations of stem cells which locate as pericytes with the endothelial cells of the vasculature (Komaki 2019). These stem cells provide for the transit ampli-fying mesenchymal progenitor cells, fibroblasts, osteoblasts and cementocytes and their respective precursor cells, which have been described with differing migratory, proliferative and matrix deposition capabilities and reside in different ana-tomical locations throughout the PDL. For further details, refer to the following reviews (de Jong et al. 2017; Komaki 2019).

Thus, the stem cells facilitate and support the differing site-specific functional characteristics of the PDL (Lekic et al. 1997). Consequently, the fibroblast population of the PDL has a synthetic role in forming new fibrous attachments, but, and uniquely,

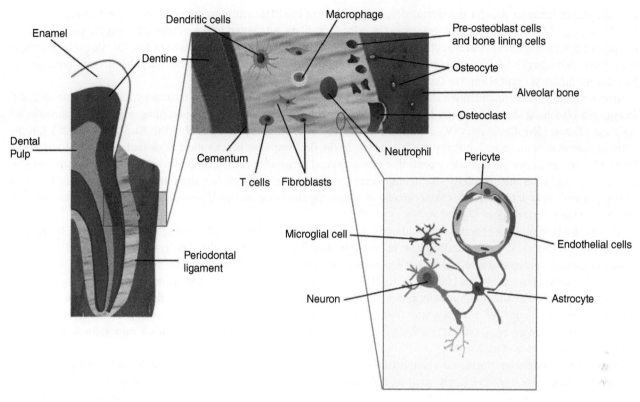

Figure 10.2 Arrangement of the periodontal ligament in supporting the tooth within the jaw and the principal cells aiding this function.

they are also capable of degrading collagen fibrils. PDL fibroblast populations, responding to extracellular signalling factors such as interleukin (IL)-1-beta, are responsible for the partial extracellular degradation and phagocytosis of collagen fragments into intracellular membrane-bound vacuoles, which are then degraded by enzymes such as acid-labile cathepsins, cysteine and aspartic proteinases (Overall et al. 1989; McCulloch and Knowles 1993; van der Pauw et al. 2001).

The PDL fibroblasts and their mesenchymal precursor cells establish themselves within a wider cellular niche, regulated by reciprocal paracrine signalling that dictates the collective biological behaviour of other cells resident within the niche. These cells include those that provide the innate immune responses, such as neutrophils, dendritic cells, macrophages, mast cells and lymphocytes. Following the application of an orthodontic force, mechanical strain is actively sensed by all cells of the PDL, via changes in interstitial fluid flow and blood flow within the vasculature (Krishnan and Davidovitch 2006). Combined with compression-induced hypoxia, this mechanical strain modulates cell signalling responses to induce an inflammatory response.

Inflammatory cytokines produced by the PDL fibroblast population are responsible for changing the signalling environment; one that evolves to increase the recruitment of proinflammatory immune cells, leading to the remodelling of the collagen-rich structures of the PDL, which ultimately orchestrate bone remodelling and orthodontic tooth movement. This response is also propagated by nerve endings that are associated with the endothelial cells of the blood vessels (Krishnan and Davidovitch 2006; Sabane et al. 2016). The release of neuropeptides such as substance P and calcitonin gene-related peptides has the potential to influence the biological activity of all cells within their respective niche. This includes the endothelial cells to increase their permeability and recruitment of further leucocytes, monocytes and macrophages to the PDL.

10.2.2 Alveolar Bone

Alveolar bone is made up of two parts: the alveolar bone proper which lines the tooth socket and the supporting alveolar bone. The supporting alveolar bone constitutes the cortical plates forming the facial and lingual surfaces with predominantly cancellous bone located between the cortical plates and the alveolar bone proper. The alveolar bone proper therefore provides the attachment sites for the extrinsic Sharpey's fibres of the PDL within a compact bone. Hence, it is also termed bundle bone and seen in clinical radiographs as the cribriform plate, attributed to the numerous foramina permitting the passage of nerves and blood vessels via the Volkmann canal network. The re-establishment of this functional architecture is essential following orthodontic tooth movement, which involves the remodelling of not only the alveolar bone proper but also the adjacent cortical bone as the tooth is moved through the alveolar process.

Alveolar bone remodelling involves the co-ordinated actions of many cells, of which mesenchymal progenitor cells, differentiated osteoblasts and osteocytes, haematopoietic progenitor cells, osteoclasts, macrophages and T lymphocytes all have established identifiable roles (Waddington et al. 2016; Loi et al. 2016; Avery et al. 2020; Guder et al. 2020). On the compression side of an orthodontically challenged tooth, the first response is activation of osteoclasts for removal of the bone. This occurs under the regulatory control of mesenchymal progenitor cells, osteoblasts and lymphocytes that synthesise RANKL and macrophage colony-stimulating factor (M-CSF), promoting the recruitment, differentiation and fusion of monocytic cells into activated osteoclasts capable of degrading the bone matrix. These cells are recruited from the PDL adjacent to the resorbing bone (Zainal Ariffin et al. 2011).

As orthodontic tooth movement is achieved and the biological events affecting bone resorption are triggered, the magnitude of the mechanical strain gradually decreases as the tooth achieves its new occlusal position. Mesenchymal progenitor cells and osteoblasts are also involved in halting the process of osteoclast differentiation by synthesising OPG, which acts as a soluble decoy preventing the binding of RANKL to its cell surface receptor, RANK, on the osteoclast cell surface. Following resolution of the inflammatory phase, mesenchymal progenitor cells, pre-osteoblasts and osteoblasts residing within the PDL and from the marrow spaces within the adjacent cancellous bone differentiate to produce osteoblasts that regenerate the alveolar bone proper, synthesising the first osteoid, which then forms into a mineralised matrix (Loi et al. 2016: Waddington et al. 2016).

However, this should be considered a simplistic view of events. Mesenchymal and immune cells within the PDL are able to secrete proinflammatory cytokines, such as IL-1, IL-6, IL-17, tumour necrosis factor (TNF)-alpha and transforming growth factor (TGF)-beta. All these cytokines have the capacity to induce osteoclast differentiation and hence bone resorption and all have reported to be elevated within compression sites during orthodontic tooth movement (Li et al. 2019; Zainal Ariffin et al. 2011) (discussed in further detail below). Further, the inflammatory response of the PDL cells should be considered against the response of the osteocytes embedded within the alveolar bone, where excessive mechanical strain can also promote bone resorption.

Osteocytes are the result of bone-synthesising osteoblasts becoming embedded within the bone matrix, to form specialised non-proliferative terminally differentiated cells (Guo and Bonewald 2009). Each osteocyte can project as many as 60 long cell processes, that pass through an extensive network of canaliculi which allow osteocytes to communicate via gap junctions, not only with each other but also with the osteoblasts lining the bone surface. How osteocytes function in bone remodelling is still unclear and hence their mechanistic contribution to orthodontic tooth movement is still built upon hypotheses (Murshid 2017). Osteocytes are proposed to respond to various mechanical stains through (1) sensing stretching and compression of the extracellular matrix, detected by cell surface adhesion molecules such as integrins, G-protein-coupled receptors; (2) geometric changes to the intracellular cytoskeleton; (3) fluid flow in the canaliculi stimulating ion channels of the cell processes; (4) changes in hydrostatic pressure where the osteocyte lacunae act as strain concentrators (Klein-Nulend et al. 2012; Boccafoschi et al. 2013; Litzenberger et al. 2010).

Mild mechanical strain applied to bone is essential to maintain osteocyte survival and response by stimulating osteoblast differentiation to form bone as protection against bone fatigue damage. A key signalling factor identified in the regulation of bone formation is sclerotin which is produced by the osteocytes and delivered to the bone lining cells via the canaliculi (Odagaki et al. 2018). Sclerostin inhibits the Wnt signalling pathways which are known to be essential for promoting osteoblast differentiation and bone synthesis. Under mild stimulation, sclerostin production is suppressed, thus removing its negative regulation on Wnt and allowing for bone formation. The secretion of signalling factors such as TGF-beta and insulin-like growth factor (IGF) by osteocytes also promotes osteoblast differentiation. However, if excessive strain is experienced, as present on compression sites following an orthodontically applied force, sclerostin and RANKL production by osteocytes is observed to increase, inhibiting osteoblast synthetic activity and promoting osteoclast bone resorption activity respectively (Shu et al. 2017). The observation that local administration of sclerostin enhances orthodontic tooth movement in a rat model evidences the strong role of this signalling factor and osteocytes in molecular and cellular events (Lu et al. 2019). The reason for the biphasic effect of mild and strong mechanical strain on sclerostin production is unclear, but it does provide a biological mechanism for how the alveolar bone proper is re-established on the compression side as the mechanical strain recedes when the tooth has moved through the dentoalveolar complex to its new occlusal position.

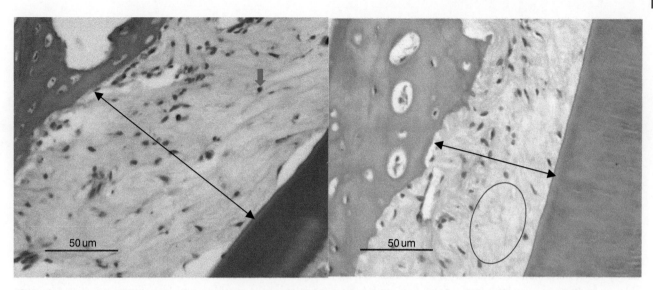

Figure 10.3 Changes in PDL due to orthodontic force. (Left) Normal PDL showing an abundance of cells (red arrow). (Right) Excessive force narrows (double arrow) the PDL space, which subsequently may cause hyalinisation (PDL areas without cells) (oval area).

In the control of bone remodelling, macrophages play important roles in regulating osteoblast activity via the expression of pro- and anti-inflammatory cytokines (Gu et al. 2017; Shapouri-Moghaddam et al. 2018). Macrophages are now recognised to broadly exist as two distinct polarised subsets. The M1 phenotype is ascribed roles in destroying pathogens and through the generation of proinflammatory cytokines, namely IL-1-beta, IL-6, IL-12, IL-23 and TNF-alpha, can propagate bone resorption and hinder bone repair. During wound healing, this M1 phenotype transitions to a M2 phenotype which, via the production of anti-inflammatory factors such as IL-10, TGF-beta, bone morphogenic protein 2 (BMP-2) and vascular endothelial growth factor (VEGF), plays important roles in tissue repair, angiogenesis and re-establishment of homeostasis. A transition from the M1 phenotype to the M2 phenotype is therefore seen as a prerequisite for initiating bone repair. A prolonged presence of M1 macrophages has the potential to extend inflammation and thus could be detrimental to successful alveolar bone rebuilding.

Orthodontic tooth movement thus initially induces on the compression side an inflammatory response generated by cells of both the PDL and the bone marrow associated with the adjacent cancellous bone, leading to osteoclast activation. With time, the inflammatory environment is resolved and bone repair ensues to restore the architecture of the alveolar process. However, high force magnitudes on the compression side can cut off the blood supply, increasing the hypoxic environment and leading to cell apoptosis and necrosis (Figure 10.3). This results in the production of hyalinised tissue and the cells of the PDL are unable to contribute to the bone resorptive process. Rather, it is only the cells within the bone marrow spaces of the adjacent cancellous bone that are activated to provide resorption of the alveolar bone proper.

Whilst the tooth is able to move into its new occlusal site, lack of a contribution from the cells of the PDL means the process usually takes longer. Conversely, on the tension side, the PDL, and the blood vessels and nerves within, are stretched and possibly damaged, causing an associated increase in blood flow and an increase in oxygen tension. This invariably has an effect on the signalling environment leading to new bone formation. A mild inflammatory environment is induced which is responsible for the recruitment of mesenchymal progenitors and angiogenesis and can be regarded as a prerequisite to efficient bone repair.

10.3 Chemical Mediators in Tooth Movement

10.3.1 Proinflammatory Cytokines

Cytokines are regarded as short-range extracellular proteins that regulate the activity of other cells and hence the various inflammatory stages. Key proinflammatory cytokines that mediate bone remodelling during orthodontic tooth movement include IL-1, IL-6, IL-17, TNF-alpha, M-CSF and RANKL.

M-CSF is a secreted cytokine that promotes haematopoietic stem cells to differentiate into macrophages or other related cell types. It is an important signalling factor for osteoclast differentiation. When orthodontic force is applied, the levels of

VEGF and M-CSF increase in the gingival crevicular fluid (Kaku et al. 2008). An optimal level of M-CSF recruits preosteoclasts into the PDL and promotes osteoclast differentiation by recruiting precursors and inhibiting apoptosis.

IL-1 and TNF-alpha are key mediators in acute-phase inflammatory reactions. At inflammatory sites, they are expressed by macrophages, fibroblasts, osteoblasts and osteoclasts. IL-1 exists in two isoforms with species differences in osteoclastic activity: IL-1-alpha and IL-1-beta (Bletsa et al. 2006). Both are encoded by distinct genes, but bind to the same receptor, IL-1R1. IL-1-alpha precursor is constitutively present, fully active and is released from the necrotic cells during early phases of inflammation. However, IL-1-beta is inactive and is cleaved by caspase 1 to release the active cytokine in extracellular space. The IL receptor antagonist, IL-1ra inhibits IL-1 activity by binding to IL-1R1 receptors to prevent signal transduction (Kalra et al. 2020).

TNF-alpha is also present in the PDL without orthodontic forces, suggesting a role in tissue homeostasis and remodelling during physiological tooth drift. In the very early stages of the inflammatory reaction of orthodontic tooth movement, TNF-alpha release increases where it plays an indirect role in bone resorption by stimulating IL-1 production. Thereafter, IL-1 production will stimulate its own synthesis in a positive feedback loop. In the later stages of inflammation, increased TNF-alpha protein levels would downregulate its further production (Bletsa et al. 2006).

IL-1 has a primary role in the early phases of orthodontic tooth movement and root resorption. In the early phase of orthodontic tooth movement, IL-1-alpha, IL-1-beta and TNF-alpha expressions are increased in both tension and compression sides as early as one day after force application, with higher secretion of the cytokines on the compressed sides. However, after mechanical stress, the induction of IL-1-beta reaches a maximum on day 3 and declines thereafter (Bletsa et al. 2006; Lalithapriya et al. 2018). IL-1-beta gene polymorphisms have been reported in subjects susceptible with external apical root resorption, though some studies found otherwise, while not only variation in IL-1-beta but also variation in IL-1RN are responsible for postorthodontic external apical root resorption (Lalithapriya et al. 2018). IL-1 also activates or sensitises the nociceptor fibres directly or indirectly via a complex signalling cascade. It is of note, IL-1-beta levels increase in the gingival crevicular fluid (GCF) and are correlated with pain levels during orthodontic tooth movement (Lalithapriya et al. 2018).

The actions of TNF-alpha and IL-1 are also regulated by IL-6 which promotes anti-inflammatory effects through its inhibitory effects on TNF-alpha and IL-1, by activation of IL-1ra and IL-10. As mentioned above, IL-1ra inhibits IL-1. Nonetheless, IL-6 also has a biphasic role of promoting inflammatory effects. IL-6 is secreted by osteoblasts to stimulate osteoclastogenesis through stromal or osteoblastic cells. As with IL-1-beta, IL-6 production peaks at day 3 on the pressure side of force application. IL-6 is expected to facilitate orthodontically induced inflammatory root resorption (OIIRR) as the cytokine levels are high in patients with severe root resorption after orthodontic treatment (Kunii et al. 2013).

IL-17 is an inflammatory cytokine produced by activated T-cells. It induces RANKL production by osteoblasts. IL-17 induced by excessive orthodontic force stimulates odontoclastogenesis through IL-6 production in PDL tissues. The T-helper 17 cell response to excessive orthodontic force leads to the progression of root resorption by increasing expression of IL-17, RANKL and RANK. Therefore, IL-17 in PDL tissues may contribute to OIIRR during orthodontic tooth movement (Nakano et al. 2015).

Osteoclastogenesis is regulated by the RANKL/RANK/OPG axis. RANKL is a key osteoclastogenic cytokine for osteoclast formation. It is also referred to as TNF-related activation-induced cytokine (TRANCE), osteoclast differentiation factor (ODF) and osteoprotegerin ligand (OPGL) and is a type II transmembrane protein belonging to the TNF superfamily. In bone, RANKL is expressed by cells of mesenchymal origin, osteoblasts, hypertrophic chondrocytes, bone marrow (BM) stromal cells and osteocytes. Its expression is regulated by factors such as parathyroid hormone (PTH) and 1,25-dihydroxy vitamin D3. Its expression is stimulated by calcium, glucocorticoids, prostaglandin E2, IL-1-alpha, IL-6, IL-11 and IL-17 while canonical Wnt signalling and TGF-beta pathways downregulate it (Iacono et al. 2013). RANKL stimulates osteoclast formation and further induces bone resorption by local osteoclasts.

M-CSF, IL-1 and TNF-alpha all promote osteoblast precursors and mature osteoblasts to produce RANKL. M-CSF downregulates OPG production and upregulates RANK receptor on osteoclast precursor cells to increase sensitivity to RANKL (Weitzmann 2013). When M-CSF binds to receptor c-fms on monocytic lineage cells, macrophage marker F4/80 and VEGF proteins are activated. RANK in turn binds to its ligand (RANKL), inducing preosteoclastic cell fusion to produce polykaryon cells that become osteoclasts (Brooks et al. 2011). Together with M-CSF, RANKL is considered the master cytokine, driving osteoclast differentiation through binding to its receptor RANK and the activation of different intracellular signalling cascades, involving an increasing number of molecules, among them TNF receptor associated factor 6 (TRAF6), NF-kappa-B, ERK1/2, JNK and p38, which ultimately result in the activation of NFATc1, a crucial transcription factor in osteoclastogenesis.

There is cross-talk between immune and bone cells through these regulatory molecules. Th1 and Th2 cells inhibit osteoclastogenesis through the production of interferon (IFN)-gamma and IL-4, while Th17 cells induce osteoclast formation and osteolysis in rheumatoid arthritis via the IL-17-mediated induction of RANKL expression on synovial fibroblasts. RANKL produced by B cells also contributes to bone resorption during periodontal infection. On the other hand, OPG acts as a decoy receptor that binds to RANKL and competes with RANK. Therefore, osteoclastogenesis is regulated by the inhibitory effect of OPG.

10.3.2 Chemokines

Chemokines are cytokines with four main subfamilies: CXC, CC, CX3C and XC, that are secreted by cells and assigned primary roles in the chemotaxis of responsive immune cells, especially directing cells of the immune system to a target site. They exert their function by binding and stimulating G-protein transmembrane receptors on their target cell. Inflammatory inducible chemokines that are secreted in response to proinflammatory stimuli such as IL-1 and TNF-alpha include, but are not restricted to, CXCL-8 (IL-8), CCL2 (macrophage inflammatory protein-1, MIP-1), CCL3 (MIP-1-alpha), CCL4 (MIP-1-beta), CCL5 (regulated on activation normal T cell expressed and secreted, RANTES), CXCL10 (IFN gamma-induced protein 10).

A number of studies have identified the presence of CCL2, CCL5S and CXCL2 (MIP-2) within the compressed periodontal tissues, where they are ascribed major roles in the regulation of immune cell infiltration and subsequent inflammatory activity (Alhashimi et al. 2004; Andrade et al. 2007, 2012; Capelli et al. 2011). Receptors for chemokines such as CXCL10 and CXCL1 have also been identified on mesenchymal stromal cells and pre-osteoblasts, where they regulate their migration, survival, proliferation and collagen synthesis for tissue repair (Yano et al. 2005).

10.3.3 Anti-inflammatory Cytokines

In the normal bone repair process, inflammation is the first crucial step and deficiencies in acute inflammation can impair bone healing. However, along the timeline of the normal bone healing progression, the associated infiltrating immune cells are also responsible for initiating the resolution of inflammation. Regulated by various anti-inflammatory cytokines such as IL-4, IL-10 and IL-13, this process can start to appear at the healing site within the first 24 to 48 hours (Maruyama et al. 2020). While the secretion of proinflammatory cytokines into the inflammatory environment continues, the increase in levels of anti-inflammatory cytokines helps to achieve 'adaptive' homeostasis that alters the cross-talk between the immune cells and the mesenchymal stromal cell population.

Within this scenario, maintaining a balance between pro- and anti-inflammatory cytokines is important for navigating through the bone remodelling process and maintaining a balance between osteoblastic and osteoclastic activity. Through this, a balance of macrophage polarisation from the proinflammatory M1 phenotype to an anti-inflammatory tissue repair M2 phenotype, which is associated with the production of IL-10 and TGF-beta, is established (Gu et al. 2017; Shapouri-Moghaddam et al. 2018). Further, IL-4 and IL-13 are associated with the stimulation of naive T helper (Th0) into Th2 cells which in turn are proposed to counter hyperosteoclastic activity inducible by Th1 and Th17. IL-10 production by Treg cells acts to suppress the general immune response to achieve self-tolerance and prevent autoimmunity (Kaiko et al. 2008; Garlet 2010).

When considering that orthodontic tooth movement requires the establishment of a chronic inflammatory environment leading to excessive bone resorption, only a few studies have investigated the presence of anti-inflammatory cytokines in gingival crevicular fluid collected from periodontal tissues during orthodontic tooth movement. It is also not surprising that for the majority of these studies, the levels of IL-4 and IL-10 fell below the detection limit for the assay used within the study (Alhashimi et al. 2004; Grant et al. 2013; van Gastel et al. 2011). It is surprising, however, that this result was observed for both the compression and the tension sides (Alhashimi et al. 2004), suggesting that neither Th2 nor M2 cells, associated with induction of tissue repair processes, develop. Where IL-10 has been detected in GCF, there was very little difference in the levels (statistically insignificant) between the orthodontically treated and untreated tooth (Karaduman et al. 2015). One study has indicated a statistically significant increase in levels of IL-10 on the tension side (Garlet et al. 2007).

Collectively, these results would suggest that anti-inflammatory cytokines only serve to interfere with the bone remodelling process required for successful orthodontic tooth movement, and the process differs from the inflammatory requirements for anti-inflammatory cytokines in normal bone healing following fracture, for example. It has been confirmed that administration of the anti-inflammatory cytokine IL-4 to a mouse orthodontic model prevented tooth movement and that was associated with a reduction in the number of tartrate-positive osteoclasts as well as reduction in root resorption (Hakami et al. 2015). Whilst the anti-inflammatory M1 phenotype predominates in the compression side, the anti-inflammatory M2 is the predominant phenotype in the tension side, and the inability to transition to the M2 phenotype is associated with increased root resorption (He et al. 2015).

10.3.4 Prostaglandins

When considering the control of bone remodelling within an inflammatory environment, prostaglandins are important signalling factors, although their precise role in regulating orthodontic tooth movement is still up for debate. Consequently, prostaglandins have been attributed roles in both the promotion and resolution of inflammation, bone formation and both promotion and inhibition of osteoclastogenesis. See the review by Kouskoura et al. (2017) for detail. Prostaglandins are lipid molecules that derive from a 20-carbon unsaturated fatty acid, arachidonic acid through the action of cyclo-oxygenase (COX) enzymes. Their synthesis is blocked by non-steroidal anti-inflammatory drugs (NSAIDs) including aspirin and ibuprofen which are inhibitors for COX-2, and administration of these drugs during active phases of tooth movement has been suggested to delay the process (Shetty et al. 2013).

Prostaglandin E2 (PGE2) has received the most attention and its elevated levels are observed in GCF collectable around the tooth during orthodontic tooth movement (Grieve et al. 1994; Shetty et al. 2013). This is most notable within the first 24 hours of force application (Ren and Vissink 2008). Their localised secretion by a variety of immune cells may be induced via the direct action of mechanical stress, the creation of a hypoxic environment or by a variety of proinflammatory cytokines including IL-1, IL-6, and TNF-alpha Tsuge et al. 2019). Therefore, a prostaglandin cytokine cross-talk is proposed to be important in regulation and maintenance of an appropriate balance of Th1/Th2/Th17 cells in chronic inflammation (Yao and Narumiya 2019).

PGE2 has also been shown to have direct effects on both promoting osteoclast formation (Collins and Chambers 1992) and inhibiting osteoclast formation (Fuller and Chambers 1989). Its differential effects on osteoclast function had for a long time been attributed to concentration effects. However, it is also apparent that these effects may be attributable to the ability of PGE2 to bind to different types of cell surface receptors. In bone formation, PGE2 binds to the EP1 receptor and stimulates osteoblast differentiation. Conversely, the binding of PGE2 to EP2 or EP4 receptors on osteoblasts stimulates secretion of the osteoclast inducing factor, i.e. RANKL (Mayahara et al. 2012). These studies would suggest that PGE2 plays an overall role in mediating many phases of bone remodelling and the inflammatory process. These can be regarded as positive effects since a number of in vivo animal studies have identified that the local administration of PGE2 can promote orthodontic tooth movement (Seifi et al. 2003; Yamasaki et al. 1982, 1984; Kale et al. 2004; Leiker et al. 1995). While this could form an innovative therapeutic intervention for manipulating the inflammatory environment to one that accelerates tooth movement and prevents root resorption, the need for repeated injections due to the short half-life of PGE2 has presented a major limitation (Kouskoura et al. 2017).

10.3.5 Growth Factors

While growth factors are generally known to be important in regulating tissue repair and formation, they can also be important participants in regulating the inflammatory process. One such example is VEGF which is well recognised for its roles in mediating angiogenesis, which is a prerequisite for tissue repair, increasing vascular permeability and facilitating migration of the immune cells. In an in vivo model, moderate increases in VEGF levels have been identified in the tension side that have been attributed to the remodelling of the vascular network and repair of the tissue (Salomão et al. 2014; Kaku et al. 2008). By contrast, intense levels of VEGF on the compression side are seen particularly over a three-day period following application of the force, which correlates with significant compression of the PDL leading to alteration in blood flow (Salomão et al. 2014).

Hypoxia, oxidative and mechanical stress, hyperglycaemia and associated acidosis have all been identified as local physiological factors that can cause an increase in VEGF (Rasila et al. 2005). Studies have identified that local injection of recombinant VEGF enhances orthodontic tooth movement (Kaku et al. 2001; Kohno et al. 2002) which has been attributed to its ability to induce osteoclast formation. Indeed, in vitro studies have identified that VEGF can enhance osteoclast formation (Taylor et al. 2012; Aldridge et al. 2005). This correlates with studies in osteopetrotic (op/op) mice where mutations to the osteoclastic inducing factor M-CSF lead to osteoclast deficiency that can be partially reversed through administration of recombinant human VEGF (Kaku et al. 2000, 2001).

Within the compressed PDL, a significant increase in the levels of fibroblast growth factor 2 (FGF-2) (also known as basic FGF) has also been reported, which also has roles in the promotion of angiogenesis, particularly in hypoxic conditions (Kardami et al. 2007). Thus, both VEGF and FGF-2 are recognised for initiating a cascade of molecular and cellular events, such as induction of chemotaxis of mesenchymal progenitor cells and macrophages and cellular proliferation (Murakami et al. 1999; Dimitriou et al. 2005). All these events contribute to a rapid remodelling of the PDL, particularly in an attempt to minimise tissue hyalinisation and the repair of necrotic tissue considered unavoidable on the compression side (Salomão et al. 2014).

TGF-beta has been acknowledged to play a pivotal role in the repair of periodontal tissues, particularly in the early stages of bone formation, stimulating proliferation of the mesenchymal progenitor cells and early differentiation to osteoprogenitor cells, although it inhibits full differentiation to fully mature bone-synthesising osteoblasts (Wu et al. 2016). Immunosuppressive roles of TGF-beta-1 include controlling initiation and resolution of inflammation (Wrzesinski et al. 2007) and preventing overstimulation of proinflammatory cytokines leading to an inappropriate immune response (Koutoulaki et al. 2010). Immuno-localisation studies have demonstrated a significant increase in TGF-beta in the tension side in PDL, particularly at 5–10 days following the application of orthodontic force (Wang et al. 2000). This demonstrates its potential role in orthodontic tooth movement for promoting repair of the PDL in accommodating stretching forces, secretion and apposition of new bone and modulating the inflammatory response.

10.3.6 Neurotransmitters

The PDL is highly innervated and the application of compressive force to this tissue results in the release of neuropeptides such as calcitonin gene-related peptides (Vandevska-Radunovic and Murison 2010; Norevall et al. 1995), vasoactive intestinal polypeptides, neuropeptide Y (Kato et al. 1996) and substance P (Yamaguchi et al. 2006; Levrini et al. 2013) from the peripheral nerve fibres. As neurons transmit signals, they induce a complex cascade of biological reactions that are responsible for pain sensation. Although cellular mechanisms remain vague, these neuropeptides are thought to stimulate a localised inflammatory response, which in turn can induce the tissue remodelling events associated with orthodontic tooth movement.

Nerves within the PDL are associated with the vascular system and the effects of the neuropeptides they produce are proposed to influence the behaviour of endothelial cells to promote vasodilation, vascular flow and permeability (Sabane et al. 2016; Krishnan and Davidovitch 2006). It has been demonstrated that substance P can act as a chemoattractant for monocytes and lymphocytes, and can enhance lymphocyte proliferation and antibody production (Maggi 1997; Santoni et al. 1999; O'Connor et al. 2004) and mobilisation of mesenchymal stem cells within peripheral blood (Hong et al. 2009). Receptors for calcitonin gene-related peptides have also been identified in monocytes, lymphocytes and mast cells stimulating the synthesis and release of inflammatory cytokines (Assas et al. 2014). It is pertinent to note that during orthodontic tooth movement, the neuropeptide calcitonin gene-related peptide has been localised to nerves and blood vessels distributed adjacent to the alveolar bone and bone resorption lacunae as well as resorption areas associated with the cementum (Vandevska-Radunovic et al. 1997). Calcitonin gene-related peptide has been demonstrated to induce osteoblast proliferation and bone formation and inhibit osteoclast activity. Slightly differing roles have been proposed for substance P which enhances both osteoblast and osteoclast activity (An et al. 2019).

Additionally, studies examining the effect of substance P on gingival fibroblasts have suggested that its action could provide a 'switch' from a proinflammatory mode that favours tissue degradation to an anabolic reparative mode (Bartold et al. 1994). Hence, neuropeptides could have a beneficial role in promoting tissue remodelling, which might be dependent upon the presence of other reparative signalling factors. This hypothesis has recently been supported by studies reporting that the systemic administration of substance P can accelerate orthodontic tooth movement and alveolar bone remodelling within a rat model (An et al. 2019).

10.3.7 Osteopontin

Osteopontin (OPN), also known as secreted phosphoprotein 1 (SPP1), is a matricellular protein that is now recognised to play a number of diverse roles in the bone remodelling process, including regulation of the immune response. OPN is synthesised by a range of cells including pre-osteoblasts, immature osteoblasts and macrophages (Singh et al. 2018; Lund et al. 2009). OPN is also regarded as a proinflammatory cytokine due to its ability to enhance the expression of proinflammatory cytokines and regulate the activity of Th1 cells, macrophages and dendritic cells (Lund et al. 2013). It has notably been identified as a negative inhibitor for osteoblast proliferation and differentiation through reducing cellular responses to the osteogenic inducing factor BMP-2 (Huang et al. 2004). It has also been identified as a potent inhibitor of mineral crystal growth, and, through binding to mineralised bone surfaces it serves to bind to $\alpha V\beta 3$ integrin cell surface receptors on osteoclasts, promoting formation of the sealing zone and activation of intracellular signalling mechanisms to promote resorptive activities (Duong et al. 2000) and reduce the expression of OPG as a decoy receptor for the osteoclastic factor RANKL (Ishii et al. 2004). Consequently, OPN becomes incorporated into cement lines, delineating new and old bone structures (McKee and Nanci 1996).

However, OPN is not a bone-specific protein as it is expressed in many different tissues. Through studies investigating its role in tumor development, OPN has been identified to play a significant role in the regulation of inflammation at several different levels (Lund et al. 2009). OPN has been identified to promote the migration, attachment and survival of immune cells to a wound healing site, most notably neutrophils (Koh et al, 2007) and macrophages (Lund et al. 2009), in facilitating their attachment to bone surfaces (McKee and Nanci, 1996).

Intracellular forms of OPN have also been identified within these immune cells where it contributes to intracellular signalling in the production of cytokines (Lund et al. 2009). Against this background, the role of OPN in the regulation of bone remodelling (Singh et al. 2018) is now attracting significant attention. Indeed, using a rodent model for orthodontic tooth movement, mechanical compression has been correlated with the upregulation of OPN in osteocytes, some osteoblasts and bone-lining cells (Fujihara et al. 2006; Terai et al. 1999). OPN induction within PDL cells has also been reported following mechanically induced compression and tensional forces, suggesting diverse roles involving different signalling pathways in bone resorption, bone remodelling and bone formation (Singh et al. 2018).

10.4 Orthodontic Pain Management and Cytokine Expression

Once applied, orthodontic forces exert their effects on paradental tissues, such as periodontal tissues and the dental pulp, resulting in a cascade of self-limiting local inflammatory reactions, including cellular, vascular, neural and immunological reactions causing orthodontic pain. Thus, orthodontic tooth movement is mechanistically linked to induce orthodontic pain. The products of local inflammation (for example, prostaglandin and bradykinin) act on sensory endings connected to the tooth to incite painful sensations (Long et al. 2016).

Generally, orthodontic pain begins 12 hours after applying the orthodontic force and reaches a peak within 24 hours. However, the pain gradually diminishes within the next 3–7 days and occasionally takes a month to return to baseline level. Upon application of the orthodontic force, the dental root starts moving in the direction of force and exerts mechanical pressure on the alveolar bone. As a result, the periodontium between the root and alveolar bone is compressed and vascular compression and local ischaemia take place. Consequently, periodontal cells, mainly fibroblasts, undergo anaerobic respiration and cause local acidosis, resulting in the production of proton ions (H^+).

The H^+ binds to ASIC3 receptors on sensory endings to generate pain. With the continuation of local ischaemia, chemokines released by mast cells and fibroblasts initiate neutrophil and monocyte recruitment at the site, causing release of an array of inflammatory mediators such as bradykinin and prostaglandin as well as cytokines such as IL-1 and TNF. Bradykinin and prostaglandin also bind and generate painful sensations. Furthermore, via anterograde transportation, sensory endings release various neurogenic mediators such as calcitonin gene-related peptides and dilate local blood vessels and enhance local inflammation, resulting in amplified local painful sensation.

NSAIDs such as ibuprofen effectively reduce pain following orthodontic treatment. As previously mentioned, NSAIDs work by inhibiting COX enzymes, which convert arachidonic acid to prostaglandin H2 (PGH2). PGH2, in turn, is converted by other enzymes to several other prostaglandins including PGE2 (which are mediators of pain, inflammation and bone remodelling; see above) and to thromboxane A2 (which stimulates platelet aggregation, leading to formation of blood clots). Ibuprofen is a non-selective COX inhibitor, in that it inhibits two isoforms of cyclo-oxygenase: COX-1 and COX-2. The analgesic, antipyretic and anti-inflammatory effects of NSAIDs operate mainly through inhibition of COX-2, which decreases the synthesis of prostaglandins involved in mediating inflammation, pain, fever and swelling. Since they act on the COX-2, which is a vital element in tooth movement, the use of NSAIDs can delay the process (Shetty et al. 2013).

Generally, NSAIDs are prescribed for up to 24 hours for orthodontic pain relief. This may not have a significant implication since the majority of ibuprofen is metabolised and eliminated within 24 hours in the urine. However, prolonged use of NSAIDs may increase treatment time. Paracetamol is a suitable alternative and equally effective for pain relief following orthodontic treatment (Monk et al. 2017). Paracetamol does not inhibit the function of any COX enzyme outside the central nervous system and is non-inflammatory. Thus, it should be considered in place of ibuprofen for non-allergic patients who require longer pain relief, since the inflammatory process is favourable for orthodontic tooth movement.

10.5 Immune Response in Osteoperforations During Accelerated Orthodontic Movement

Generally, orthodontic treatment would take about 18 to 24 months to complete an average case. Longer treatment times are expected in more complicated cases, which can take up to a few years.

The regional acceleratory phenomenon (RAP) (Frost 1983) is a tissue reaction to different noxious stimuli. The condition is characterised by an acceleration of normal ongoing processes of the soft and hard tissues. A RAP can be stimulated by a noxious stimulus, which is directly proportional to the magnitude and nature of the stimulus. Once induced, the vital processes accelerate above normal values. The metabolism and activities of differentiated cells, activities of precursor cells, differentiation of cells and bone remodelling activities are affected by the RAP (Verna 2016). The RAP can occur after a tooth extraction, fractures and surgical procedures of the alveolar bone, implant placement, in periodontal disease and during orthodontic treatment. In orthodontics, the mechanical stimulus of RAP occurs mainly under specific loading circumstances.

Corticotomy causes an increase in the chemoattractant of macrophages. These macrophages contribute to the early disappearance of the hyaline zone, which leads to acceleration of tooth movement around the corticated alveolar area. In human bones, RAP usually lasts for about 4 to 6 months. Animal studies have shown that the amount of tooth movement doubles during RAP (Li et al. 2018).

Orthodontic tooth movement is seen as a modified skeletal wound healing and adaptation, typified by an increased bone remodelling response in addition to elevated formation of woven bone. Within this principle, RAP has been explored as a means to speed up orthodontic treatment. An intentional surgical injury to the bone starts a cascade of physiological events, leading to an increase in bone turnover with concomitant demineralisation and new bone formation at the site of the bone injury. A few modes of injury have been proposed, from extractions, to corticisions, corticotomies and minimally invasive micro-osteoperforations. Various surgical techniques have shown promising results with regard to the acceleration of tooth movement (Al-Khalifa and Baeshen 2021).

Osteoperforations have been shown to increase osteoclastic activity (Teixeira et al. 2010). The animal study found that the procedure induces inflammatory response with high expressions of cytokines such as markers of lymphocytes (CCL20, CCR1), T cells (LTa, IL-3, CCL5, CCR5, CX3CR1, IL-18rb, IL-1r1), monocytes (IL-1, IL-6, IL-11, IL-18, IL-6ra) and macrophages (IL-1, TNF, IL-6, IL-11, IL-18, IL13ra1, CCL2, CCL9, CCL12, CCR5, IL-6ra) within 24 hours after shallow perforations of the cortical plate in response to orthodontic forces. These cytokines are key mediators for osteoclast recruitment and bone remodelling.

This is supported by systematic reviews, which have found that corticotomy prior to orthodontic treatment accelerates dental movement and reduces treatment time (Fernández-Ferrer et al. 2016). Meanwhile, meta-analysis has shown that, over a short observation, there is no evidence that micro-osteoperforations have a clinically significant effect to accelerate orthodontic tooth movement. However, it remains unclear whether repeated micro-osteoperforations over the entire treatment duration may lead to clinically significantly accelerated orthodontic tooth movement (Sivarajan et al. 2020).

10.6 Root Resorption in Orthodontics

The term orthodontically induced inflammatory root resorption (OIIRR) was based on the observed root resorption (Figure 10.4) resulting from the orthodontic treatment initiated by tooth movement and subsequent inflammation (Brezniak and Wasserstein 2002). Orthodontic tooth movement has been conceptually accepted as a sterile inflammatory process as it involves inflammatory mediators and neurotransmitters such as calcitonin gene-related peptides (CGRP) and substance P (SP) without the manifestation of classic inflammatory responses such as redness, swelling, and heat (Meikle 2006).

Therefore, mechanical forces during orthodontic treatment to stimulate tooth movement can induce resorption of the cemental and dentinal layers of the root tissues. The pathology of root resorption is thought to similarly follow bone resorption process by osteoclasts. The resorbing cells of the root tissues are mainly the odontoclasts, which have similar properties to the osteoclasts.

The incidence of root resorption can be up to 100% (Brezniak and Wasserstein 1993). The prevalence of incisor resorption in adults increases from 15% before orthodontic treatment to 73% after treatment. Prevalence of OIIRR of incisors with moderate to severe resorption increases from 2% before treatment to 24.5% after treatment (Lupi et al. 1996).

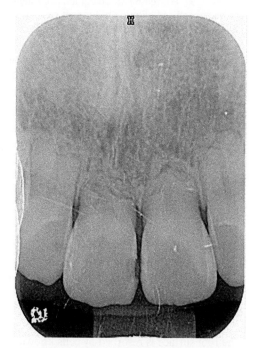

Figure 10.4 Severe root resorption of more than one-third of the original root length. Completely developed roots of the central incisors are usually between two and three times the length of the crown height.

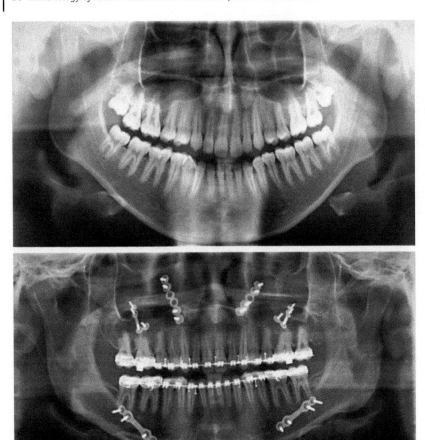

Figure 10.5 Pretreatment radiograph (top) showing fully formed roots with pointed tips. A mid-treatment radiograph (bottom) shows generalised blunting of the root tips due to root resorption. *Source:* Radiographs curtesy of Dr Mohd Zambri Mohamed Makhbul.

Orthodontically induced inflammatory root resorption could progress further if found within the first 6 to 9 months of treatment. Approximately 12% of roots with irregular contour and 38% of roots that had minor resorption detected at 6 to 9 months of treatment would progress to severe resorption at the end of treatment, while 80% of teeth with severe resorption at the initial stages would resorb extremely at the end of orthodontic treatment (Levander et al. 1994). On average, the maximum single root shortening in adolescents is 1.54 (SD = 1.11) mm with 16.5% exhibiting root resorption of more than 2.5 mm (Linge and Linge 1991). In adults, the mean most severely resorbed tooth is 2.99 (SD = 1.43) mm while 40% have resorption of 2.5 mm or more (Mirabella and Artun 1995). Figure 10.5 shows a patient before orthodontic treatment and during fixed appliance therapy.

The degree of root loss is usually transient while for some, there can be blunting of the root apices. The root loss can be detected using radiographs and classified from (i) irregular outline; (ii) loss of up to 2 mm; (iii) loss 2 mm to one-third of the root; (iv) more than one-third of the root loss. In extreme cases, detection of more than one-third root loss can be worrying for the patient (Figure 10.6).

There is still lack of understanding on the immunology that differentiates cellular and tissue responses between orthodontic tooth movement and that which causes root resorption. The next section describes what is currently known about OIIRR.

10.6.1 Mechanism of Root Resorption

The root surface is resorbed by cells known as odontoclasts. Odontoclasts are mono- and multinucleated TRAP-secreting cells located in the resorption lacunae of the root surface (Brudvik and Rygh 1993a; Farrell et al. 1990). Odontoclasts are also be found in the dental pulp of the inner surface of exfoliating teeth and may have ruffled borders towards the dentine surface of the resorption lacunae (Domon et al. 2006).

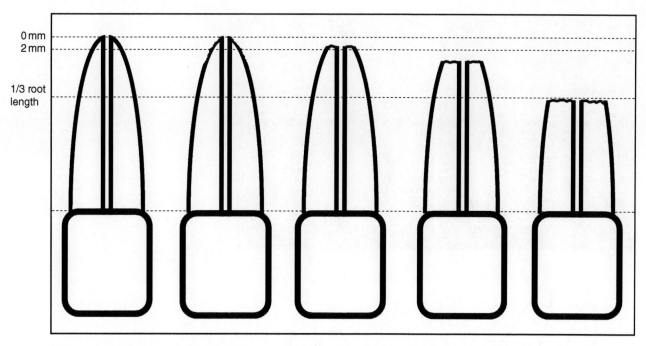

Figure 10.6 Root resorption assessment index by Levander and Malmgren (1988). From left: grade 0 (complete roots), grade 1 (irregular root contour), grade 2 (apical root resorption of less than 2 mm), grade 3 (root resorption between 2 mm up to one-third root length) and grade 4 (root resorption of more than one-third root length).

Odontoclasts are cytochemically similar to osteoclasts as they express similar molecular products. RANKL expression has been detected in odontoclasts and adjacent stromal cells in resorbing root dentine (Sasaki 2003). Precursor cells of osteoclasts and odontoclasts, small osteoclasts and odontoclasts have been found to express cathepsin K and MMP-9 (collagenase B) but large, mature osteoclasts expressed only cathepsin K with significantly less expression of MMP-9. Both osteoclasts and odontoclasts share a common mechanism during the cellular resorption of mineralised tissue (Sasaki 2003). Similar to osteoclasts, odontoclasts were suggested to demineralise the hydroxyapatite crystals of dental hard tissues by H^{+}-ATPase action and degrade the dentine matrix by secretion of proteolytic enzymes.

During orthodontic tooth movement, the biological mechanism by which the tissues discriminate between bone remodelling and root resorption is not fully understood. However, the differences may be in the overexpression of certain signals like caspase-1. When the PDL is compressed, the PDL undergoes ischaemia, increased cAMP and release of pro-inflammatory cytokines (Yan et al. 2009). The fibroblast-like, mononucleated macrophage-like cells and multinucleated giant cells in the PDL are also stimulated to produce a protease known as caspase-1 (Yan et al. 2009). Increased caspase-1 activity intensifies the inflammatory response, in particular the proinflammatory cytokine IL-1-beta to induce odontoclast differentiation, which in turn promotes side-effects such as irreversible root resorption, that results from a local excessive inflammatory response (Yan et al. 2009). Caspase-1 activity can be inhibited by medicines such as pralnacasan and VX-765, which may be useful for avoiding serious root resorption due to the local, excessively severe inflammatory response (Yan et al. 2009).

It has been proposed that the trigger mechanism of external root resorption is a root surface that lacks the protective blastic layer. The lack of protection can be the result of damage to the cementoblastic layer. For resorption to progress, stimuli such as constant application of intense orthodontic force are required and must generate inflammatory changes such as the liberation of prostaglandins and interleukins (Villa et al. 2005). Figure 10.7 is an example of a periodontally compromised case which resulted in overeruption of the central incisors. The intrusion mechanics which caused localised compressive forces on the apices to align the teeth were followed by external root resorption.

Continued progression of root resorption could be influenced by root breakdown products. As odontoclasts dissolve the mineralised tissue of the exposed dentine surface, matrix proteins of the dentine are endocytosed along the ruffled border, transcytosed through the cells and released at the basolateral membrane facing the extracellular space, away from the resorbing surface (Nesbitt and Horton 1997). Molecules released from mineralised tissues such as the bone, cementum and dentine may act as chemotactic and activator signals for cells within the periodontium (Ogata et al. 1997). Dentine extracts

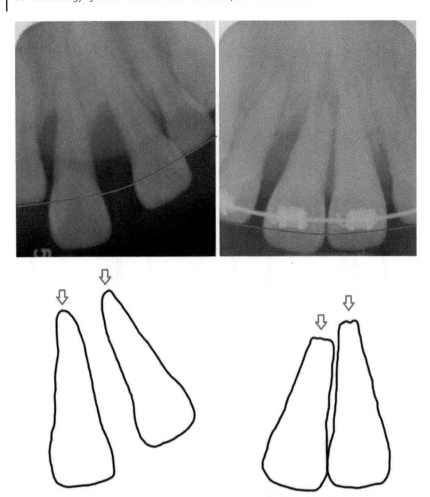

Figure 10.7 Root resorption after fixed appliance therapy. Intraoral radiographs (top) and the outlines (bottom) show overerupted central incisors (left), which had intruded with fixed appliances therapy (right) into the line of the arch (red line). The red arrows show the resorption of the root apices, especially the right incisor which had more resorption from a further movement for intrusion compared to the left incisor. *Source:* Radiographs curtesy of Dr Mohd Zambri Mohamed Makhbul.

such as dentine phosphoprotein (DPP) and dentine sialoprotein (DSP) could induce neutrophil chemotaxis in a time- and dose-dependent manner via the release of inflammatory mediators such as IL-1-beta and TNF-alpha by macrophages (Silva et al. 2004, 2005). It is possible that this in turn could influence the course of root resorption. For example, the released TNF-alpha may induce stimulation of osteoclast cell proliferation and differentiation independent of the RANK-RANKL pathway and in the presence of IL-1-alpha maintain the function of osteoclasts (Kobayashi et al. 2000). Because IL-1-beta could induce RANKL expression on PDL cells, it could therefore also stimulate osteoclastogenesis (Nukaga et al. 2004). Therefore, dentine crude extracts, DPP and DSP may indirectly maintain the function and induce further formation of osteoclast and odontoclast cells, which in turn resorb the mineralised tissues. Indeed, cessation of orthodontic forces would eliminate the inflammatory effects associated with treatment. Figure 10.8 shows a superimposition outline of a patient who had root resorption which stabilised after removal of the orthodontic fixed appliances.

10.6.2 Cellular Response in the Initiation of Root Resorption

Local overcompression of the PDL by orthodontic forces induces the formation of hyalinised zones within the stressed area (Brudvik and Rygh 1993a). Root resorption commences in the periphery of the necrotic hyalinised tissue by the removal of the precementum layer by non-clast fibroblasts and cementoblast-like cells and removal of the mineralised acellular cementum by odontoclast cells. This is followed by root resorption towards the central parts of the hyalinised zone (Brudvik and Rygh, 1993a, 1993b).

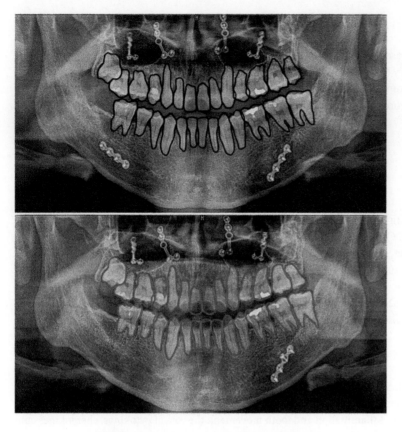

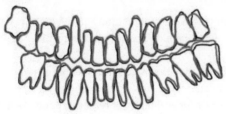

Figure 10.8 Root resorption after prolonged fixed appliance therapy. The radiographs show the outlines of the dentition after debonding and three years of monitoring in a patient who had prolonged fixed appliance therapy and orthognathic surgery. Superimposition of the outlines of the teeth showed no significant root resorption since the orthodontic forces had ceased.

   Beneath the main hyalinised tissue, the majority of cells involved in removal of the necrotic tissue and resorption of superficial cementum are multinucleated giant cells without ruffled borders and mononucleated macrophage-like cells (Brudvik and Rygh, 1994a, 1994b). After much of the hyaline tissue has been removed, odontoclasts actively resorb the root surface, especially near the persisting hyaline layer. Their activity ceases when orthodontic forces are terminated (Brudvik and Rygh 1995).

10.6.3   Metabolic Response in Orthodontically Induced Root Resorption

Since the root tissue does not undergo physiological remodelling, as is seen in bone, loss of dental tissue is an indication of root resorption. The GCF contains an array of cellular and biochemical factors to indicate the metabolic status of the periodontium, which is suitable to detect and quantify amount of tissue destruction (Embery and Waddington 1994) during root resorption. Teeth under orthodontic forces with root resorption secrete proteins such as DPP, DSP and dentine matrix protein-1 (DMP1) (Balducci et al. 2007; Kereshanan et al. 2008; Mah and Prasad 2004; Wan Hassan et al. 2012), that are widely found in dentine (Qin et al. 2002, 2003), indicating pathological root dentine breakdown.

10.7 Conclusion

Orthodontic treatment takes advantage of the aseptic inflammatory response to move the teeth to correct the underlying malocclusion. Understanding this inflammatory behaviour and influence in regulating resorption and repair of the periodontal tissue will thus be key to addressing current aims for clinical improvements such as accelerating orthodontic movement. Nonetheless, this is balanced against continued heavy force that may induce side-effects of excessive immune response to result in root resorption.

References

Aldridge, S.E., Lennard, T.W., Williams, J.R. and Birch, M.A. (2005). Vascular endothelial growth factor acts as an osteolytic factor in breast cancer metastases to bone. *Br. J. Cancer* 92: 1531–1537.

Alhashimi, N., Frithiof, L., Brudvik, P. and Bakhiet, M. (2004). Chemokines are upregulated during orthodontic tooth movement. *J. Interferon Cytokine Res.* 19: 1047–1052.

Alikhani, M., Sangsuwon, C., Alansari, S., Nervina, J.M. and Teixeira, C.C. (2018). Biphasic theory: breakthrough understanding of tooth movement. *J. World Fed. Orthodont.* 7: 82–88.

Al-Khalifa, K.S. and Baeshen, H.A. (2021). Micro-osteoperforations and its effect on the rate of tooth movement: a systematic review. *Eur. J. Dent.* 15: 158–167.

An, S., Zhang, Y., Chen, Q. et al. (2019). Effect of systemic delivery of Substance P on experimental tooth movement in rats. *Am. J. Orthod. Dentofacial Orthop.* 155: 642–649.

Andrade, I. Jr, Silva, T.A., Silva, G.A., Teixeira, A.L. and Teixeira, M.M. (2007). The role of tumor necrosis factor receptor type 1 in orthodontic tooth movement. *J. Dent. Res.* 86: 1089–1094.

Andrade, I., Taddei, S.R.A. and Souza, P.E.A. (2012). Inflammation and tooth movement: the role of cytokines, chemokines, and growth factors. *Semin. Orthodon.* 18: 257–269.

Asiry, M.A. (2018). Biological aspects of orthodontic tooth movement: a review of literature. *Saudi J. Biol. Sci.* 25: 1027–1032.

Assas, B.M., Pennock, J.I. and Miyan, J.A. (2014). Calcitonin gene-related peptide is a key neurotransmitter in the neuro-immune axis. *Front. Neurosci.* 8: 23.

Avery, S.J., Ayre, W.N., Sloan, A.J. and Waddington, R.J. (2020). Interrogating the osteogenic potential of implant surfaces in vitro: a review of current assays. *Tissue Eng. Part B Rev.* 26: 217–229.

Balducci, L., Ramachandran, A., Hao, J. et al. (2007). Biological markers for evaluation of root resorption. *Arch. Oral Biol.* 52: 203–208.

Bartold, P.M., Kylstra, A. and Lawson, R. (1994). Substance P: an immunohistochemical and biochemical study in human gingival tissues. A role for neurogenic inflammation? *J. Periodontol.* 65: 1113–1121.

Bletsa, A., Berggreen, E. and Brudvik, P. (2006). Interleukin-1alpha and tumor necrosis factor-alpha expression during the early phases of orthodontic tooth movement in rats. *Eur. J. Oral Sci.* 114: 423–429.

Boccafoschi, F., Mosca, C., Ramella, M., Valente, G. and Cannas, M. (2013). The effect of mechanical strain on soft (cardiovascular) and hard (bone) tissues: common pathways for different biological outcomes. *Cell Adh. Migr.* 7: 165–173.

Brezniak, N. and Wasserstein, A. (1993). Root resorption after orthodontic treatment: Part 1. Literature review. *Am. J. Orthod. Dentofacial Orthop.* 103: 62–66.

Brezniak, N. and Wasserstein, A. (2002). Orthodontically induced inflammatory root resorption. Part I: The basic science aspects. *Angle Orthod.* 72: 175–179.

Brooks, P.J., Heckler, A.F., Wei, K. and Gong, S.G. (2011). M–CSF accelerates orthodontic tooth movement by targeting preosteoclasts in mice. *Angle Orthod.* 81: 277–283.

Brudvik, P. and Rygh, P. (1993a). The initial phase of orthodontic root resorption incident to local compression of the periodontal ligament. *Eur. J. Orthod.* 15: 249–263.

Brudvik, P. and Rygh, P. (1993b). Non-clast cells start orthodontic root resorption in the periphery of hyalinized zones. *Eur. J. Orthod.* 15: 467–480.

Brudvik, P. and Rygh, P. (1994a). Multi-nucleated cells remove the main hyalinized tissue and start resorption of adjacent root surfaces. *Eur. J. Orthod.* 16: 265–273.

Brudvik, P. and Rygh, P. (1994b). Root resorption beneath the main hyalinized zone. *Eur. J. Orthod.* 16: 249–263.

Brudvik, P. and Rygh, P. (1995). Transition and determinants of orthodontic root resorption-repair sequence. *Eur. J. Orthod.* 17: 177–188.

Capelli, J. Jr, Kantarci, A., Haffajee, A., Teles, R.P., Fidel, R. Jr and Figueredo, C.M. (2011). Matrix metalloproteinases and chemokines in the gingival crevicular fluid during orthodontic tooth movement. *Eur. J. Orthod.* 33: 705–711.

Collins, D.A. and Chambers, T.J. (1992). Prostaglandin E2 promotes osteoclast formation in murine hematopoietic cultures through an action on hematopoietic cells. *J. Bone Miner. Res.* 7: 555–561.

De Jong, T., Bakker, A.D., Everts, V. and Smit, T.H. (2017). The intricate anatomy of the periodontal ligament and its development: lessons for periodontal regeneration. *J. Periodont. Res.* 52: 965–974.

Dimitriou, R., Tsiridis, E. and Giannoudis, P.V. (2005). Current concepts of molecular aspects of bone healing. *Injury* 36: 1392–1404.

Domon, T., Taniguchi, Y., Fukui, A. et al. (2006). Features of the clear zone of odontoclasts in the Chinook salmon (Oncorhynchus tshawytscha). *Anat. Embryol.* 211: 87–93.

Duong, L.T., Lakkakorpi, P., Nakamura, I. and Rodan, G.A. (2000). Integrins and signaling in osteoclast function. *Matrix Biol.* 19: 97–105.

Embery, G. and Waddington, R. (1994). Gingival crevicular fluid: biomarkers of periodontal tissue activity. *Adv. Dent. Res.* 8: 329–336.

Farrell, L., Yen, E., Brudvik, P., Rygh, P. and Suga, D. (1990). Identification of orthodontically induced root resorptive cells using TRAP stain. *J. Dent. Res.* 69: 201.

Fernández-ferrer, L., Montiel-Company, J.M., Candel-Martí, E., Almerich-Silla, J.M., Peñarrocha-Diago, M. and Bellot-Arcís, C. (2016). Corticotomies as a surgical procedure to accelerate tooth movement during orthodontic treatment: a systematic review. *Med. Oral Patol. Oral Cir. Bucal.* 21: e703–e712.

Frost, H.M. (1983). The regional acceleratory phenomenon: a review. *Henry Ford Hosp. Med. J.* 31: 3–9.

Fujihara, S., Yokozeki, M., Oba, Y., Higashibata, Y., Nomura, S. and Moriyama, K. (2006). Function and regulation of osteopontin in response to mechanical stress. *J. Bone Miner. Res.* 21: 956–964.

Fuller, K. and Chambers, T.J. (1989). Effect of arachidonic acid metabolites on bone resorption by isolated rat osteoclasts. *J. Bone Miner. Res.* 4: 209–215.

Garlet, G.P. (2010). Destructive and protective roles of cytokines in periodontitis: a re-appraisal from host defense and tissue destruction viewpoints. *J. Dent. Res.* 89: 1349–1363.

Garlet, T.P., Coelho, U., Silva, J.S. and Garlet, G.P. (2007). Cytokine expression pattern in compression and tension sides of the periodontal ligament during orthodontic tooth movement in humans. *Eur. J. Oral Sci.* 115: 355–362.

Grant, M., Wilson, J., Rock, P. and Chapple, I. (2013). Induction of cytokines, MMP9, TIMPs, RANKL and OPG during orthodontic tooth movement. *Eur. J. Orthod.* 35: 644–651.

Grieve, W.G. 3rd, Johnson, G.K., Moore, R.N., Reinhardt, R.A. and Dubois, L.M. (1994). Prostaglandin E (PGE) and interleukin-1 beta (IL-1 beta) levels in gingival crevicular fluid during human orthodontic tooth movement. *Am. J. Orthod. Dentofacial Orthop.* 105: 369–374.

Gu, Q., Yang, H. and Shi, Q. (2017). Macrophages and bone inflammation. *J. Orthop. Translat.* 10: 86–93.

Guder, C., Gravius, S., Burger, C., Wirtz, D.C. and Schildberg, F.A. (2020). Osteoimmunology: a current update of the interplay between bone and the immune system. *Front. Immunol.* 11: 58.

Guo, D. and Bonewald, L.F. (2009). Advancing our understanding of osteocyte cell biology. *Ther. Adv. Musculoskelet. Dis.* 1: 87–96.

Hakami, Z., Kitaura, H., Kimura, K. et al. (2015). Effect of interleukin-4 on orthodontic tooth movement and associated root resorption. *Eur. J. Orthod.* 37: 87–94.

He, D., Kou, X., Luo, Q. et al. (2015). Enhanced M1/M2 macrophage ratio promotes orthodontic root resorption. *J. Dent. Res.* 94: 129–139.

Hong, H.S., Lee, J., Lee, E. et al. (2009). A new role of substance P as an injury-inducible messenger for mobilization of CD29(+) stromal-like cells. *Nat. Med.* 15: 425–435.

Huang, W., Carlsen, B., Rudkin, G. et al. (2004). Osteopontin is a negative regulator of proliferation and differentiation in MC3T3-E1 pre-osteoblastic cells. *Bone* 34: 799–808.

Iacono, N., Pangrazio, A., Abinun, R. et al. (2013). RANKL cytokine: from pioneer of the osteoimmunology era to cure for a rare disease. *J. Immunol. Res.* 2013: Article ID 412768.

Ishii, T., Ohshima, S., Ishida, T. et al. (2004). Osteopontin as a positive regulator in the osteoclastogenesis of arthritis. *Biochem. Biophys. Res. Commun.* 316: 809–815.

Kaiko, G.E., Horvat, J.C., Beagley, K.W. and Hansbro, P.M. (2008). Immunological decision-making: how does the immune system decide to mount a helper T-cell response? *Immunology* 123: 326–338.

Kaku, M., Niida, S., Kawata, T., Maeda, N. and Tanne, K. 2000. Dose- and time-dependent changes in osteoclast induction after a single injection of vascular endothelial growth factor in osteopetrotic mice. *Biomed. Res.* 21: 67–72.

Kaku, M., Kohno, S., Kawata, T. et al. (2001). Effects of vascular endothelial growth factor on osteoclast induction during tooth movement in mice. *J. Dent. Res.* 80: 1880–1883.

Kaku, M., Motokawa, M., Tohma, Y. et al. (2008). VEGF and M-CSF levels in periodontal tissue during tooth movement. *Biomed. Res.* 29: 181–187.

Kale, S., Kocadereli, I., Atilla, P. and Aşan, E. (2004). Comparison of the effects of 1,25 dihydroxycholecalciferol and prostaglandin E2 on orthodontic tooth movement. *Am. J. Orthod. Dentofacial Orthop.* 125: 607–614.

Kalra, S., Gupta, P., Tripathi, T. and Rai, P. (2020). External apical root resorption in orthodontic patients: molecular and genetic basis. *J. Family Med. Prim. Care* 9: 3872–3882.

Karaduman, B., Uraz, A., Altan, G.N. et al. (2015-. Changes of tumor necrosis factor-α, interleukin-10, and tartrate-resistant acid phosphatase5b in the crevicular fluid in relation to orthodontic movement. *Eur. J. Inflamm.* 13: 3–13.

Kardami, E., Detillieux, K., Ma, X. et al. (2007). Fibroblast growth factor-2 and cardioprotection. *Heart Fail. Rev.* 12: 267–277.

Kato, J., Wakisaka, S. and Kurisu, K. (1996). Immunohistochemical changes in the distribution of nerve fibers in the periodontal ligament during an experimental tooth movement of the rat molar. *Acta Anat.* 157: 53–62.

Kereshanan, S., Stephenson, P. and Waddington, R. (2008). Identification of dentine sialoprotein in gingival crevicular fluid during physiological root resorption and orthodontic tooth movement. *Eur. J. Orthod.* 30: 307–314.

Klein-Nulend, J., Bacabac, R.G. and Bakker, A.D. (2012). Mechanical loading and how it affects bone cells: the role of the osteocyte cytoskeleton in maintaining our skeleton. *Eur. Cell Mater.* 24: 278–291.

Kobayashi, K., Takahashi, N., Jimi, E. et al. (2000). Tumor necrosis factor alpha stimulates osteoclast differentiation by a mechanism independent of the ODF/RANKL-RANK interaction. *J. Exp. Med.* 191: 275–286.

Kohno, T., Matsumoto, Y., Kanno, Z., Warita, H. and Soma, K. (2002). Experimental tooth movement under light orthodontic forces: rates of tooth movement and changes of the periodontium. *J. Orthod.* 29: 129–135.

Komaki, M. (2019). Pericytes in the periodontal ligament. *Adv. Exp. Med. Biol.* 1122: 169–186.

Kouskoura, T., Katsaros, C. and Von Gunten, S. (2017). The potential use of pharmacological agents to modulate orthodontic tooth movement (OTM). *Front. Physiol.* 8: 67.

Koutoulaki, A., Langley, M., Sloan, A.J., Aeschlimann, D. and Wei, X.Q. (2010). TNFalpha and TGF-beta1 influence IL-18-induced IFNgamma production through regulation of IL-18 receptor and T-bet expression. *Cytokine* 49: 177–184.

Krishnan, V. and Davidovitch, Z. (2006). Cellular, molecular, and tissue-level reactions to orthodontic force. *Am. J. Orthod. Dentofacial Orthop.* 129: 469.e1–e32.

Kunii, R., Yamaguchi, M., Tanimoto, Y. et al. (2013). Role of interleukin-6 in orthodontically induced inflammatory root resorption in humans. *Korean J. Orthod.* 43: 294–301.

Lalithapriya, S., Rajasigamani, K. and Bhaskar, V. (2018). Role of interleukin-1 beta in orthodontics. *Int. J. Health Sci. Res.* 8: 270–278.

Leiker, B.J., Nanda, R.S., Currier, G.F., Howes, R.I. and Sinha, P.K. (1995). The effects of exogenous prostaglandins on orthodontic tooth movement in rats. *Am. J. Orthod. Dentofacial Orthop.* 108: 380–388.

Lekic, P.C., Pender, N. and Mcculloch, C.A. (1997). Is fibroblast heterogeneity relevant to the health, diseases, and treatments of periodontal tissues? *Crit. Rev. Oral Biol. Med.* 8: 253–268.

Levander, E. and Malmgren, O. (1988). Evaluation of the risk of root resorption during orthodontic treatment: a study of upper incisors. *Eur. J. Orthodont.* 10 (1): 30–38.

Levander, E., Malmgren, O. and Eliasson, S. (1994). Evaluation of root resorption in relation to two orthodontic treatment regimes. A clinical experimental study. *Eur. J. Orthod.* 16: 223–228.

Levrini, L., Sacerdote, P., Moretti, S., Panzi, S. and Caprioglio, A. (2013). Changes of substance P in the crevicular fluid in relation to orthodontic movement preliminary investigation. *Sci. World J.* 2013: 896874.

Li, M., Zhang, C. and Yang, Y. (2019). Effects of mechanical forces on osteogenesis and osteoclastogenesis in human periodontal ligament fibroblasts: a systematic review of in vitro studies. *Bone Joint Res.* 8: 19–31.

Li, Y., Jacox, L.A., Little, S.H. and Ko, C.C. (2018). Orthodontic tooth movement: the biology and clinical implications. *Kaohsiung J. Med. Sci.* 34: 207–214.

Linge, L. and Linge, B.O. (1991). Patient characteristics and treatment variables associated with apical root resorption during orthodontic treatment. *Am. J. Orthod. Dentofacial Orthop.* 99: 35–43.

Litzenberger, J.B., Kim, J.B., Tummala, P. and Jacobs, C.R. (2010). Beta1 integrins mediate mechanosensitive signaling pathways in osteocytes. *Calcif. Tissue Int.* 86: 325–332.

Loi, F., Córdova, L.A., Pajarinen, J., Lin, T.H., Yao, Z. and Goodman, S.B. (2016). Inflammation, fracture and bone repair. *Bone* 86: 119–130.

Long, H., Wang, Y., Jian, F., Liao, L.N., Yang, X. and Lai, W.L. (2016). Current advances in orthodontic pain. *Int. J. Oral Sci.* 8: 67–75.

Lu, W., Zhang, X., Firth, F. et al. (2019). Sclerostin injection enhances orthodontic tooth movement in rats. *Arch. Oral Biol.* 99: 43–50.

Lund, S.A., Giachelli, C.M. and Scatena, M. (2009). The role of osteopontin in inflammatory processes. *J. Cell Commun. Signal.* 3: 311–322.

Lund, S.A., Wilson, C.L., Raines, E.W., Tang, J., Giachelli, C.M. and Scatena, M. (2013). Osteopontin mediates macrophage chemotaxis via α4 and α9 integrins and survival via the α4 integrin. *J. Cell Biochem.* 114: 1194–1202.

Lupi, J.E., Handelman, C.S. and Sadowsky, C. (1996). Prevalence and severity of apical root resorption and alveolar bone loss in orthodontically treated adults. *Am. J. Orthod. Dentofacial Orthop.* 109: 28–37.

Maggi, C.A. (1997). The effects of tachykinins on inflammatory and immune cells. *Regul. Pept.* 70: 75–90.

Mah, J. and Prasad, N. (2004). Dentine phosphoproteins in gingival crevicular fluid during root resorption. *Eur. J. Orthod.* 26: 25–30.

Maruyama, M., Rhee, C., Utsunomiya, T. et al. (2020). Modulation of the inflammatory response and bone healing. *Front. Endocrinol.* 11: 386.

Mayahara, K., Yamaguchi, A., Takenouchi, H., Kariya, T., Taguchi, H. and Shimizu, N. (2012). Osteoblasts stimulate osteoclastogenesis via RANKL expression more strongly than periodontal ligament cells do in response to PGE(2). *Arch. Oral Biol.* 57: 1377–1384.

McCulloch, C.A. and Knowles, G.C. (1993). Deficiencies in collagen phagocytosis by human fibroblasts in vitro: a mechanism for fibrosis? *J. Cell. Physiol.* 155: 461–471.

McKee, M.D. and Nanci, A. (1996). Osteopontin: an interfacial extracellular matrix protein in mineralized tissues. *Connect. Tissue Res.* 35: 197–205.

Meikle, M.C. (2006). The tissue, cellular, and molecular regulation of orthodontic tooth movement: 100 years after Carl Sandstedt. *Eur. J. Orthod.* 28: 221–240.

Menicanin, D., Bartold, P.M., Zannettino, A.C. and Gronthos, S. (2010). Identification of a common gene expression signature associated with immature clonal mesenchymal cell populations derived from bone marrow and dental tissues. *Stem Cells Dev.* 19: 1501–1510.

Mirabella, A.D. and Artun, J. (1995). Prevalence and severity of apical root resorption of maxillary anterior teeth in adult orthodontic patients. *Eur. J. Orthod.* 17: 93–99.

Monk, A.B., Harrison, J.E., Worthington, H.V. and Teague, A. (2017). Pharmacological interventions for pain relief during orthodontic treatment. *Cochrane Database Syst. Rev.* 11: CD003976.

Murakami, S., Takayama, S., Ikezawa, K. et al. (1999). Regeneration of periodontal tissues by basic fibroblast growth factor. *J. Periodont. Res.* 34: 425–430.

Murshid, S.A. (2017). The role of osteocytes during experimental orthodontic tooth movement: a review. *Arch. Oral Biol.* 73: 25–33.

Nakano, Y., Yamaguchi, M., Shimizu, M. et al. (2015). Interleukin-17 is involved in orthodontically induced inflammatory root resorption in dental pulp cells. *Am. J. Orthod. Dentofacial Orthop.* 148: 302–309.

Nesbitt, S.A. and Horton, M.A. (1997). Trafficking of matrix collagens through bone-resorbing osteoclasts. *Science* 276: 266–269.

Norevall, L.I., Forsgren, S. and Matsson, L. (1995). Expression of neuropeptides (CGRP, substance P) during and after orthodontic tooth movement in the rat. *Eur. J. Orthod.* 17: 311–325.

Nukaga, J., Kobayashi, M., Shinki, T. et al. (2004). Regulatory effects of interleukin-1beta and prostaglandin E2 on expression of receptor activator of nuclear factor-kappaB ligand in human periodontal ligament cells. *J. Periodontol.* 75: 249–259.

O'Connor, T.M., O'Connell, J., O'Brien, D.I., Goode, T., Bredin, C.P. and Shanahan, F. (2004). The role of substance P in inflammatory disease. *J. Cell. Physiol.* 201: 167–180.

Odagaki, N., Ishihara, Y., Wang, Z. et al. (2018). Role of osteocyte-PDL crosstalk in tooth movement via SOST/sclerostin. *J. Dent. Res.* 97: 1374–1382.

Ogata, Y., Niisato, N., Moriwaki, K., Yokota, Y., Furuyama, S. and Sugiya, H. (1997). Cementum, root dentin and bone extracts stimulate chemotactic behavior in cells from periodontal tissue. *Comp. Biochem. Physiol. B Biochem. Mol. Biol.* 116: 359–365.

Overall, C.M., Wrana, J.L. and Sodek, J. (1989). Independent regulation of collagenase, 72-kDa progelatinase, and metalloendoproteinase inhibitor expression in human fibroblasts by transforming growth factor-beta. *J. Biol. Chem.* 264: 1860–1869.

Qin, C., Brunn, J.C., Cadena, E. et al. (2002). The expression of dentin sialophosphoprotein gene in bone. *J. Dent. Res.* 81: 392–394.

Qin, C., Brunn, J.C., Cadena, E., Ridall, A. and Butler, W.T. (2003). Dentin sialoprotein in bone and dentin sialophosphoprotein gene expressed by osteoblasts. *Connect. Tissue Res.* 44 Suppl 1: 179–183.

Rasila, K.K., Burger, R.A., Smith, H., Lee, F.C. and Verschraegen, C. (2005). Angiogenesis in gynecological oncology-mechanism of tumor progression and therapeutic targets. *Int. J. Gynecol. Cancer* 15: 710–726.

Ren, Y. and Vissink, A. (2008). Cytokines in crevicular fluid and orthodontic tooth movement. *Eur. J. Oral Sci.* 116: 89–97.

Sabane, A., Patil, A., Swami, V. and Nagarajan, P. (2016). Biology of tooth movement. *BMJ Med. Res.* 16: 1–10.

Salomão, M.F., Reis, S.R., Vale, V.L., Machado, C.V., Meyer, R. and Nascimento, I.L. (2014). Immunolocalization of FGF-2 and VEGF in rat periodontal ligament during experimental tooth movement. *Dental Press. J. Orthod.* 19: 67–74.

Santoni, G., Perfumi, M.C., Spreghini, E., Romagnoli, S. and Piccoli, M. (1999). Neurokinin type-1 receptor antagonist inhibits enhancement of T cell functions by substance P in normal and neuromanipulated capsaicin-treated rats. *J. Neuroimmunol.* 93: 15–25.

Sasaki, T. (2003). Differentiation and functions of osteoclasts and odontoclasts in mineralized tissue resorption. *Microsc. Res. Tech* 61: 483–495.

Seifi, M., Eslami, B. and Saffar, A.S. (2003). The effect of prostaglandin E2 and calcium gluconate on orthodontic tooth movement and root resorption in rats. *Eur. J. Orthod.* 25: 199–204.

Shapouri-Moghaddam, A., Mohammadian, S., Vazini, H. et al. (2018). Macrophage plasticity, polarization, and function in health and disease. *J. Cell. Physiol.* 233: 6425–6440.

Shetty, N., Patil, A.K., Ganeshkar, S.V. and Hegde, S. (2013). Comparison of the effects of ibuprofen and acetaminophen on PGE2 levels in the GCF during orthodontic tooth movement: a human study. *Prog. Orthod.* 14: 6.

Shu, R., Bai, D., Sheu, T. et al. (2017). Sclerostin promotes bone remodeling in the process of tooth movement. *PLoS One* 12: e0167312.

Silva, T.A., Lara, V.S., Silva, J.S., Garlet, G.P., Butler, W.T. and Cunha, F.Q. (2004). Dentin sialoprotein and phosphoprotein induce neutrophil recruitment: a mechanism dependent on IL-1beta, TNF-beta, and CXC chemokines. *Calcif. Tissue Int.* 74: 532–541.

Silva, T.A., Lara, V.S., Silva, J.S., Oliveira, S,H., Butler, W.T. and Cunha, F.Q. (2005). Macrophages and mast cells control the neutrophil migration induced by dentin proteins. *J. Dent. Res.* 84: 79–83.

Singh, A., Gill, G., Kaur, H., Amhmed, M. and Jakhu, H. (2018). Role of osteopontin in bone remodeling and orthodontic tooth movement: a review. *Prog. Orthod.* 19: 18.

Sivarajan, S., Ringgingon, L.P., Fayed, M.M.S. and Wey, M.C. (2020). The effect of micro-osteoperforations on the rate of orthodontic tooth movement: a systematic review and meta-analysis. *Am. J. Orthod. Dentofacial Orthop.* 157: 290–304.

Sodek, J. (1977). A comparison of the rates of synthesis and turnover of collagen and non-collagen proteins in adult rat periodontal tissues and skin using a microassay. *Arch. Oral Biol.* 22: 655–665.

Taylor, R.M., Kashima, T.G., Knowles, H.J. and Athanasou, N.A. (2012). VEGF, FLT3 ligand, PlGF and HGF can substitute for M-CSF to induce human osteoclast formation: implications for giant cell tumour pathobiology. *Lab. Invest.* 92: 1398–1406.

Teixeira, C.C., Khoo, E., Tran, J. et al. (2010). Cytokine expression and accelerated tooth movement. *J. Dent. Res.* 89: 1135–1141.

Terai, K., Takano-Yamamoto, T., Ohba, Y. et al. (1999). Role of osteopontin in bone remodeling caused by mechanical stress. *J. Bone Miner. Res.* 14: 839–849.

Tsuge, K., Inazumi, T., Shimamoto, A. and Sugimoto, Y. (2019). Molecular mechanisms underlying prostaglandin E2-exacerbated inflammation and immune diseases. *Int. Immunol.* 31: 597–606.

Van der Pauw, M.T., van den Bos, T., Everts, V. and Beertsen, W. (2001). Phagocytosis of fibronectin and collagens type I, III, and V by human gingival and periodontal ligament fibroblasts in vitro. *J. Periodontol.* 72: 1340–1347.

Vandevska-Radunovic, V. and Murison, R. (2010). Emotional stress and orthodontic tooth movement: effects on apical root resorption, tooth movement, and dental tissue expression of interleukin-1 alpha and calcitonin gene-related peptide immunoreactive nerve fibres in rats. *Eur. J. Orthod.* 32: 329–335.

Vandevska-Radunovic, V., Kvinnsland, S. and Kvinnsland, I.H. (1997). Effect of experimental tooth movement on nerve fibres immunoreactive to calcitonin gene-related peptide, protein gene product 9.5, and blood vessel density and distribution in rats. *Eur. J. Orthod.* 19: 517–529.

Van Gastel, J., Teughels, W., Quirynen, M. et al. (2011). Longitudinal changes in gingival crevicular fluid after placement of fixed orthodontic appliances. *Am. J. Orthod. Dentofacial Orthop.* 139: 735–744.

Verna, C. (2016). Regional acceleratory phenomenon. *Front. Oral Biol.* 18: 28–35.

Villa, P.A., Oberti, G., Moncada, C.A. et al. (2005). Pulp-dentine complex changes and root resorption during intrusive orthodontic tooth movement in patients prescribed nabumetone. *J. Endod.* 31: 61–66.

Waddington R.J., Jones, Q. and Moseley, R. (2016). Assessing the potential of mesenchymal stem cells in craniofacial bone repair and regeneration. In: *Tissue Engineering and Regeneration in Dentistry: Current Strategies* (eds R. Waddington and A. Sloan). Chichester: Wiley Blackwell.

Wang, L.L., Zhu, H. and Liang, T. (2000). Changes of transforming growth factor beta 1 in rat periodontal tissue during orthodontic tooth movement. *Chin. J. Dent. Res.* 3: 19–22.

Wan Hassan, W.N., Stephenson, P.A., Waddington, R.J. and Sloan, A.J. (2012). An ex vivo culture model for orthodontically induced root resorption. *J. Dent.* 40: 406–415.

Weitzmann, M.N. (2013). The role of inflammatory cytokines, the RANKL/OPG axis, and the immunoskeletal interface in physiological bone turnover and osteoporosis. *Scientifica* 2013: 125705.

Wrzesinski, S.H., Wan, Y.Y. and Flavell, R.A. (2007). Transforming growth factor-beta and the immune response: implications for anticancer therapy. *Clin. Cancer Res.* 13: 5262–5270.

Wu, M., Chen, G. and Li, Y.P. (2016). TGF-β and BMP signaling in osteoblast, skeletal development, and bone formation, homeostasis and disease. *Bone Res.* 4: 16009.

Yamaguchi, M., Yoshii, M. and Kasai, K. (2006). Relationship between substance P and interleukin-1beta in gingival crevicular fluid during orthodontic tooth movement in adults. *Eur. J. Orthod.* 28: 241–246.

Yamasaki, K., Shibata, Y. and Fukuhara, T. (1982). The effect of prostaglandins on experimental tooth movement in monkeys (Macaca fuscata). *J. Dent. Res.* 61: 1444–1446.

Yamasaki, K., Shibata, Y., Imai, S., Tani, Y., Shibasaki, Y. and Fukuhara, T. (1984). Clinical application of prostaglandin E1 (PGE1) upon orthodontic tooth movement. *Am. J. Orthod.* 85: 508–518.

Yan, X., Chen, J., Hao, Y., Wang, Y. and Zhu, L. (2009). Changes of caspase-1 after the application of orthodontic forces in the periodontal tissues of rats. *Angle Orthod.* 79: 1126–1132.

Yano, S., Mentaverri, R., Kanuparthi, D. et al. (2005). Functional expression of beta-chemokine receptors in osteoblasts: role of regulated upon activation, normal T cell expressed and secreted (RANTES) in osteoblasts and regulation of its secretion by osteoblasts and osteoclasts. *Endocrinology* 146: 2324–2335.

Yao, C. and Narumiya, S. (2019). Prostaglandin-cytokine crosstalk in chronic inflammation. *Br. J. Pharmacol.* 176: 337–354.

Zainal Ariffin, S.H., Yamamoto, Z., Zainol Abidin, I.Z., Megat Abdul Wahab, R. and Zainal Ariffin, Z. (2011). Cellular and molecular changes in orthodontic tooth movement. *Sci. World J.* 11: 1788–1803.

11

Sex Hormone Modulation in Periodontal Inflammation and Healing

Aruni Tilakaratne

Department of Oral Medicine and Periodontology, Faculty of Dental Sciences, University of Peradeniya, Sri Lanka
Department of Restorative Dentistry, Faculty of Dentistry, University of Malaya, Kuala Lumpur, Malaysia

11.1 Periodontal Disease and Its Inflammatory Nature

The hallmark of periodontal disease is initial inflammation of the gingiva following microbial insult by oral micro-organisms which are encased in a well-organised structure called dental plaque biofilm. Initiation of periodontal disease is characterised by episodic bursts of inflammation triggered by micro-organisms in the biofilm. Primarily, periodontal diseases can be categorised into two broad groups: periodontitis and gingivitis.

Inflammation of the gingiva is called gingivitis which is reversible if effective plaque removal is instituted by daily tooth brushing. The clinical features of gingivitis are gingival redness, swelling and bleeding, with notable changes in gingival topography due to altered surface characteristics of the gingiva along with reduced tissue adaptation to the teeth. If gingivitis is unresolved, it may lead to an infection in the deep tooth-supporting tissues.

11.2 Periodontitis

Unresolved gingivitis may result in deep infection in the periodontal supporting tissues, namely the periodontal ligament, cementum and alveolar bone. This infection is called periodontitis and it is usually chronic in nature and characterised by prolonged damage to the tooth-supporting tissues. Periodontitis, characterised by inflammation in deep periodontal structures, may lead to episodic attachment loss of periodontal ligament and alveolar bone. Periodontal attachment loss risks potential tooth loss, if timely interventional measures are not made. Gingivitis may be a prerequisite for periodontitis, although the actual mechanism for transition from gingivitis to periodontitis is yet to be agreed upon.

11.3 Periodontal Treatment and Modulators of Periodontal Healing

The mainstay in controlling gingivitis and periodontitis is mechanical removal of dental plaque biofilm. Effective removal of supragingival plaque reduces the formation of subgingival plaque which appears to play a major role in the progression of disease from gingivitis to periodontitis. The primary aim of periodontal treatment is to control the infection through mechanical debridement methods, thereby to stop the disease progression and enable maintenance of a healthy, functional periodontal support for the tooth. Professional mechanical debridement methods aiming at removal of supra- and deep subgingival biofilm, together with adequate daily plaque removal, are considered standard periodontal therapy. Deep subgingival debridement aims for a significant reduction in total bacterial counts, importantly of pathological micro-organisms.

After the initial phase of plaque control measures, mechanical subgingival debridement involving scaling and root debridement, elimination of plaque-retentive factors followed by surgical methods of treatment for tissue and bone remodelling have provided significant promise that the clinician's main objective of controlling periodontal infection is possible.

However, with a growing body of knowledge regarding the beneficial aspects of sex steroid metabolism on periodontal healing responses, the metabolites of sex hormones are considered as vital and innate biological agents of periodontal healing. This adjunctive role of sex hormones is further established as research provides evidence regarding the ability of oestradiol and progesterone to mediate androgen metabolic responses in human periodontal tissues.

Oestradiol-induced stimulation of production of the potent androgen 5-alpha dihydro-testosterone (DHT) in gingival tissue could indicate a possible mechanism for instigation of repair and healing relevant to the inflamed periodontium. Most research supports the view that androgen metabolic response to oestrogen in the gingiva may contribute to an understanding of repair in gingival tissues. In vitro studies have demonstrated that fibroblasts in gingival tissue could respond to growth factors in a similar manner when incubated with androgen substrates. Other cell types, such as macrophages and platelets found in gingival tissue, could also contribute to this metabolic activity, although these cells constitute a smaller proportion than fibroblasts within gingival tissues.

As a result of sex steroids, periodontal treatment outcomes are improved due to instigated periodontal healing responses mediated via sex steroid metabolic pathways. These healing effects are true for inflamed perodontium in both sexes, since the physiological levels of all the steroid hormones are relevant to both males and females at a cellular level, with variation in the ratios of androgens, oestrogen and progesterone between the two sexes.

11.4 Sex Steroid Hormones in Periodontal Tissues

From a general health perspective, it is well understood that if biological functions in the male are taken as the norm, the female is considered to be exactly the same except for reproductive functions. Given the potential roles of sex hormones in periodontal inflammation and healing, there is a growing need to study the implications of gender differences in periodontal tissues. Although teeth are gender free, the supporting tissues of the periodontium are vulnerable to physiological variations in the levels of circulating steroid hormones in males and females. Thus, the clinical manifestations and severity of periodontal disease may be a reflection of the existing sex hormone profile of an individual.

11.5 Effects of Female Sex Steroids on Periodontal Tissues

The primary female sex hormones which influence the periodontal supporting tissues are oestrogen and progesterone. Both are known to influence the organs and systems in the body. Oestrogens influence cellular differentiation of stratified squamous epithelium and fibrous collagen of connective tissue and are involved in the synthesis and maintenance of collagen. Therefore, the gingival and periodontal supporting tissues which are rich in stratified epithelial cells and fibrous collagenous connective tissue are known target tissues of oestrogen and progesterone.

The two theories that have been brought forward for the actions of oestrogen and progesterone on these cells are altered effectiveness of the epithelial barrier to bacterial insult and the effects on collagen maintenance and repair. Elevated levels of oestrogen and progesterone, particularly during pregnancy, could affect the microvascular system in gingival and periodontal tissues. Such hormonal variations play a significant part in the pathogenic process of periodontal disease. Similarly, other physiological conditions with variations in female sex steroids are evident in puberty, the menstrual cycle and menopause where gingivitis and inflammatory changes in the periodontal supporting tissues have been identified.

11.6 Effects of Male Sex Steroids on Periodontal Tissues

Testosterone is a sex hormone that exhibits many functions beyond reproduction. Like oestrogen, testosterone can exert marked anabolic effects in tissues. It can augment the rate of connective tissue turnover and the osteogenic capacity of the periodontium. It regulates bone metabolism and has biological effects that contribute to repair of connective tissue and bone matrices. Testosterone modulates bone loss, and this action is mediated at least in part through androgen receptor expression. As periodontitis is a microbial-mediated chronic inflammatory disease characterised by overproduction of innate immune cytokines, such as interleukin (IL)-1-beta, IL-6, and tumour necrosis factor (TNF), the exaggerated inflammatory reaction in periodontal tissues can be counteracted by the anabolic responses of testosterone in target tissue.

Functions attributed to androgens are now recognised as partly mediated by oestrogens. The metabolic activities of testosterone occur mainly in fibroblasts and osteoblasts. The matrix repair of gingiva and other periodontal tissues could be attributed to target tissue functions mediated by hormonal metabolic pathways. Many of the effects of oestrogens are seen in the male, as a result of local production of oestrogen. The balance between the actions of androgens and oestrogen is of importance at many oestrogen target sites. Conversion of testosterone into a more potent metabolite, DHT, gives rise to more anabolic responses in target tissues of androgen. Modulation of androgen action by oestrogen with direct effects on target tissue activity has been demonstrated in in vitro studies. This evidence suggests its relevance for reparatory events in the inflamed periodontium in both males and females.

11.7   Effects of Puberty on Periodontal Tissues

Puberty is defined as sexual maturation of an individual with changes in physical appearance and behaviour that are related to rising levels of sex steroid hormones, i.e. testosterone in males and oestradiol in females. Puberty gingivitis is characterised by florid inflammation of gingiva along with interdental papilla. Gingival bleeding is also a cardinal feature in puberty gingivitis. It is widely known that children entering puberty could demonstrate increased gingival inflammation, leading to pubertal gingivitis. The peak ages of pubertal gingivitis are 12–13 years in girls and around 13–14 years in boys.

The increase in gingivitis during puberty has been linked to an alteration of subgingival microbial ecology. *Prevotella intermedia* is a key micro-organism which can utilise oestrogen and progesterone for its growth as a substitute for vitamin K which is an essential growth factor. However, the severity of puberty gingivitis is directly related to the build-up of plaque biofilm and the hormonal influence is only an exaggerating factor.

11.8   Effects of Menstrual Cycle on Periodontal Tissues

The 25–30-day menstrual cycle is controlled by the secretion of sex hormones. It has two phases: the proliferative phase and the secretory phase. The two phases are analogous with pre- and postovulatory events in the ovaries respectively. The proliferative phase is characterised by a gradual increase in the production of oestrogens due to follicular stimulating hormone (FSH) which is a gonadotropin. At ovulation, there is a sudden and marked rise in the production of gonadotropin and oestrogens. Research has found a gradual low-grade increase in gingival exudation in females towards the day of ovulation, while the secretory phase is characterised by a gradual decrease in gingival exudation. In further research evidence, gingival exudate increased by at least 20% during ovulation in about 75% of females. However, it has been noted that during the menstrual cycle of a woman who is free of clinical gingivitis, no increase in gingival exudate was noted whereas in those with clinically evident gingivitis, an increase in gingival exudate was apparent. Therefore, the increased sex hormones during the menstrual cycle appears to modulate the development of localised gingival inflammation. Studies from premenopausal women reveal that an increase in gingival inflammation could be observed around the time of ovulation, even if their plaque scores remained constant throughout the other parts of the menstrual cycle.

In general, it is hypothesised that increased sex hormone levels at different phases of a woman's menstrual cycle could modulate development of localised gingival inflammation. Both oestradiol and progesterone in different concentrations could further mediate inflammatory processes by enhancing production of other inflammatory mediators such as prostaglandins.

11.9   Effects of Pregnancy on Periodontal Tissues and Clinical Manifestations

Pregnancy is accompanied by a significant rise in both oestrogen and progesterone. This is a result of continuous production of the two hormones by the corpus luteum. Peak plasma concentrations of 6 ng/ml for oestrogen and 100 ng/ml for progesterone are evident by the end of the third trimester of pregnancy. The fold increase is 30 for oestrogen and 10- for progesterone when compared with the levels observed during the menstrual cycle.

The most common oral manifestation of elevated levels of gestational hormones is gingivitis. Gingivitis is accompanied by an increase in gingival exudatory fluid, which in turn could alter the characteristic gingival topography seen in healthy gingiva. The resultant gingivitis can be minimised by establishing low plaque levels during pregnancy. The other basic oral changes during pregnancy have been identified as increased levels of oestrogen and progesterone in the saliva, florid and prominent inflammatory features in gingiva and periodontal ligament, high tendency for gingival bleeding and susceptibility to progression of periodontal and oral infections. Susceptibility to infections, especially during the early gestation period, has been attributed to alterations in the immune system due to hormonal changes in pregnancy. Suppression of T-cell activity, decreased neutrophil chemotaxis and phagocytosis, altered lymphocyte response and depressed antibody production have been evident in the early gestation period.

Pregnancy gingivitis is exceedingly common, affecting 30–100% of all pregnant women in different populations. During pregnancy, gingival inflammation increases significantly from the first to the third trimester, with a maximum increase in the second trimester and a decrease after three months post partum.

Pregnancy gingivitis is characterised by an increase in probing depths, bleeding on probing and increased gingival crevicular fluid flow. In addition to the gingival changes seen during pregnancy, about 1–10% of pregnant women may experience localised gingival enlargement consistent with pyogenic granuloma or pregnancy epulis (Figure 11.1). Pregnancy epulis, though benign and generally painless, could pose significant discomfort and interference with function, especially when the epulis is large in size. Pregnancy epulis can present as an exophytic mass that has either a sessile or pedunculated base extending from the gingival margin or the interdental papillae. Pregnancy epulis is usually a result of an exaggerated inflammatory response to factors of irritation such as calculus or ill-contoured tooth restoration. Pregnancy epulis bleeds easily and it may enlarge rapidly up to about 2 cm in diameter, but rarely grows any larger.

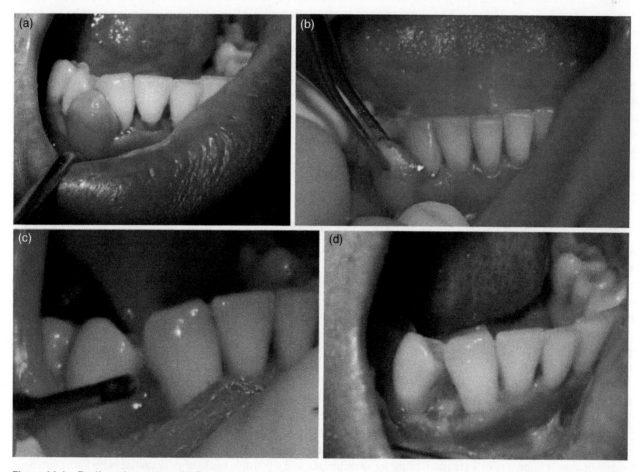

Figure 11.1 Epulis and treatment. (a) Pregnancy epulis. (b) Surgical resection of epulis. (c) Periodontal treatment following surgical resection of epulis. (d) One week following surgical resection of epulis.

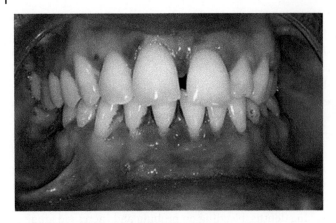

Figure 11.2 Gingival overgrowth (interdental papillae of mandibular incisor region) during hormonal contraceptive therapy.

11.10 Effects of Hormonal Contraceptives on Periodontal Tissues and Clinical Manifestations

Gestational hormones, progesterone and oestrogen are incorporated into oral contraceptive pills. Therefore, hormonal contraceptives resemble a 'false pregnancy' status in terms of the female sex hormone profile. Oral hormonal contraceptives which contain low doses of oestrogen and progesterone are introduced to the body on a daily basis, and the gingival crevicular fluid contains elevated levels of oestrogen and progesterone in hormonal contraceptive users. When in close proximity with microbial colonies, these hormones may act as growth factors, contributing towards an exacerbation of plaque-associated gingivitis. It has also been identified that, similar to that in pregnant women, those on oral hormonal contraceptives could harbour increased counts of specific bacterial species known as key periodontal pathogens which are capable of instigating the inflammatory process.

Oral contraceptives act to establish hormone levels of pregnancy and they may elicit similar clinical effects on tissues. Unlike the effects of pregnancy which last for 40 weeks, the effects of oral contraceptives on the periodontal tissues may last much longer.

During oral contraceptive therapy, exacerbation of inflammatory responses has been reported in the gingival and other periodontal tissues. However, the resultant gingival and periodontal inflammation can be minimised by establishing low plaque levels from the beginning of oral contraceptive therapy. Regular use of contraceptive pills for 12 months could increase the amount of gingival exudate and thereby cause a significant increase in gingival inflammation. Hormonal contraceptive therapy for durations greater than two years has resulted in hyperplastic gingivitis or gingival overgrowth (similar to pregnancy epulis) as well as loss of periodontal attachment (Figure 11.2). Most recently prescribed oral contraceptive pills consist of low doses of oestrogens and progestins, in contrast to early formulations which contained higher concentrations of these hormones. As a result of the new combination in oral contraceptives, if low plaque levels are established and maintained during the period of hormonal contraceptive usage, effects on the periodontium could be minimised.

11.11 Effects of Menopause on Periodontal Tissues and Clinical Manifestations

The menopause, which leads to dwindling levels of ovarian sex steroid hormones, is known to promote significant changes in connective tissue. Although the exact mechanisms for tissue change are not clear, they are thought to be related to the action of oestradiol on the connective tissue. While the menopause causes a wide range of changes in women's bodies, there are important changes in the oral tissues as well. Although elevated levels of ovarian hormones, as seen in pregnancy and oral contraceptive usage, can lead to an increase in gingival inflammation, during the menopause, the absence of ovarian sex steroids has been related to deterioration in gingival health. This suggests a protective effect of ovarian hormones in maintaining gingival and periodontal health. Hormonal replacement therapy is known to help in counteracting the waning protective effects of ovarian hormones and minimising any negative effects on the oral tissues.

Oestrogen deficiency leads to an increase in immune function, which culminates in increased production of TNF by activated T cells. TNF increases osteoclast formation and bone resorption both directly and by augmenting the sensitivity of maturing osteoclasts to the essential osteoclastogenic factor RANKL.

Commonly reported oral manifestations of menopause are dry mouth, thinning or desquamation of the oral and gingival epithelium and gingivitis. Unresolved gingivitis may lead to periodontitis and eventual tooth loss. Oestrogen deficiency in the menopause is known to be a common cause for osteoporosis and a possible cause of periodontal bone loss. Oestrogen plays an important role in the growth and maturation of bone as well as in the regulation of bone turnover in the adult. During bone growth, oestrogen is needed for proper closure of epiphyseal growth plates in both females and males. Oestrogen deficiency has been identified as a possible cause of bone loss and insufficient skeletal development in men. In the young skeleton, oestrogen deficiency leads to increased osteoclast formation and enhanced bone resorption. In the menopause, oestrogen deficiency induces cancellous as well as cortical bone loss. Highly increased bone resorption in cancellous bone leads to general bone loss and destruction of local bone architecture due to penetrative resorption and microfractures.

11.12 Sex Steroid Receptor Expression and Modulatory Effects in Periodontal Tissues

It is well accepted that human gingiva has receptors for oestrogen and progesterone. These receptors provide evidence that the gingiva is a target tissue for both gestational hormones. The expression of androgen receptors has also been detected in a high proportion of periodontal and gingival tissue as well as in fibroblasts derived from the same sources. Androgen receptor expression is an important factor which determines the ability of a cell type to respond to sex steroids.

Evidence from metabolic studies indicates that androgens, oestrogens and progesterone are actively metabolised in the gingival tissues of humans and animals, and the presence of inflammation can increase the level of activity of the enzymes involved in the metabolic conversion of these hormones. Therefore, it is believed that the presence of inflammation may alter the expression of steroid hormone receptors, partly mediated by inflammatory cytokines, which can modulate the metabolism of circulating steroids and their effects on target tissues. The modulatory effects of androgen, oestrogen and progesterone are also known to be instrumental in triggering acute-phase protein turnover characteristic of inflamed tissue. This metabolic activity of testosterone is known to be heightened in inflamed gingival tissue when compared with healthy tissue.

Research studies have revealed that the potent androgen metabolite, DHT and oestradiol-17-beta promote periosteal bone formation in animal models. While androgens, more particularly DHT, and oestradiol demonstrate anabolic responses on tissue matrices, progesterone is considered as a hormone with potential catabolic effects. However, the catabolic effects of progesterone in tissues occur in a dose-dependent manner, where higher concentrations appear to exert catabolic effects. However, physiological concentrations of circulating sex steroids are known to be adequate to influence formation of connective tissue and bone matrices.

11.13 Mechanisms of Action of Sex Steroid Hormones in Periodontal Tissues

11.13.1 Cellular Proliferation

Sex steroid hormones can directly or indirectly influence cellular proliferation, differentiation and growth in target tissues, including keratinocytes and fibroblasts in the gingiva. Two theories regarding the action of sex hormones on cells have been proposed: a possible change in the effectiveness of the epithelial barrier in response to bacterial insult and the effects on collagen maintenance and repair.

Oestradiol can induce cellular proliferation while depressing protein production in cultures of human gingival fibroblasts derived from premenopausal women. The proliferation is believed to be the result of a specific population of cells within the parent culture that responds to physiological concentrations of oestradiol. In contrast to the stimulatory effects of oestrogen on gingival fibroblast proliferation, both collagen and non-collagen protein production is reduced in the presence of physiological concentrations of oestradiol.

11.13.2 Folate Metabolism

Sex steroid hormones have been shown to increase the rate of folate metabolism in oral mucosa. Since folate is required for tissue maintenance, increased metabolism may deplete folate stores and inhibit tissue repair.

11.13.3 Tissue Vasculature

Oestrogen is the main sex steroid hormone responsible for alterations in blood vessels of target tissues in females, stimulating endometrial blood flow during the rise in plasma oestrogen seen in the follicular phase. In contrast, progesterone has been shown to have little effect on the vasculature of systemic target tissues. However, in gingival and other oral soft tissues, there is evidence that progesterone affects the local vasculature more than oestrogen. Progesterone causes increased vascular permeability, resulting in infiltration of polymorphonuclear leucocytes and raised levels of prostaglandin E2 in the crevicular fluid. In addition, it has been shown to reduce corpuscular flow rate, with an influx of inflammatory cells and increase in cell proliferation.

During pregnancy, a slight increase in tooth mobility may be observed. This initial tooth mobility is due to increased vascularisation and vascular volume within the periodontal ligament space. Exposure to high concentrations of female sex hormones for longer periods may result in hyperaemia and increased permeability in the periodontal vascular system. Slight inflammatory oedema in the periodontal ligament space could result in slight extrusion of the tooth, manifested as increased tooth mobility.

11.13.4 Immune Reactivity

Progesterone and oestrogens have been shown to affect the immune system. Human periodontal ligament cells possess immune reactivity towards oestrogen receptors. Although oestrogenic effects in periodontal ligament cells are mediated via oestrogen receptors, no immune reactivity is expressed in these periodontal ligament cells for progesterone receptors. This may imply that progesterone does not have a direct effect on periodontal ligament cell function. Hormone-induced immunological factors and responses can alter antigen expression and presentation, cytokine production, expression of apoptotic factors and cell death. The presence of oestrogen receptors in various immune cells and the presence of androgen receptors in T and B lymphocytes have been demonstrated in animal models.

Experimental evidence suggests that oestrogen prevents bone loss by regulating T-cell function and immune cell–bone interactions. During the menopause, oestrogen deficiency could predispose to bone loss, the mechanism of which remains unclear. However, oestrogen deficiency leads to an increase in immune function, which culminates in an increased production of TNF by activated T cells. TNF increases osteoclast formation and bone resorption both directly and by augmenting the sensitivity of maturing osteoclasts to the essential osteoclastogenic factor RANKL.

Significant progress is being made in understanding the cross-talk between the immune system and bone, and in uncovering the mechanism by which sex steroids, inflammation and infection could lead to bone loss by disrupting the regulation of T-lymphocyte function.

11.13.5 Inflammatory Mediators

Sex steroid hormones appear to modulate the production of cytokines. Progesterone has been shown to downregulate IL-6 production in human gingival fibroblasts. Of the sex steroids, progesterone in particular is known to stimulate production of the inflammatory mediator prostaglandin E2 and enhance accumulation of polymorphonuclear leucocytes in the gingival crevice. Progesterone has also been found to enhance the chemotaxis of polymorphonuclear leucocytes, while low concentrations of oestradiol have been demonstrated to reduce polymorphonuclear leucocyte chemotaxis.

11.13.6 Change in Microbial Ecology

Some micro-organisms, such as *Aggregatibacter actinomycetemcomitans*, *Porphyromonas gingivalis* and *Prevotella intermedia*, are known to synthesise steroid metabolising enzymes required for steroid synthesis and catabolism. Steroid metabolites may supply nutritional requirements for pathogenic micro-organisms. Culture supernatants of these micro-organisms have been shown to enhance the expression of 5-alpha-reductase enzyme activity in human gingiva and in cultured gingival fibroblasts resulting in the formation of DHT from androgen substrates. DHT can influence protein synthetic activity in these pathogens, through a variety of applications such as formation of surface capsular protein which in turn could contribute to evasion of host elimination mechanisms such as phagocytosis.

5-Alpha-reductase activity can be activated in a phospholipidic environment. Increased amounts of phospholipases are synthesised by periodontal pathogens such as spirochaetes. Phospholipase C is released from leucocytes during cell lysis and in addition to degrading gingival crevicular epithelium it is also known to stimulate 5-alpha-reductase enzyme activity.

The ratio of subgingival bacterial anaerobes to aerobes is reported to be increased with high proportions of *Bacteroides melaninogenicus* and *Prevotella intermedia* during pregnancy along with high concentrations of oestradiol and progesterone in plaque samples taken from pregnant women. At the same time, progesterone in the presence of bacterial endotoxins could promote production of prostaglandins which trigger alveolar bone loss. The onset of pregnancy gingivitis appears to coincide with the selective growth of periodontal pathogens such as *Prevotella intermedia* in subgingival plaque from the third to fourth month of pregnancy. However, the overall evidence from experimental studies suggests conflicting results, where some experiments report that pregnancy gingivitis is associated with limited microbial changes, while others report that hormonal changes during pregnancy may result in a more than 50-fold increase in *Bacteroides* species in periodontal samples.

As for hormonal contraceptive use, a significant increase in *Prevotella intermedia* and an increase in the population of *Bacteroides* by several fold has been reported in women using hormonal contraceptives.

11.14   Altered Metabolism of Sex Steroids

High concentrations of progesterone common in late pregnancy could lower the metabolism of progesterone in tissues. The lowered metabolism results in accumulation of high levels of progesterone, which may lead to the characteristic manifestations of pregnancy gingivitis or pregnancy epulis. Although testosterone has to be metabolised to become biologically active, progesterone becomes inactivated through metabolism. In its active form, progesterone stimulates synthesis of prostaglandins, contributing to increased vascular permeability in chronically inflamed periodontal tissues. The catabolic role of progesterone in the presence of plaque-induced inflammation has been well documented.

11.15   Clinical Applications

The clinical situations with altered sex hormone profile are pregnancy, hormonal contraceptive therapy, puberty, menstrual cycle and menopause. There is adequate evidence that altered sex hormone profile could result in changes in clinical periodontal parameters as well as biochemical markers such as inflammatory cytokines in gingival crevicular fluid.

Reinforcement of oral hygiene practices with improved plaque control is a crucial factor in reducing clinical signs of gingivitis and periodontitis. Experimental studies have reported that those who had good plaque control and maintained low plaque scores achieved continued gingival and periodontal health irrespective of the changing sex hormone levels. While most studies have revealed that there is an increasing tendency to periodontal inflammation during the three trimesters of pregnancy, it is apparent that the inflammatory reaction is induced by bacteria in relation to heightened sex hormone load. The overall research evidence supports the view that pregnancy has limited influence on gingival inflammation when good plaque control is maintained, and no change in clinical attachment level was detected during the follow-up periods of study in pregnant women. It is known that increase in periodontal pocket during pregnancy is caused by enlargement of gingival tissue rather than any periodontal destruction, and that long-term inflammatory state of the gingiva is necessary to cause clinical attachment loss.

The basis of hormonal contraceptive therapy is to simulate a pregnancy status to prevent the occurrence of ovulation. Many studies have pointed out that physiological hormonal imbalances could occur during puberty, the menstrual cycle and pregnancy, and these physiological changes are capable of instigating gingivitis, manifested clinically as gingival inflammation, gingival enlargement and bleeding on probing.

Most studies have demonstrated that probing depths and gingival bleeding are increased in women who are on hormonal contraceptive therapy, for around one year. Studies which used matched control groups have demonstrated that women taking hormonal contraceptive pills had similar oral hygiene levels as women who did not. However, a significantly higher level of gingival inflammation was observed in women taking pills. The findings also showed that women who took pills for 2–4 years had higher clinical attachment loss than control subjects. However, most gingival and periodontal changes which are associated with sex hormones are related to gingival hyperplasia or false pocketing, rather than destruction of supporting periodontal tissues.

All forms of mechanical debridement such as scaling and root surface debridement benefit patients and improve their plaque control ability, thereby achieving an improved treatment response during and after periodontal care. Therefore, in the clinical management of patients who are subjected to the influence of variations in sex steroids, the following tenets of care may be recommended.

- Thorough periodontal assessments (both clinical and investigations such as radiographs, while being cautious of safety in individual circumstances).
- Carrying out all preventive care procedures with special emphasis on improvement of daily plaque control.
- Correcting all possible risk factors which may hinder an individual's plaque control ability and subsequent exacerbation of the existing periodontal condition.
- Carrying out all non-surgical treatment procedures which are less invasive based on the individual patient's condition.
- Monitoring progress and planning future care which may include more invasive interventions based on the individual care needs.
- Long-term maintenance to minimise the chances of relapse or recurrence of disease.

11.16 Conclusion

Female sex hormones are neither necessary nor sufficient to produce gingival changes by themselves. However, they may alter gingival and periodontal tissue responses to microbial plaque, thus indirectly contribute to periodontal disease. Instituting proper periodontal care would minimise the occurrence of sex steroid-associated inflammatory periodontal diseases. The most important message for both the clinician and the patient is raising awareness of the link between sex steroids and periodontal health, applying evidence-based knowledge to clinical practice and determining the best approach for clinical care in individual circumstances.

Further Reading

Ali, I., Patthi, B., Singla, A. et al. (2016). Oral health and oral contraceptive. Is it a shadow behind broad daylight? A systematic review. *J. Clin. Diagn. Res.* 10: ZE01–ZE06.

Becerik, S., Ozcaka, O., Nalbantsoy, A. et al. (2010). Effects of menstrual cycle on periodontal health and gingival crevicular fluid markers. *J. Periodontol.* 81 (5): 673–681.

Bhardwaj, A. and Bhardwaj, S.V. (2012). Effects of menopause on women's periodontium. *J. Midlife Health* 3 (1): 5–9.

Domingues, R.S., Ferraz, F.R., Greghi, S.L.A., De Rezende, L.R. and Sant'ana, A.C.P. (2012). Influence of combined oral contraceptives on the periodontal condition. *J. Appl. Oral Sci.* 59 (2): 253–259.

Markou, E., Eleana, B., Lazaros, T. and Antonios, K. (2009). The influence of sex steroid hormones on gingiva of women. *Open Dentist. J.*, 3: 114–119.

Nebel, D. (2012). Review– functional importance of estrogen receptors in the periodontium. *Swedish Dent. J.* 221: 11–66.

Rathore, S., Khuller, N., Dev, Y.P., Singh, P., BaSavaraj, P. and Gera, K. (2015). Effects of scaling and root planing on gingival status during menstrual cycle – a cross-sectional analytical study. *J. Clin. Diagn. Res.* 9 (10): ZC35–ZC39.

Soory, M. (2000). Targets for steroid hormone mediated actions of periodontal pathogens, cytokines and therapeutic agents: some implications on tissue turnover in the periodontium. *Curr. Drug Targets* 1 (4): 309–325.

Steffens, J.P., Coimbra, L.S., Rossa, C., Kantarci, A., Dyke, T.E.V. and Spolidorio, L.C. (2015). Androgen receptors and experimental bone loss – an in vivo and in vitro study. *Bone* 81: 683–690.

Tilakaratne, A. and Soory, M. (2014). Anti-inflammatory actions of adjunctive tetracyclines and other agents in periodontitis and associated comorbidities. *Open Dentist. J.* 8: 109–124.

Tilakaratne, A., Soory, M., Ranasinghe, A.W., Corea, S.M.X., Ekanayake, S.L. and De Silva, M. (2000). Effects of hormonal contraceptives on the periodontium in a rural population of Sri Lankan women. *J. Clin. Periodontol.* 27: 753–757.

Tilakaratne, A., Soory, M., Ranasinghe, A.W., Corea, S.M.X., Ekanayake, S.L. and De Silva, M. (2000). Periodontal disease status during pregnancy and 3-months post-partum in a rural population of Sri Lankan women. *J. Clin. Periodontol.* 27: 787–792.

Wu, M., Chen, S. and Jiang, S. (2015). Relationship between gingival inflammation and pregnancy. *Mediators Inflamm.* 2015: ID 623427.

Wu, M., Chen, S., Su, W. et al. (2016). Sex hormones enhance gingival inflammation without affecting IL-1β and TNF-α in periodontally-healthy women during pregnancy. *Mediators Inflamm.* 2016: ID 4897890.

12

Dental Alloy-associated Innate Immune Response

Dessy Rachmawati[1] and Cornelis J. Kleverlaan[2]

[1] Department of Dental Biomedical Science, Faculty of Dentistry, University of Jember, Jember, Indonesia
[2] Department of Dental Materials Science, Academic Centre for Dentistry Amsterdam (ACTA), Amsterdam, The Netherlands

12.1   Introduction

The number of metals to which humans are exposed has sharply increased during the 20th century. In dentistry, usually alloys are a mixture of two or more metals. Alloying allows for combining different metals in order to get the best properties for particular purposes, e.g. inlays, long span bridges, removable partial denture framework, full denture bases and implants. Pure metals are rarely used in dentistry since these lack sufficient physical and mechanical resistance against masticatory forces. Precious metals such as gold, palladium and platinum have been used for decades in high noble or noble alloys as materials for dental constructions due to their corrosion and tarnish resistance as well as their relatively good biocompatibility (Anusavice et al. 2013).

Classification of dental alloys has recently been renewed after the introduction of titanium (Ti) and Ti alloys (Table 12.1). The latter have been located in between high noble and noble alloys because of their excellent biocompatibility which makes these particularly suitable for dental implants and prostheses (ADA 2003). The costs of such alloys are, however, still relatively high compared to other alloys with similar physical and mechanical properties such as nickel chromium (Ni-Cr) and cobalt chromium (Co-Cr) alloys (Sakaguchi and Powers 2012). The development of these predominantly base metal-based alloys (non-noble or non-precious alloys) has increased in the last twenty years, not only because of cost-effectiveness concerns but also because of the need to develop dental alloys with better physical and mechanical properties (Al-Hiyasat and Darmani 2005).

Base metal alloys contain no or less than 25% noble metal, i.e. gold (Au), silver (Ag), platinum (Pt) and palladium (Pd) (ADA 2003). Compositions have now been defined that make alloys not only cheaper but also corrosion and colour resistant, with hardness and elasticity twice as high as most precious metal alloys. However, the incidence of metal allergies and other side-effects from these alloys is reportedly higher than from noble alloys (Anusavice et al. 2013).

In this chapter, the effects of a broad panel of orally applied metals and alloys on the human immune system are described, with a focus on innate responsiveness and early inflammatory events. Of note, these might eventually facilitate the understanding of allergy and autoimmunity. Knowledge of the relation between oral metal exposure and allergy or autoimmunity are of public health interest and is valuable for our understanding of mechanisms of action of metal immunotoxicity in general. Reviews and research reports on individual metals and their relations to specific allergies and/or autoimmune diseases (AIDs) can be found, but an overview on innate immune responses to clinically relevant transition metals, in particular those neighbouring nickel in the Periodic Table (chromium [Cr], iron [Fe], cobalt [Co], copper [Cu], zinc [Zn], gold [Au], mercury [Hg], palladium [Pd]) (Figure 12.1), is lacking. Here we aim to provide such an overview.

Immunology for Dentistry, First Edition. Edited by Mohammad Tariqur Rahman, Wim Teughels and Richard J. Lamont.
© 2023 John Wiley & Sons Ltd. Published 2023 by John Wiley & Sons Ltd.

Table 12.1 Classification of dental alloys based on ADA classifications (adapted from ADA 2003).

Classification	Composition	Type of alloy	Usage
High noble alloys	≥60% (Au + Pt group[a]) or ≥40% Au	Au-Pt	Metal-ceramic restorations
		Au-Pd	Crowns, bridges
		Au-Cu-Ag	Crowns, bridges
Titanium alloys	≥85% Ti	cpTi (commercial pure titanium)	Implants
		Ti-6A1-4V (Ti alloys)	metal-ceramic FDPs
Noble alloys	≥25% (Au + Pt group[a])	Ag-Au-Cu	Crowns, bridges
		Pd-Cu	Crowns, bridges
		Ag-Pd	Crowns, bridges
Predominantly base alloys	<25% (Au + Pt group[a])	Ni-Cr	Crowns, bridges, orthod. braces
		Co-Cr	Crowns, bridges
		Stainless steel	Paediatric crowns, orthod. braces

[a] Pt group: platinum, palladium, rhodium, iridium, osmium and ruthenium.

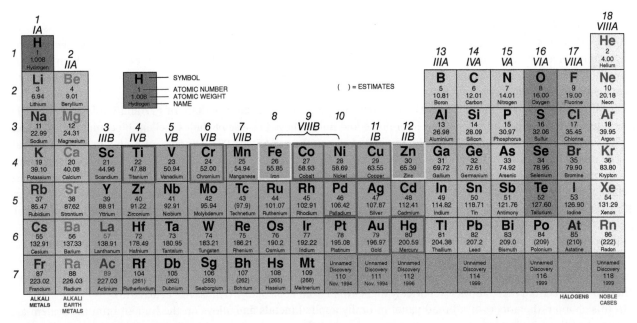

Figure 12.1 Periodic Table of Elements. Metals shown in boxes are commonly used in dentistry. The red outlines show the metals which are known as sensitisers whereas the yellow ones show non-allergenic metals.

12.2 Metals and Their Application in Dental Alloys

Most elements in the middle part of the Periodic Table (Figure 12.1) are metals, which in dentistry are frequently alloyed together for many purposes, such as fillings, posts/cores, crowns, bridges and orthodontic devices. Thus, more than 25 elements in the Periodic Table are used in dental alloys, but the most prominent metals are Ti, Cr, Fe, Co, Ni, Cu, Zn, Pd, Au and Hg (Wataha 2000).

Each metal has its own role, e.g. adding hardness, corrosion resistance, etc. when alloyed with other metals to create dental constructions. Whereas nickel has been recognised as an important sensitiser for many decades, the neighbouring elements have notorious health effects, e.g. cobalt, palladium and, to a lesser extent, copper (Fage et al. 2014; Yoshihisa et al. 2015). Interestingly, other metals, e.g. Zn, Fe, are known as typical non-sensitisers. The sensitising level of metals depends on many factors such as their capacity to associate with proteins, i.e. their chemical characteristics and at the other end the available T-cell repertoire in the host (Esser et al. 2014). In recent years the importance of their capacity to trigger early, innate immune responsiveness has become clear (Martin 2015). Here, general properties of the selected metal panel are outlined first, after which immunological aspects will be addressed.

Titanium (Ti) is a noble metal. Titanium and titanium alloys, in line with their physical and chemical properties, are clinically suitable for dental implants and prostheses. Due to their biocompatibility, mechanical properties and corrosion resistance, Ti alloys are widely accepted as a material for endosseous implant devices, crown and bridge prostheses. However, careful selection of processing methods and laboratory skills are required to guarantee success because titanium is a very hard metal. Ti is generally considered as 'biologically inert' although recent research has shown that Ti-based implants undergo biocorrosion and release metal ions and particles into surrounding tissues. Indeed, potential immuno-toxicological reactions to Ti have received increasing attention (ADA 2003; Hosoki et al. 2009; Anusavice et al. 2013; Syed et al. 2015).

Chromium (Cr) is widely used in dentistry since it increases the strength of the alloy product, adds durability against corrosion and oxidation, and acts in combination with carbon (about 0.1%) as a hardener. It is usually alloyed together with Ni and/or Co to produce a good quality of alloy. On the other hand, Cr is also known as the most frequent metal sensitiser, after nickel and cobalt (Thyssen and Menne 2010; Yoshihisa and Shimizu 2012). Sensitisation is mostly caused by trivalent (3+) metal ions, which can arise from both metallic and hexavalent (6+) chromium by oxidation and reduction processes, respectively. Chromium is a commonly used in metal industries and its protein-binding capacity is still exploited in third-world leather industries.

Iron (Fe) is an essential micronutrient, vital to metabolically active and proliferating cells. It functions as an oxygen carrier, an electron acceptor and donor and as a co-factor for several enzymes. In the oral cavity, Fe is mostly used in gold-platinum-based porcelain fused to metal (PFM) alloys. It is used as a strengthener and promotes formation of a porcelain-bonding oxide layer. Importantly, its application in stainless steel alloys is rapidly on the rise. Stainless steel alloys are composed of iron, carbon, chromium, nickel, manganese and other metals. The term 'stainless steel' is used when the chromium contents exceeds 11% (usually a range of 12–30%). Little is known about the possible effects of Fe exposure on allergy and autoimmunity.

Cobalt (Co) is, like iron, abundantly found in soil, dust and sea water. In dentistry, cobalt has been alloyed with Cr since the 1920s, resulting in lower costs and better mechanical and physical properties. This alloy is still commonly used in metal-ceramic crowns and partial denture frameworks. Its immunotoxicological disrepute connects to that of nickel. Contact with cobalt can result in allergic reactions involving cobalt-specific allergic contact dermatitis next to irritant dermatitis. Nevertheless, allergic reactions to Co alloys may not only be caused by cobalt sensitisation since these alloys almost always also contain nickel and/or chromium.

Nickel (Ni) is a very important transition element essential for many dental alloys. Nickel-based (non-precious) alloys are used in the dental industry for all types of restorative work (fillings, crowns, bridges, partial dentures) and orthodontic appliances (wires, bands, brackets, etc.). Nowadays, nickel is still being used in dentistry for several reasons, e.g. corrosion resistance and low cost. Small amounts of nickel improve gold hardness. It is used in dental constructions ranging from a few percent to over 50%. The use of nickel casting alloys for long-term restorations in dentistry has long been controversial since nickel is considered the most frequent metal sensitiser in humans (Rustemeyer and Frosch 2000). In sensitised individuals, a low dose of nickel (about 300 µg or 10 µM) is able to induce skin inflammatory reactions (Spiewak et al. 2007).

Copper (Cu) is an essential nutrient that in living matter occurs in two oxidation states: cuprous ($Cu1^+$) and cupric ($Cu2^+$) ions. Cu is found in various kinds of food and in drinking water. In dentistry, it is used mostly in crowns and bridges together with gold. Its main role is hardening and strengthening the alloy. In one review, it was concluded that copper is a relatively weak sensitiser compared to other metals, although in some individuals it may provoke severe allergic reactions (Fage et al. 2014). Since copper can cross-react with nickel (Pistoor et al. 1995), it is still unknown to what extent it can act as a sensitiser on its own.

Zinc (Zn) Similar to Fe and Cu, Zn is an essential micronutrient, with known functions in several parts of the immune system. In dentistry, it is used in crown and bridge alloys, predominantly as an oxygen scavenger. It excludes oxygen and prevents gas porosity during the casting process. It also has a role in hardening and strengthening the alloy. In PFM, zinc also lowers the melting range, increases strength and hardness, and raises the thermal expansion. Zinc plays a central role in the immune system as an essential micronutrient for both cellular and humoral immune responses. It is known as a non-sensitiser, although one severe case of systemic contact dermatitis was reported due to zinc-containing dental fillings (Yoshihisa et al. 2015). Such sensitising capacity, however, still needs to be confirmed.

Palladium (Pd) is also a noble metal and belongs to the platinum group of metals (PGMs) which have similar chemical and physical properties. Exposure to Pd occurs through dental appliances, jewellery, food, inhalation and in some regions through mining pollution. In dentistry, Pd has been used widely as a substitute for platinum and gold. It is hard, very strong, white and has a high melting point. It has a very high modulus of elasticity and is also known to provide corrosion resistance. Therefore, Pd is increasingly used for alloying with Au as they complement each other. However, Pd is also increasingly observed to cause sensitisation, up to 10% among the general population in several studies (Hosoki et al. 2009; Faurschou et al. 2011; Muris et al. 2015). Pd is clearly an important sensitiser on its own, but sensitisation rates are increased further due to its cross-reactivity with Ni (Pistoor et al. 1995; Muris et al. 2015).

Gold (Au) is a precious, noble metal, one of the oldest dental restorative materials and still used for crowns by dentists today. It was assumed to be inert, resisting corrosion. However, it is now known that gold can cause immunotoxicological reactions including sensitisation and allergic reactivity (Moller 2002; Nonaka et al. 2003). Au is soft, ductile and yellow coloured with a low melting point. Thus, the pure metal lacks adequate strength to stand up to the forces generated in the oral cavity. It cannot be bonded to porcelain. Therefore it should first be alloyed with other metals.

Mercury (Hg) has been widely used in dentistry for more than 150 years, due to low cost, ease of application, ideal mechanical properties and durability in the oral cavity. Despite reduced use of mercury in dental applications, the release of inorganic Hg from dental amalgam is still the most important source of Hg exposure in the Western world. Allergic reactions to amalgam fillings are rare but widely confirmed (Schmalz 2002; Aminzadeh and Etminan 2007; Anusavice et al. 2013; Bergdahl et al. 2013; Syed et al. 2015). For several decades possible immunotoxicities of mercury have received much attention, although it is still not clear whether it is causing allergy, toxicity and/or autoimmunity. Of all Hg exposures, the safety of Hg in amalgam dental restorations has especially received much attention in the scientific literature as well as politics and lay press. Notably, in a study on Swedish women, of the total blood Hg, 25% was inorganic, correlating with the number of amalgam fillings, and 75% was organic, correlating with fish consumption (Oskarsson et al. 1996).

12.3 Metal Ion Release from Dental Alloys

Dental alloys for dental prostheses have been routinely used in clinical dentistry since the 1800s. Compared to more recently introduced dental materials, e.g. ceramics, composites and polymers, metals provide superior mechanical and physical properties characterised by high strength, ductility, hardness and fracture toughness, needed to withstand chewing stress in the oral cavity (Upadhyay et al. 2006). Next to mechanical properties, patient safety is a critical factor since dental alloys interact for prolonged times with oral mucosa tissues (periodontal tissues, gingival and alveolar bone) which provide a wet environment facilitating metal ion release (Wataha 2000; Schmalz 2002; Elshahawy et al. 2009). Metal ion release is facilitated by corrosion which is defined as the gradual destruction of materials (usually metals) by chemical reaction with their environment, e.g. oxygen. Corrosion degrades the useful properties of materials and structures, including strength and appearance, and can be concentrated locally to form pits or crevices. Since corrosion may cause adverse effects, knowledge of the biocompatibility of alloys is of great importance to avoid health problems (Elshahawy et al. 2009; Muris et al. 2014).

Noble metal-based alloys have the longest history of use in dentistry. High noble and noble alloys, in particular gold, platinum and palladium, were increasingly used because of their physical and mechanical properties. As a most precious metal, gold was assumed to be relatively inert, resisting corrosion. However, pure gold is weak and therefore needs to be alloyed with other metals. Indeed, mixing gold with copper and other less noble metals resulted in strong, effective filling, crown or bridge alloys. Metal ion release from these alloys remains low and adverse reactions to noble alloys are infrequent. Nevertheless, gold-allergic symptoms have been reported both in patients with contact dermatitis and in those with oral disease (Kanerva et al. 2001; Nonaka et al. 2003; Khamaysi et al. 2006; Ditrichova et al. 2007; Davis et al. 2011; Steele et al. 2012; Kim et al. 2015).

Due to the dramatic increase in the price of gold, base metal alloys were introduced for dental constructions in the early 1930s. They have largely replaced the noble metal-based alloys for dental prostheses (Nelson et al. 1999; Wataha 2000; Anusavice et al. 2013). When compared with high noble/noble alloys, base metal alloys perform even better as to physical and mechanical properties, e.g. high modulus of elasticity which allows thinner metals to be used, and thus minimal tooth destructions during preparation of crown/bridge prostheses (Roach et al. 2000).

Alloying conditions and compositions have been explored intensively over recent decades and were optimised for minimal metal leakage and maximal physico-mechanical properties (Lin et al. 2008; Ma and Wu 2011). Nevertheless, doubts remain as to the biocompatibility of the base metal alloys such as Ni-Cr and Co-Cr which tend to have more elevated corrosion rates than the noble alloys. Leakage of metal ions from base metal alloys is also strongly facilitated by handling of the alloys during processing such as casting, heat treatment and porcelain firing. In particular, recasting of alloys was found to be related to increased metal release. Recasting alloys has been introduced to decrease costs, and involves combining previously cast metal parts, e.g. previously melted buttons or sprues removed from casting process, with up to 50% new metal (Al-Hiyasat and Darmani 2005; Imirzalioglu et al. 2012). Microstructural changes can affect the development of protective surface oxides, altering the corrosion behaviour of these alloys (Qiu et al. 2011). In brief, base metal alloys are cheap but more difficult to handle and susceptible to corrosion.

Metal release from dental alloys can be tested by classic chemical methods or modern atomic spectroscopic techniques such as inductively coupled plasma mass spectroscopy (ICP-MS) (Milheiro et al. 2015). In vitro, basic measurements are usually made with alloy specimens in water, culture media or artificial saliva. Virtually all dental mental alloys tested show distinct release rates of metals, generally in the nanogram to microgram range per cm^2 exposed surface area per day (Table 12.2). As expected, different alloy types show markedly different release rates, whereas these rates are not simply correlated with the composition of the alloys (Schmalz et al. 1999; Dimic et al. 2014). Moreover, extrinsic factors can increase release rates substantially. In particular, low pH values as frequently found in saliva have been shown to accelerate metal release (Dimic et al. 2014).

The biological response to released metal ions does not simply depend on their concentrations but also on the duration of exposure and susceptibility of the host cells (Wataha 2000; Schmalz 2002). Studies on tissue–dental alloy interactions therefore involve in vitro testing with culture systems utilising primary cells or cell lines. Here, the most frequently used assays are based on cytotoxicity measurements. Of course, in vivo studies may provide the most useful data but require appropriate animal models or trial conditions in a clinical setting. Apparently, few animal models have been found of use (mouse, guinea pig, rat) in this regard, whereas important clinical data on metal release rates have become available. Here, measurements have focused on saliva, blood and urine (Sicilia et al. 2008; Elshahawy et al. 2013; Matusiewicz 2014). Also biopsies have been studied from gingival tissues adjacent to metallic restorations showing accumulation of metals in the neighbouring tissues (Garhammer et al. 2003).

Comparing metal ion release from dental alloys in vitro and in vivo is difficult since huge variations are found in reported metal ion release data. Clinical variations are most probably due to the fact that numerous factors can affect release, such as conditions in the oral cavity created by temperature, pH, saliva, exogenous agents like tobacco and alcohol, ongoing immune reactions, combined presence of different metals as well as the shape and surface treatment of the dental alloys. Also micro-organisms or bacterial factors can provide important contributions to corrosion of dental metal alloys. Bacteria inhabit all structures of the oral cavity and easily adhere to alloys (Subramani et al. 2009). On the surfaces of metallic materials, they may alter interfacial electrochemical processes, which can lead to increased corrosion and release of small metal particles or metal salts (Chaturvedi 2013). In addition to this plethora of extrinsic factors, personal individual factors, e.g. dietary habits and life style (Chaturvedi 2009; Mikulewicz et al. 2015), may determine reactions to released metals.

In our studies, 125 to 750 µM for most metals and 250 to 750 nM for Hg were found as optimal concentration in triggering innate immune responses in vitro. Thus, the amounts of metal ion released from dental appliances in the oral cavity and subsequently absorbed in the gastrointestinal tract are very small. Still, several secondary factors may facilitate the development of systemic complaints (Wataha et al. 2013; Yu et al. 2015). Apparently the wide range of extrinsic factors can act synergistically by enhancing corrosion and metal ion leakage resulting in locally and possibly systemically health-disturbing metal exposure. Whether this leads to substantial local irritancy and/or systemic allergic reactivity may depend on other co-factors, notably concomitant microbial pressure by oral bacteria (de Kivit et al. 2014). Moreover, while the release of metal ions may be subliminal, it should be realised that it often continues for months or years (Wataha et al. 1999).

Table 12.2 Reported metal ion release in vitro/in vivo from dental alloys.

| Type of alloy | | Methods and conditions of exposure[a] | | | Release/day | | | Reference[b] |
	(name/brand)	Device/specimen quantification	Fluid volume	Duration	μg/cm²	Ppb (μg/l)	nM	
Ti	Ti-6Al-4V (Zimmer®)	dental implant Ø 22 × 2mm	MEM 100 ml	28 days	<<	<<	<<	(Höhn and Virtanen 2015)
	Ti (Ormco®)	20 orthodontic brackets 4 buccal molar tubes (in vitro)	MEM 30 ml	30 days	NA	0.18	3.73	(Ortiz et al. 2011)
Cr	Stainless steel (Ultraminitrim®, Dentaurum®)	20 orthodontic brackets 4 molar tubes (in vitro)	MEM 30 ml	30 days	NA	0.3	5.76	(Ortiz et al. 2011)
	Ni-Cr (Remanium CS®)	cast alloy specimen Ø 5 × 3 mm (in vitro)	AS 11.5 ml	60 days	0.0001	0.01	0.192	(Oyar et al. 2014)
	Ni-Cr (Vera Bond II®)	cast alloy specimen + electrolysis 40 × 20 × 3 mm (in vitro)	AS 50 ml	2 days	0.085	33.25	639.42	(Galo et al. 2012)
	Co-Cr-Mo (Wironit®)	cast alloy specimen Ø 8 × 3.2mm (in vitro)	AS pH 7.5 ǀ AS pH 4 5 ml	6 weeks	0.036 0.042	13.09 15.47	251.73 297.5	(Dimic et al. 2014)
	Co-Cr (Remanium)	cast alloy specimen + electrolysis 40 × 20 × 3 mm (in vitro)	AS 50 ml	2 days	0.5	18.95	364.5	(Galo et al. 2012)
	Stainless steel (Preform® arch wires, Ortho-Organizers®)	orthodontic wire 0.017 × 0.025 inch 100 mm length (in vitro)	As 100 ml	28 days	0.018	0.39	7.57	(Gopikrishnan et al. 2015)
	Stainless steel (American Orthodontics, 3M Unitek)	2 orthodontic wires 20 orthodontic brackets 2 ligatures (in vitro)	AS 0.5 ml/min 19.41 L (flow)	28 days	NA	0.01	0.192	(Mikulewicz et al. 2014)
Co	Stainless steel (Ultraminitrim, Dentaurum)	20 orthodontic brackets 4 molar tubes (in vitro)	MEM 30 ml	30 days	NA	0.05	0.84	(Ortiz et al. 2011)
	Co-Cr-Mo (Wironit)	cast alloy specimen Ø 8 × 3.2 mm (in vitro)	AS pH 7.5 ǀ AS pH4 5 ml	6 weeks	0.04 0.096	15 34.76	254.23 589.12	(Dimic et al. 2014)
	Co-Cr (Remanium)	cast alloy specimen + electrolysis 40 × 20 × 3 mm (in vitro)	AS 50 ml	2 days	0.01	4.65	78.81	(Galo et al. 2012)
Ni	Ni-Cr (Remanium CS)	cast alloy specimen Ø 5 × 3 mm (in vitro)	AS 11.5 ml	60 days	0.004	0.35	5.93	(Oyar et al. 2014)
	Stainless steel (Ultraminitrim, Dentaurum)	20 orthodontic brackets 4 molar tubes (in vitro)	MEM 30 ml	30 days	NA	13.9	231.66	(Ortiz et al. 2011)
	Ni-Cr (Remanium CS)	cast alloy specimen Ø 5 × 3.2 mm (in vitro)	AS 11.5 ml	60 days	0.018	1.38	23	(Oyar et al. 2014)

Element	Material	Specimen	Medium	Duration				Reference
	Ni-Cr (Vera Bond II)	cast alloy specimen + electrolysis 40 × 20 × 3 mm (in vitro)	AS 50 ml	2 days	0.265	103.5	1.75	(Galo et al. 2012)
	Stainless steel (Preform arch wires, Ortho-Organizers)	orthodontic wire 0.017 × 0.025 inch 100 mm length (in vitro)	AS 100 ml	28 days	0.01	0.21	3.5	(Gopikrishnan et al. 2015)
	Stainless steel (American Orthodontics, 3M Unitek)	2 orthodontic wires 20 ortho brackets 2 ligatures (in vitro)	AS (0.5 ml/min) 19.41 L	28 days	NA	0.035	0.58	(Mikulewicz et al. 2014)
Cu	Stainless steel (American Orthodontics, 3M Unitek)	2 orthodontic wires 20 ortho brackets 2 ligatures (in vitro)	AS (0.5 ml/min) 19.41 L	28 days	NA	0.057	0.904	(Mikulewicz et al. 2014)
	Pd-Cu (Orion Vesta®)	cast alloy specimen 2.06 cm² (in vitro)	lactic acid/NaCl; pH 2.3 | 5 ml	7 days	0.37	149.71	2376	(Milheiro et al. 2016)
	Pd-Ag (Orion Argos®)	cast alloy specimen 2.06 cm² (in vitro)	lactic acid/NaCl; pH 2.3 | 5 ml	7 days	0.007	2.86	45.39	(Milheiro et al. 2016)
	Amalgam (Tytin®)	discs Ø 10 × 2 mm (in vitro)	0% H_2O_2 | 1% H_2O_2 20 ml	24 hrs	0.003 / 0.016	0.38 / 1.73	6.03 / 27.46	(Al-Salehi et al. 2007)
Zn	Type IV Au	dental crown (in vivo)	Saliva 2 ml	3 months	NA	0.022	0.349	(Elshahawy et al. 2013)
	Au-Pt based (a.o. Biocclus 4®)	cast alloy specimen plate 10 × 10 × 0.5 mm (in vitro)	H_2O Sprite light®; pH 2.8 20 ml	2 hrs	0.366 / 2.0	40.3 / 220	610.6 / 3330	(Johnson et al. 2010)
Pd	Type IV Au	dental crown (in vivo)	Saliva 2 ml	3 months	NA	3.42	51.81	(Elshahawy et al. 2013)
	Pd-Cu (Orion Vesta)	cast alloy specimen 2.06 cm² (in vitro)	lactic acid/NaCl; pH 2.3 | 5 ml	7 days	0.096	39.43	371.98	(Milheiro et al. 2016)
	Pd-Ag (Orion Argos)	cast alloy specimen 2.06 cm² (in vitro)	lactic acid/NaCl; pH 2.3 | 5 ml	7 days	0.047	19.43	183.3	(Milheiro et al. 2016)
Au	Type IV Au	dental crown (in vivo)	Saliva | 2 ml	3 months	NA	0.022	0.207	(Elshahawy et al. 2013)
	Au-Pt based (Biocclus 4®)	cast alloy specimen 10 × 10 × 0.5 mm (in vitro)	H_2O Sprite light®; pH 2.8 | 20 ml	2 hrs	0.009 / 0.068	0.95 / 7.5	4.84 / 38.26	(Johnson et al. 2010)
Hg	Type IV Au	dental crown (in vivo)	Saliva | 2 ml	3 months	NA	0.022	0.112	(Elshahawy et al. 2013)
	Amalgam (Tytin)	discs (in vitro) Ø 10 × 2 mm	0% H_2O_2 / 1% H_2O_2	24 hrs	0.0008 / 0.14	0.11 / 15	0.54 / 74.63	(Al-Salehi et al. 2007)
	Amalgam	dental filling (in vivo)	Urine	5 years	NA	0.44	2.19	(Dunn et al. 2008)

[a] Unless otherwise stated, experiments were performed with polished alloys, at 37°, and at a neutral pH.

[b] References published from 2005 to 2015.

<, not detectable; A, artificial saliva; MEM, minimal essential medium; NA, cannot be calculated or not applicable.

12.4 Local and Systemic Adverse Reactivity to Metal Alloys

Despite the fact that the gastrointestinal tract is known as a tolerogenic entry route for foreign proteins and chemicals, oral exposure to dental alloys has often been associated with local or even systemic adverse reactions. The release of metal ions from dental alloys may be slow but is in fact unstoppable. Depending on their concentration, metal ions can have toxic, inflammatory, allergenic or even mutagenic effects. Out of these, metal allergies with oral and/or distant lesions are the most well known. The precise pathogenesis of the adverse reactions to metals is, however, often unclear since systemic complaints may be highly unspecific and interpretation of oral lesions is not always easy. In the following paragraphs local and systemic adverse reactions will be described in more detail.

12.4.1 Local Adverse Reactions (Table 12.3)

Table 12.3 Oral problems associated with dental metal alloys.

No	Material	Principal elements	Usage	Oral symptoms	Reference
1	Titanium alloys: Ti-Al-V Ti-Al-Nb	± Ti 6%, Al 4–7%, 4% V, 0.25% Fe, 0.3% O	All metal prostheses, metal-ceramic prostheses, denture frameworks	Allergy, CFS, headache, PGCG	(Sicilia et al. 2008; Penarrocha-Diago et al. 2012; Brown et al. 2015)
2	Ni-Cr alloys: Ni-Cr-Mo-Be Ni-Cr-Mo	± Ni 62%, Cr 19.1%, Mo 7.1%, Ga 2%	All metal prostheses, metal-ceramic prostheses, denture frameworks	Allergy, AID, burning mouth, cheilitis and perioral dermatitis, CSF, gingivitis, OLP, orofacial granulomatosis, stomatitis	(Sterzl et al. 1999; Khamaysi et al. 2006; Torgerson et al. 2007; Stejskal 2014)
3	Co-Cr alloy: Co-Cr-Mo	± Co 63%, Cr 27%, Mo 6%, Other 4%	All metal prostheses, metal-ceramic prostheses, denture frameworks	Allergy, burning mouth, cheilitis and perioral dermatitis, orofacial granulomatosis, OLL/OLP	(Khamaysi et al. 2006; Torgerson et al. 2007)
4	Palladium alloys: Pd-Cu-Ga Pd-Ag-Ga	± Pd 75–61%, Cu 7%, Ag 24–66% In 6.3%, Ga 6%, Ru<1%	Metal-ceramic prostheses	Allergy, burning mouth, cheilitis and perioral dermatitis, gingivitis, NPG, OLL/OLP	(Koch and Bahmer 1999; Torgerson et al. 2007; Muris et al. 2015)
5	Stainless steel	± Ni 13–15.5%, Cr 17–19%, Mo 2–4%	Paediatric crown, orthodontic braces	Allergy, angular cheilitis, burning sensation, numbness, NPGP, papular perioral rash, stomatitis from mild to severe, erythema	(Rahilly and Price 2003; Genelhu et al. 2005; Kolokitha and Chatzistavrou 2009; Chakravarthi et al. 2012)
6	Amalgam	± Hg (50%), Ag (~22–32%), tin (14%), cu (8%), and other trace metals	Fillings	Allergy, AID, burning mouth, cheilitis and perioral dermatitis, CFS, dry mouth, fibromyalgia Headache, dizziness, OLP, OLL, stomatitis	(Koch and Bahmer 1999; Sterzl et al. 1999; Dunsche et al. 2003; Khamaysi et al. 2006; McParland and Warnakulasuriya 2012; Stejskal 2014)
7	Gold alloy Au-Ag-Pd Au-Pd-Cu-Ag	± Au 45–86%, Pd 3–38%, Pt 11.5–12%, Cu 25–10%, Ag 15–14%, Zn 1.6 %, In, Rh, Fe each <1%	All metal prostheses, metal-ceramic prostheses, denture frameworks	Allergy, burning mouth, cheilitis and perioral dermatitis, fibromyalgia, gingivitis, OLP, OLL, orofacial granulomatosis, stomatitis	(Koch and Bahmer 1999; Khamaysi et al. 2006; Torgerson et al. 2007; Stejskal 2014; Muris et al. 2015)

CFS, chronic fatigue syndrome; OLP/OLL, oral lichen planus/oral lichenoid lesions; NPG, non-plaque-related gingivitis; PGCG, peripheral giant cell granuloma.

12.4.1.1 Oral Lichen(oid) Lesions

Oral lichen(oid) lesions are common in the general population, with a prevalence of 1–2% (Bouquot and Gorlin 1986). They are often observed in association with oral metal exposure, e.g. to amalgam, Au or Pd (Laeijendecker and Van 1994; Koch and Bahmer 1999; Ahlgren et al. 2002; Moller 2002; Laeijendecker et al. 2004). In that case, lesions are mostly unilateral, non-symmetrical and localised on the palate, buccal mucosa or tongue where the lining mucosa comes into contact with restorations. These lesions are referred to as oral lichenoid lesions (OLL). Oral lichen planus (OLP), on the other hand, is putatively caused by an autoimmune reaction involving keratinocytes as the target. The lesions are usually symmetrical and systemic manifestations may also occur (Thornhill et al. 2003; Cawson and Odell 2008). However, the clinical and histopathological aspects of OLP and OLL are indistinguishable, showing a variable clinical presentation with white reticular lesions, patches, papules, erosion or ulceration and, when biopsied, dense T-cell infiltrates in the oral mucosa underlying the lesions.

Although a substantial part of the lichenoid lesions is caused by allergy to dental materials (Cawson and Odell 2008), the pathogenesis of the majority of lichenoid reactions, even if a putative triggering agent has been identified, is not fully understood. It is plausible that direct immunotoxicity of dentally applied alloys causing local irritant inflammatory reactions plays an important role (Muris et al. 2014).

Most clinicians do not discriminate between OLP and OLL. In cases of persistent complaints, replacing restorations adjacent to the lesion is needed to achieve lesion resolution. In addition, patch tests are the gold standard to diagnose possible involvement of allergy (Thornhill et al. 2003; Issa et al. 2005). The potential premalignant character of metal allergic mucositis is a recent finding (Hougeir et al. 2006; Ismail et al. 2007; van der Meij et al. 2007) and stresses the importance of careful diagnostics and follow-up of patients with such lesions (Ditrichova et al. 2007).

12.4.1.2 Gingivitis/Perioral Lesions

Typical signs of gingivitis/perioral lesions are redness and swelling that may involve any part of the mouth including the tongue, roof of the mouth, cheeks and lips (cheilitis). There is occasional formation of blisters and/or ulcers. Affected individuals may complain of a burning sensation and mouth sensitivity on consumption of or exposure to food, drugs and other substances (such as metals). These reversible conditions and symptoms resolve once the cause is removed (Dunsche et al. 2003; Ditrichova et al. 2007; Torgerson et al. 2007).

12.4.1.3 Metal-specific Allergy

The most common local adverse reaction to metal exposure is metal-specific hypersensitivity. This allergy to metals is usually of the delayed type (type IV in the classification by Gell and Coombs). It is called 'delayed' because when metals are applied to the skin of allergic persons, as is done in the diagnostic patch test, the skin becomes red, indurated and inflamed for 24–48 hours, normalising after 3–4 days. Based on such patch test reactivity, the dermatologist will diagnose the patient as being allergic to a certain metal or chemical.

This type of reactivity is most relevant for the dental clinic, since exposure via the oral mucosa should be considered as a challenge of allergic responsiveness. Oral application of Ni-containing constructions in a Ni-allergic individual may thus cause local inflammation in and around the oral mucosa but, interestingly, also flaring of former reaction sites even at a distance, e.g. flare of former hand eczema (Feilzer et al. 2013).

Allergy to orally applied metals such as Ni, Co and Cr is well known, while other metals like gold and palladium have attracted attention as important allergens, in particular in patients with oral adverse reactions (Nonaka et al. 2003; Muris et al. 2014). Some other metals (e.g. Zn, Fe) are not known as contact allergens. Table 12.4 shows the frequency of metal allergies in patients with oral disease. Of the metals tested, Ni, Cr and Au cause most frequently positive reactions in this population (up to 58.5%, 29% and 38.1% respectively). Khamaysi et al. (2006) examined 134 patients who were patch tested with a dental screen, and evaluated the extent to which the clinical manifestations (perioral reactions, burning mouth, OLL and other oral complaints) correlated with the allergens for which the patients had positive patch tests. However, no obvious association was found between clinical presentation and particular allergens.

Important for the diagnostic and therapeutic work-up of a patient with adverse skin reactions possibly related to dentally applied alloys is a detailed anamnesis, with focus on allergic reactions and metal exposure, followed by skin testing. Knowledge of the composition of the suspected alloy is essential in this process (Muris and Feilzer 2006). In vitro assays with blood samples have been introduced but although they might add an objective parameter for sensitisation in difficult cases, their sensitivity and specificity are still inferior compared to skin testing (Menne 1981; Skoglund 1994; Rustemeyer et al. 2004).

Table 12.4 The frequency of metal allergy in the population with oral disease.[a]

Metal	Frequency	Median frequency	Reference
Ti	– 0% (0/151)[b]	1.1%	(Torgerson et al. 2007)
	– 2.2% (2/92)		(Davis et al. 2011)
Cr	– 29% (9/31)	13.85%	(Minang et al. 2006)
	– 3.2% (1/183)		(Ditrichova et al. 2007)
	– 0.5% (1/182)		(Torgerson et al. 2007)
	– 10.7% (3/28)		(Steele et al. 2012)
	– 17% (85/500)		(Davis et al. 2011)
	– 22.7% (10/44)		(Kim et al. 2015)
Co	– 38.7% (12/31)	10.2%	(Minang et al. 2006)
	– 4.9% (6/121)		(Khamaysi et al. 2006)
	– 9.7% (3/183)		(Ditrichova et al. 2007)
	– 5.2% (16/307)		(Torgerson et al. 2007)
	– 9.5% (88/931)		(Nonaka et al. 2011)
	– 10.7 (3/28)		(Steele et al. 2012)
	– 14.9% (143/959)		(Davis et al. 2011)
	– 15.9% (7/44)		(Kim et al. 2015)
Ni	– 54.8% (19/31)	19.8%	(Minang et al. 2006)
	– 13.2% (16/121)		(Khamaysi et al. 2006)
	– 12.9% (4/183)		(Ditrichova et al. 2007)
	– 12.5% (40/320)		(Torgerson et al. 2007)
	– 58.5% (148/253)		(Nonaka et al. 2011)
	– 28.6% (8/28)		(Steele et al. 2012)
	– 14.6% (243/1693)		(Kanerva et al. 2001)
	– 25% (11/44)		(Kim et al. 2015)
Cu	– 3.6% (1/28)	3.53%	(Steele et al. 2012)
	– 3.53% (94/2660)		(Wohrl et al. 2001)
	– 0.2% (6/2611)		(Kanerva et al. 2001)
Zn	– 0% (0/903)	0.6%	(Kanerva et al. 2001)
	– 0.6% (1/180)		(Torgerson et al. 2007)
	– 3.5% (34/963)		(Davis et al. 2011)
Pd	– 4.2% (107/2405)	9.7%	(Kanerva et al. 2001)
	– 7.4% (9/121)		(Khamaysi et al. 2006)
	– 12.9% (4/183)		(Ditrichova et al. 2007)
	– 9.7% (19/196)		(Torgerson et al. 2007)
	– 35% (7/25)		(Muris et al. 2015)
	– 25% (7/28)		(Steele et al. 2012)
	– 6.8% (3/44)		(Kim et al. 2015)
Au	– 7.7% (345/4508)	12.8%	(Kanerva et al. 2001)
	– 14% (17/121)		(Khamaysi et al. 2006)
	– 6.4% (2/183)		(Ditrichova et al. 2007)
	– 11.6% (34/293)		(Torgerson et al. 2007)
	– 38.1% (21/55)		(Nonaka et al. 2011)
	– 28.6% (8/28)		(Steele et al. 2012)
	– 28% (306/1092)		(Davis et al. 2011)
	– 4.5% (2/44)		(Kim et al. 2015)
Hg	– 8.9% (139/1568)	9.7%	(Kanerva et al. 2001)
	– 10% (12/121)		(Khamaysi et al. 2006)
	– 19.3% (6/183)		(Ditrichova et al. 2007)
	– 2% (4/198)		(Torgerson et al. 2007)
	– 20.4% (11/54)		(Nonaka et al. 2011)
	– 10.7% (3/28)		(Steele et al. 2012)
	– 9.4% (104/1103)		(Davis et al. 2011)
	– 4.5% (2/44)		(Kim et al. 2015)

[a] Reports on patch testing of major types of metals from dental alloys; the list may not be exhaustive.
[b] Positive patch tests/total patients tested.

12.4.2 Systemic Adverse Reactions (Figure 12.2)

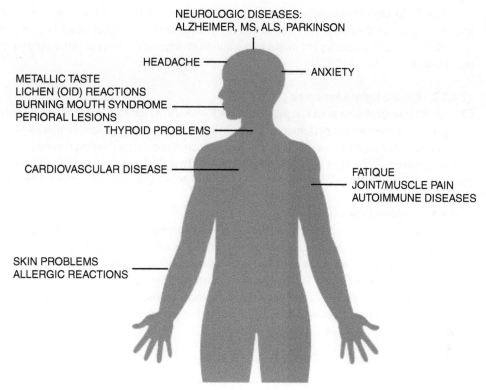

Figure 12.2 Clinical symptoms that can manifest in different organs of the body that could be linked to dental alloys.

NEUROLOGIC DISEASES:
ALZHEIMER, MS, ALS, PARKINSON

HEADACHE

ANXIETY

METALLIC TASTE
LICHEN (OID) REACTIONS
BURNING MOUTH SYNDROME
PERIORAL LESIONS
THYROID PROBLEMS

CARDIOVASCULAR DISEASE

FATIQUE
JOINT/MUSCLE PAIN
AUTOIMMUNE DISEASES

SKIN PROBLEMS
ALLERGIC REACTIONS

12.4.2.1 Autoimmune Diseases

Genetic and environmental factors play a role in the pathogenesis of AID. Metal exposure could be considered as one of the latter. Still, robust pathogenic studies have mainly been performed in animal models whereas in humans, much controversy exists about the role of metal exposure in the development of autoimmunity.

Several studies suggest a causal relation between exposure to transition metals and autoimmune manifestations in the skin, oral cavity, joints, brain and thyroid gland. Affected individuals may display multiple subjective symptoms associated with several organ systems, the most common being fatigue, fibromyalgia, dizziness and headache. Intraoral symptoms include burning sensations, taste disturbances and dry mouth (Carocci et al. 2014; Giacoppo et al. 2014; Stejskal 2014).

A direct causative role of metal exposure in the development of AID is, however, difficult to prove. Most studies are epidemiological, relating metal exposure to the frequency of, often subjective, AID manifestations. Hg and Ni exposure were thus considered as potential risk factors for fatigue and autoimmunity (Sterzl et al. 1999). Also Pd has been associated with systemic complaints, such as chronic fatigue and urine Pd levels with thyroid disease (Helm 2002; Torgerson et al. 2007; Muris et al. 2015). A pathogenic role of amalgam in AID is similarly controversial, and a meta-analysis on multiple sclerosis (Aminzadeh and Etminan 2007) was not conclusive. Still, some indirect evidence for involvement of metal exposure in autoimmune manifestations is available, since removal of metal constructions may reportedly improve subjective and incidentally objective autoimmune manifestations (Langworth et al. 2002; Lygre et al. 2003; Sjursen et al. 2015).

12.4.2.2 Neurotoxicity

For many years, neurotoxic effects such as headache, anxiety and disorientation have been ascribed to metal exposure. Metals may also be involved in the pathogenesis of neurodegenerative diseases (Alzheimer, Parkinson, amyotrophic lateral sclerosis and multiple sclerosis), since Mg, Al, Cd, Co, Cu, Zn and Pb levels were all found to be increased in the CSF of these patients compared to blood plasma, indicating mechanisms of accumulation (Roos et al. 2013). Exactly how the entrance and accumulation of the different metal ions into the central nervous system is effected still needs to be elucidated (Modgil et al. 2014). Nevertheless, hypothetically, the development of neurodegenerative diseases could be facilitated by augmented metal release from dental alloys in the oral cavity with metals reaching the brain and causing activation of brain microglia cells.

To date, little attention has been given to the effects on human brain of the combination of bacteria or bacterial products and metal alloys in the oral cavity. Interaction between bacteria and metal alloys not only facilitates corrosion of the latter and subsequent metal release, but might also result in synergy at the level of inflammation induction, as described in more detail below.

12.4.2.3 Chronic Fatigue Syndrome

Chronic fatigue syndrome is an idiopathic disease for which, as for most other idiopathic illnesses, such as autism or fibromyalgia, many theories are presented to explain the pathogenesis. Exposure to metals is one of the factors which may be involved. Chronic mercury toxicity is one of the most common factors believed to be a cause of, or contributor to, chronic fatigue syndrome (Sterzl et al. 1999; Stejskal 2014). Besides Hg exposure, Cd and Ni have been associated with this syndrome (Sterzl et al. 1999; Pacini et al. 2012; Stejskal 2014), but conclusive studies are still lacking.

12.4.2.4 Cardiovascular Disease

The risk of cardiovascular disease was studied in Swedish women in relation to mercury exposure from amalgam and fish consumption. Interestingly, increased blood levels of Hg predicted a low risk of death and myocardial infarction (Bergdahl et al. 2013). Blood Cd levels, on the other hand, turned out to correlate with the incidence of heart failure in another Swedish study (Borne et al. 2015). The risk of exposure to other metals for developing cardiovascular disease was reviewed by Hampel et al. (2015). They concluded that long-term exposure to transition metals, due to air pollution or industrial contacts, may result in increased systemic inflammation, eventually facilitating cardiovascular events.

12.5 Immunological Aspects of Oral Metal Exposure

12.5.1 Oral Immune Responses to Metals

Many different substances and micro-organisms enter the body via the oral cavity. Only a minority of these are pathogenic and should be prevented from outgrowth and invasion. This is a delicate job for the immune system, which on one hand has to be very sensitive to recognise all pathogens that can inflict harm; on the other hand, when the immune system is too sensitive, it will see harmless substances like metals as foreign, resulting in allergy, or see self antigens as pathogens, resulting in autoimmune disease.

Metal alloys in the oral cavity constantly interact with the environment, resulting in continuous release of metal ions, contacting the mucosal epithelium and the oral mucosa-associated immune system. Generally, oral antigen contact, in contrast to skin contact, will lead to immunological tolerance: thus, nickel-containing braces were shown to reduce the risk of developing Ni allergy later in life (van Hoogstraten et al. 1991). However, adverse immunological effects of oral metal exposure can occur due to local conditions or previous sensitising skin contacts. These vary from direct immunotoxicity to metal-specific allergy and possibly autoimmune disease.

The immune response is classically divided into innate and adaptive immunity. The innate immune system provides a fast, unspecific defence mechanism, but cannot always eliminate infectious organisms. The lymphocytes of the adaptive immune system provide a more specific defence and, in addition, create a specific amplification memory so that subsequent exposure to the same pathogens can be handled more efficiently. The two key features of the adaptive immune response are thus specificity and memory. The innate and adaptive immune systems work together at all levels of the immune response. As outlined below, many metals can evoke both innate and adaptive immune responses.

12.5.2 Innate Immune Response to Metals

Innate immunity is the body's first line of protection against potential microbial, viral and environmental attacks, whereas the skin and oral mucosa provide the most powerful barriers that we rely on to stay well. In the oral cavity, saliva, containing mucus, enzymes and various antibacterial agents, covers the mucosal epithelium and thus contributes largely to this barrier function. Other cellular components of the innate immunity include phagocytes, e.g. neutrophils and monocytes/macrophages, dendritic cells, mast cells, basophils, eosinophils and natural killer cells. They all 'sense' pathogens by distinct receptors and contribute to elimination of the pathogen.

The key molecular players in innate immunity are the pattern recognition receptors (PRRs) that recognise molecules broadly shared by pathogens, the so-called pattern-associated molecular patterns (PAMPs). Activation of PRR signalling pathways triggers the nuclear translocation of various transcription factors, including NF-kappa-B, AP-1, IRFs and C/EBP-beta. This leads to the production of inflammatory mediators to co-ordinate the elimination of pathogens and infected cells. PRRs include Toll-like receptors (TLRs), C-type lectin receptors (CLRs) and intracellular nucleotide-binding and oligomerisation domain (NOD)-like receptors (NLRs). In addition, there are retinoid acid-inducible gene I (RIG-I)-like receptors (RLRs) and other, not yet grouped receptors like the cytosolic nucleic acid sensors AIM2 (absent in melanoma 2) and DAI (DNA-dependent activator of INF regulatory factors) (Murphy 2012).

Chemicals are extremely diverse in the mechanisms that facilitate and trigger immune responses. The capacity of metals to trigger the innate immune system was first reported by Schmidt et al. (2010) for Ni. They showed that Ni ions could trigger innate immune responses in humans via TLR4 binding, the receptor for bacterial lipopolysaccharide (LPS). An additional paper (Raghavan et al. 2012) showed that Co could also trigger TLR4. Little is still known about other dental metals and about potential triggering of other PRRs by metals.

The first cells in the oral cavity that come into contact with micro-organisms are the keratinocytes. Keratinocytes (KCs) express TLRs, thus providing a first layer of defence in skin and mucosa (Baker et al. 2003; Mempel et al. 2003). Accumulation of metal ions from alloys in oral tissues might thus affect the keratinocytes and induce the release of inflammatory mediators. It is, however, still not known how mucosal keratinocytes differ from skin keratinocytes with respect to functional TLR expression. In the skin, KCs are known to play a role in all phases of allergic contact dermatitis, from the early initiation phase with the elaboration of inflammatory cytokines, that play a role in Langerhans cell (LC) migration and T-cell trafficking, through the height of the inflammatory phase with direct interactions with epidermotrophic T cells, to the resolution phase of allergic contact dermatitis with the production of anti-inflammatory cytokines and regulatory antigen presentation to effector T cells (Gober and Gaspari 2008; Kosten et al. 2015).

The dendritic cells (DCs) reside in between the epithelial cells as a network, ready to pick up potential antigens. They need 'danger signals', such as PAMPs, to be mobilised and become fully active by maturation. While maturing, the DCs migrate to the draining lymph nodes (LNs), where they present the peptides derived from pathogens or from metal–protein complexes to specific T cells. One of the cytokines most abundantly produced by DCs upon stimulation is interleukin (IL)-8. In vitro, IL-8 is secreted by DCs in response to allergens and not irritants (Toebak et al. 2006). IL-8 is a chemokine which attracts neutrophils and naive T cells. IL-8 release is widely used as a biomarker for the NF-kappa-B pathway. To induce accurate and efficient pathogen-specific immunity, DCs adjust their immune response to the type of pathogen. Importantly, the profile of innate PRR signalling largely determines the quality of the DCs and thus the type of subsequent adaptive immune response.

Microglia are the resident innate cells of the brain, derived from monocytes early in development, and make up approximately 10% of the white matter. In contrast to the short half-life of macrophages, microglia can remain for a lifetime. They clear the brain of debris after neurological injury and are readily activated by pathogens. Like DCs, they express PRRs like TLRs and also bear MHC class II (Arroyo et al. 2011), enabling them to function as antigen-presenting cells (APCs) (Kettenmann et al. 2013). The mRNA of TLR 1-9 has been found to be present in human microglia, and at the protein level, the presence of TLR 2, 3 and 4 has been demonstrated (Gambuzza et al. 2014; Das et al. 2015). When the microglia cells are stimulated, they release matrix metalloproteinases, reactive oxygen species and other inflammatory factors (Kauppinen et al. 2008), such as IL-8.

The activation of microglia is advantageous under most circumstances. However, if they are overactivated, they can damage host tissue, thereby promoting neural death in both cerebral ischaemia and neurodegenerative disorders (Klegeris et al. 2007; Kauppinen et al. 2008; Amor et al. 2014). Hypothetically, the development of neurodegenerative disease such as ALS could thus be facilitated by metal release from dental material in the oral cavity (Mou et al. 2012; Roos et al. 2013).

12.5.3 Adaptive Immune Response to Metals

Metal ions, like low molecular weight organic chemicals, have to be protein reactive to become immunogenic and evoke adaptive immune responses. Since metals are too small to function as haptens themselves, covalent bonding with cellular and matrix proteins, containing preferably cysteine (Cys) and histidine (His) residues, creates epitopes that can be recognised by T cells. Such epitopes will thus always consist partly of self molecules. To become fully immunogenic, the free metal ions and/or metal-containing complexes should also provide innate immune danger signals to the PRR of the APCs, leading to local production of proinflammatory cytokines that induce DC maturation and mobilisation to the draining lymph nodes. Here, the metal (containing complex) is presented by APCs in combination with HLA class I or II molecules to metal-specific T-cells (Figure 12.3).

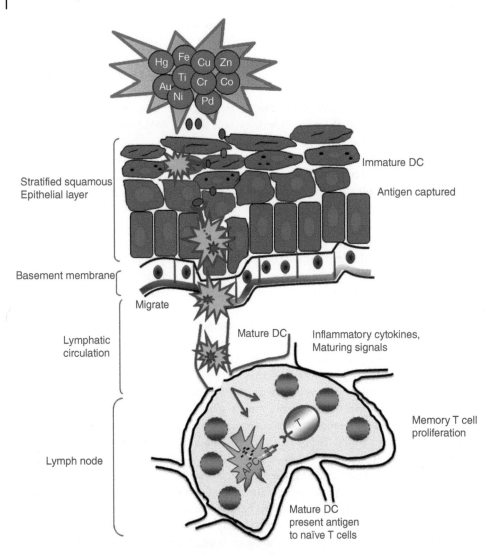

Figure 12.3 Innate activation by metals resulting in an adaptive immune response.

Specificity is one of the key features of adaptive immunity and is mediated by T cells. B cells and antibodies are adapted to recognition of more foreign molecules, e.g. containing unusual sugar residues as present in bacteria, and do not seem to play a role in metal-specific immune responses. If the TCR of a certain T cell recognises metal-modified peptides on the surface of APCs, the T cell can respond with clonal expansion and cytokine production (Figure 12.4) (Rudolph et al. 2006; Stockinger et al. 2006).

The initiation of a primary T-cell response, i.e. triggering of naive T cells, depends on co-stimulatory signals given by the APC. These involve both cytokine production and expression of surface adhesion molecules, upregulated during maturation, and enable a close, stimulatory contact between APCs and specific T cells. The character of the resulting T-cell response (inflammatory or regulatory, mucosa or skin seeking) depends on these co-stimulatory signals as well as on the local microenvironment in the lymph node where sensitisation takes place.

Once naive T cells have been triggered and expanded, memory T cells are generated and released into the circulation. As a consequence, the frequency of metal-specific memory T cells in the blood will increase; the individual is now 'sensitised' or 'hypersensitive' and will respond promptly with the production of inflammatory mediators upon all further metal contacts. Such allergic reactions can be elicited in the skin but may also take place in the oral mucosa of sensitised patients. Upon contact with the relevant metal, T lymphocytes induce an inflammatory response causing tissue damage, seen as contact dermatitis or mucositis, i.e. intraoral diffuse, red zones, blisters or ulceration with pain and burning sensation.

Metal hypersensitivity nowadays is diagnosed by epicutaneous patch testing with a panel of potentially relevant metal salts in non-toxic concentrations. Skin reactions are read after 48 and 72 hours, since T-cell-mediated reactions, visible in

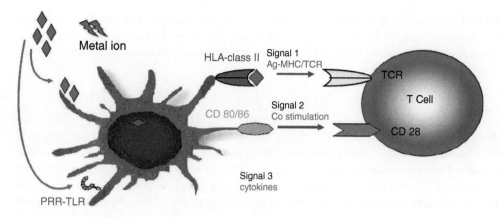

Figure 12.4 Metal-mediated T-cell activation: role of dendritic cells.

the skin as erythema, blistering and induration, then reach their maximum. By far, patch testing is the gold standard method for detecting metal sensitisation, since it is simple and has minimal adverse reactions. However, the accuracy of this method strongly depends on the experience of the dermatologist who interprets the results. Sometimes irritant reactions are difficult to discriminate from true allergic reactions, resulting in 'false-positive' readouts. On the other hand, false-negative patch tests may occur for metals like Ni (46%) (Rustemeyer et al. 2004) and Pd (7.9 %) (Muris et al. 2012) and can be due to suboptimal formulation of the test salts (Muris et al. 2012) or slow penetration. This relative lack of accuracy of the skin test together with the fact that each allergen contact may facilitate or boost sensitisation stimulated the search for blood-based in vitro assays (Moed et al. 2005; Muris et al. 2012).

The presence of recirculating metal-specific T cells can indeed be demonstrated in vitro using peripheral blood lymphocytes. Upon culturing with metal salts, metal-specific lymphocytes will proliferate and produce cytokines, such as IL-5. For diagnosing metal allergy, in vitro tests have some advantages compared to patch tests: they do not interfere with the patient's immune response, they are objective and can be used in clinical situations where patch testing is contraindicated. However, the quality of the results depends on the number of lymphocytes tested, the metal salt solubility and laboratory expertise. In the diagnostics of metal allergy, patch tests remain the gold standard, whereas in vitro tests are helpful in doubtful cases or when skin testing is contraindicated.

12.6 Sensitising Capacity of Metals

12.6.1 Allergenicity

The capacity of chemicals to induce an adaptive immune response, referred to as allergenicity, depends on the chemical characteristics as well as on the available T-cell repertoire in the host (Table 12.5). The most important chemical characteristics are solubility, capacity to penetrate skin or mucosa, protein binding capacity and the 'danger signals' they provide to the PRR of DCs, allowing the latter to mature and prime T cells as outlined above. The T-cell repertoire in the host is

Table 12.5 Crucial factors for sensitisation to metal alloys.

	Factor
1.	Exposure to the metal
2.	Metal ion release
3.	Penetration of skin or mucosae by metal (ions)
4.	Protein-binding capacity of the metal (ions)
5.	Innate triggering by metal (ions)
6.	Availability of T cells recognising the metal–peptide complex
7.	Microenvironment in the draining lymph node

determined in the thymus, where T lymphocytes are educated to optimally recognise pathogen-modified self molecules. Many different models and test protocols have been developed to predict allergenicity of chemicals, all aiming at a maximal correlation with clinical data from allergic patients. Such data sets have been published, and for dentally applied metals the frequency of positive patch tests is shown in Table 12.4.

12.6.2   In vivo Allergenicity Testing

For many years, guinea pigs were the experimental models of choice for testing the skin-sensitising potential of chemicals (Magnusson and Kligman 1969; Maurer et al. 1975). These in vivo test systems evaluated whether a chemical can induce an adaptive immune response, as detected by a skin challenge 2–4 weeks later. In 1989, however, the use of mice was introduced as a rapid and cost-effective alternative (Kimber et al. 1989a). Soon, the resulting local lymph node assay (LLNA) with focus on the induction phase became the preferred animal model for allergenicity testing. In the LLNA, chemicals are applied in vivo but the readout is based on lymphocyte proliferation in the draining lymph nodes and measured in vitro (Kimber et al. 1989b; Dean et al. 2001), Although these models generally predict the sensitising capacity of chemicals well, reflecting allergic reactivity in humans, some common human sensitisers like Ni showed only very weak sensitisation in mice. Interestingly, this species dependency could be explained by the findings of Schmidt et al. (2010), who showed that the triggering of DCs by Ni via TLR4 requires non-conserved histidines at distinct positions, which were not found in the mouse TLR4. Human cells or tissues would of course provide optimal test material for in vitro allergenicity testing of new metal alloys.

Since 2013, in vivo screening methods for cosmetic compounds have been banned, for ethical and legislative reasons. This has resulted in renewed interest in quantitative structure-activity relationship (QSAR) models and in vitro tests for allergenicity.

12.6.3   Quantitative Structure-Activity Relationship (QSAR)

Low molecular weight chemicals, including metals, must bind to carrier molecules to become antigenic and be recognised by the immune system. The rate of protein binding is considered a major determinant of allergenic potency (Chipinda et al. 2011). Whereas small organic allergens usually form covalent bonds with nucleophilic centres on proteins, metals rather bind to proteins through disulfide exchange or co-ordinate covalent bonds. Based on the assumption that all allergens are protein reactive, screening assays have been developed to predict allergenicity. Such assays use cysteine, lysine, glutathione or model peptides as carrier molecules and efforts are under way to validate them as alternative in chemico methods for screening skin sensitisers (Gerberick et al. 2004; Roberts et al. 2006). The protein-binding capacity, together with other chemical characteristics such as size and solubility (octanol/water partitioning) of the compounds, are used for combined risk analyses of chemicals in so-called QSAR models.

12.6.4   Cell-based Allergenicity Testing

A crucial step in the sensitisation process is the induction of DC maturation by allergens. This innate stimulatory capacity of chemicals can be tested in vitro by exposing immature blood monocyte-derived DCs (MoDCs) to non-toxic concentrations of chemicals. The resulting in vitro maturation of the DCs can be evaluated by measuring the release of cytokines by ELISA (IL-8, IL-6, etc.) or by monitoring the upregulation of cell surface expression of CD40, CD80 and CD86 by flow cytometry. Nowadays, new technologies such as microarray or pepchip analysis might also be used to determine allergen-driven DC activation.

Indeed, it was shown that allergens, but not irritants, could induce maturation of immature MoDCs as measured by IL-8 production and upregulation of adhesion molecules (Toebak et al. 2006; Szameit et al. 2008). Also transition metals (Ni> Co> Cu> Pd> Cr) were thus found to stimulate DCs (Spiekstra et al. 2005), although the underlying mechanisms were still obscure at that time.

Next to MoDCs, various cell lines have been explored as potential DC surrogates, including THP-1, a human monocytoid cell line (Miyazawa et al. 2007), to avoid donor-to-donor variability in the assays. Moreover, the use of cell lines would allow for robust high-throughput screening of potential allergens.

In vivo, DCs are always surrounded by keratinocytes and fibroblasts, which are also known to produce cytokines upon allergenic stimuli (Ouwehand et al. 2008, 2010; Haniffa et al. 2013), thereby contributing to the microenvironment in which the DCs mature. Therefore, ideally, culture systems for allergenicity testing should involve all three cell types (keratinocytes, fibroblasts and DCs) (Ouwehand et al. 2011).

References

ADA (2003). Titanium applications in dentistry. *J. Am. Dent. Assoc.* 134: 347–349.

Ahlgren, C., Ahnlide, I., Bjorkner, B. et al. (2002). Contact allergy to gold is correlated to dental gold. *Acta Derm. Venereol.* 82: 41–44.

Al-Hiyasat, A.S. and Darmani, H. (2005). The effects of recasting on the cytotoxicity of base metal alloys. *J. Prosthet. Dent.* 93: 158–163.

Al-Salehi, S.K., Hatton, P.V., McLeod, C.W. and Cox, A.G. (2007). The effect of hydrogen peroxide concentration on metal ion release from dental amalgam. *J. Dent.* 35: 172–176.

Aminzadeh, K.K. and Etminan, M. (2007). Dental amalgam and multiple sclerosis: a systematic review and meta-analysis. *J. Public Health Dent.* 67: 64–66.

Amor, S., Peferoen, L.A., Vogel, D.Y., van Breur, M. Baker, V.D. and van Noort, J.M. (2014). Inflammation in neurodegenerative diseases – an update. *Immunology* 142: 151–166.

Anusavice, K.J., Shen, C. and Rawls, H.R. (2013). *Phillip's Science of Dental Materials*. Philadelphia: Saunders.

Arroyo, D.S., Soria, J., Gaviglio, E., Rodriguez-Galan, M. and Iribarren, P. (2011). Toll-like receptors are key players in neurodegeneration. *Int. Immunopharmacol.* 11: 1415–1421.

Baker, B.S., Ovigne, J., Powles, A., Corcoran, S. and Fry, L. (2003). Normal keratinocytes express Toll-like receptors (TLRs) 1, 2 and 5: modulation of TLR expression in chronic plaque psoriasis. *Br. J. Dermatol.* 148: 670–679.

Bergdahl, I.A., Ahlqwist, M., Barregard, L. et al. (2013). Mercury in serum predicts low risk of death and myocardial infarction in Gothenburg women. *Int. Arch. Occup. Environ. Health* 86: 71–77.

Borne, Y., Barregard, L., Persson, M., Hedblad, B., Fagerberg, B. and Engstrom, G. (2015). Cadmium exposure and incidence of heart failure and atrial fibrillation: a population-based prospective cohort study. *BMJ Open* 5: e007366.

Bouquot, J.E. and Gorlin, R.J. (1986). Leukoplakia, lichen planus, and other oral keratoses in 23,616 white Americans over the age of 35 years. *Oral Surg. Oral Med. Oral Pathol.* 61: 373–381.

Brown, A.L., de Camargo, M., Sperandio, M. et al. (2015). Peripheral giant cell granuloma associated with a dental implant: a case report and review of the literature. *Case Rep. Dent.* 2015: 697673.

Carocci, A., Rovito, N., Sinicropi, M. and Genchi, G. (2014). Mercury toxicity and neurodegenerative effects. *Rev. Environ. Contam. Toxicol.* 229: 1–18.

Cawson, R.A. and Odell, E.W. (2008). *Cawson's Essentials of Oral Medicine and Pathology*. London: Churchill Livingstone.

Chakravarthi, S., Padmanabhan, S. and Chitharanjan, A. (2012). Allergy and orthodontics. *J. Orthod. Sci.* 1: 83–87.

Chaturvedi, T. (2009). An overview of the corrosion aspect of dental implants (titanium and its alloys). *Indian J. Dent. Res.* 20: 91–98.

Chaturvedi, T. (2013). Allergy related to dental implant and its clinical significance. *Clin. Cosmet. Invest. Dent.* 5: 57–61.

Chipinda, I., Hettick, J. and Siegel, P. (2011). Haptenation: chemical reactivity and protein binding. *J. Allergy* 2011: 839682.

Das, A., Chai, J., Kim, S. et al. (2015). Transcriptome sequencing of microglial cells stimulated with TLR3 and TLR4 ligands. *BMC Genomics* 16: 517.

Davis, M.D., Wang, M., Yiannias, J. et al. (2011). Patch testing with a large series of metal allergens: findings from more than 1,000 patients in one decade at Mayo Clinic. *Dermatitis* 22: 256–271.

de Kivit S., Tobin, M., Forsyth, C., Keshavarzian, A. and Landay, A. (2014). Regulation of intestinal immune responses through TLR activation: implications for pro- and prebiotics. *Front. Immunol.* 5: 60.

Dean, J.H., Twerdok, L., Tice, R. et al. (2001). ICCVAM evaluation of the murine local lymph node assay. Conclusions and recommendations of an independent scientific peer review panel. *Regul. Toxicol. Pharmacol.* 34: 258–273.

Dimic I.D., Cvijovic-Alagic I., Kostic I.T. et al. (2014). Metallic ion release from biocompatible cobalt-based alloy. *Chem. Industr. Chem. Engin.* Q 20: 571–577.

Ditrichova, D., Kapralova, S., Tichy, M. et al. (2007). Oral lichenoid lesions and allergy to dental materials. *Biomed. Pap. Med. Fac. Univ Palacky. Olomouc. Czech. Repub.* 151: 333–339.

Dunn, J.E., Trachtenberg, F., Barregard, L., Bellinger, D., and McKinlay, S. (2008). Scalp hair and urine mercury content of children in the Northeast United States: the New England Children's Amalgam Trial. *Environ. Res.* 107: 79–88.

Dunsche, A., Kastel, I., Terheyden, H., et al. (2003). Oral lichenoid reactions associated with amalgam: improvement after amalgam removal. *Br. J. Dermatol.* 148: 70–76.

Elshahawy, W., Watanabe, I. and Koike, M. (2009). Elemental ion release from four different fixed prosthodontic materials. *Dent. Mater.* 25: 976–981.

Elshahawy, W., Ajlouni, R., James, W., Abdellatif, H. and Watanabe, I. (2013). Elemental ion release from fixed restorative materials into patient saliva. *J. Oral Rehabil.* 40: 381–388.

Esser, P.R., Kimber, I. and Martin, S.F. (2014). Correlation of contact sensitiser potency with T cell frequency and TCR repertoire diversity. *EXS* 104: 101–114.

Fage, S.W., Faurschou, A. and Thyssen, J. (2014). Copper hypersensitivity. *Contact Dermatitis* 71: 191–201.

Faurschou, A., Menne, T., Johansen, J. and Thyssen, J. (2011). Metal allergen of the 21st century – a review on exposure, epidemiology and clinical manifestations of palladium allergy. *Contact Dermatitis* 64: 185–195.

Feilzer, A.J., Kleverlaan, C. Prahl, C. and Muris, J. (2013). [Systemic reactions to orally applied metal alloys]. *Ned. Tijdschr. Tandheelkd.* 120: 335–341.

Galo, R., Ribeiro, R., Rodrigues, R., Rocha, L. and de Mattos, M. (2012). Effects of chemical composition on the corrosion of dental alloys. *Braz. Dent. J.* 23: 141–148.

Gambuzza, M.E., Sofo, V., Salmeri, F., Soraci, L., Marino, S. and Bramanti, P. (2014). Toll-like receptors in Alzheimer's disease: a therapeutic perspective. *CNS Neurol. Disord. Drug Targets* 13: 1542–1558.

Garhammer, P., Schmalz, G., Hiller, K. and Reitinger, T. (2003). Metal content of biopsies adjacent to dental cast alloys. *Clin. Oral Invest.* 7: 92–97.

Genelhu, M.C., Marigo, M., Alves-Oliveira, L., Malaquias, L. and Gomez, R. (2005). Characterisation of nickel-induced allergic contact stomatitis associated with fixed orthodontic appliances. *Am. J. Orthod. Dentofacial Orthop.* 128: 378–381.

Gerberick, G.F., Vassallo, J., Bailey, R., Chaney, J., Morrall, S. and Lepoittevin, J. (2004). Development of a peptide reactivity assay for screening contact allergens. *Toxicol. Sci.* 81: 332–343.

Giacoppo, S., Galuppo, M., Calabro, R. et al. (2014). Heavy metals and neurodegenerative diseases: an observational study. *Biol. Trace Elem. Res.* 161: 151–160.

Gober, MD. and Gaspari, A.A. (2008). Allergic contact dermatitis. *Curr. Dir. Autoimmun.* 10: 1–26.

Gopikrishnan, S., Melath, A., Ajith, V. and Mathews, N.B. (2015). A comparative study of bio degradation of various orthodontic arch wires: an in vitro study. *J. Int. Oral Health* 7: 12–17.

Hampel, R., Peters, A., Beelen, R. et al. (2015). Long-term effects of elemental composition of particulate matter on inflammatory blood markers in European cohorts. *Environ. Int.* 82: 76–84.

Haniffa, M., Collin, M. and Ginhoux, F. (2013). Ontogeny and functional specialization of dendritic cells in human and mouse. *Adv. Immunol.* 120: 1–49.

Helm, D. (2002). Association between palladium urinary concentrations and diseases of the thyroid and the immune system. *Sci. Total Environ.* 299: 247–249.

Höhn, S. and Virtanen, S. (2015). Biocorrosion of TiO2 nanoparticle coating of Ti–6Al–4V in DMEM under specific in vitro conditions. *Appl. Surface Sci.* 329: 356–362.

Hosoki, M., Bando, E., Asaoka, K., Takeuchi, H. and Nishigawa, K. (2009). Assessment of allergic hypersensitivity to dental materials. *Biomed. Mater. Eng.* 19: 53–61.

Hougeir, F.G., Yiannias, J., Hinni, M., Hentz, J. and el-Azhary, R. (2006). Oral metal contact allergy: a pilot study on the cause of oral squamous cell carcinoma. *Int. J. Dermatol.* 45: 265–271.

Imirzalioglu, P., Alaaddinoglu, E., Yilmaz, Z., Oduncuoglu, B., Yilmaz, B. and Rosenstiel, S. (2012). Influence of recasting different types of dental alloys on gingival fibroblast cytotoxicity. *J. Prosthet. Dent.* 107: 24–33.

Ismail, S.B., Kumar, S. and Zain, R. (2007). Oral lichen planus and lichenoid reactions: etiopathogenesis, diagnosis, management and malignant transformation. *J. Oral Sci.* 49: 89–106.

Issa, Y., Duxbury, A., Macfarlane, T. and Brunton, P. (2005). Oral lichenoid lesions related to dental restorative materials. *Br. Dent. J.* 198: 361–366.

Johnson, A., Shiraishi, T. and Al-Salehi, S. (2010). Ion release from experimental Au-Pt-based metal-ceramic alloys. *Dent. Mater.* 26: 682–687.

Kanerva, L., Rantanen, T., Aalto-Korte, K. et al. (2001). A multicenter study of patch test reactions with dental screening series. *Am. J. Contact Dermat.* 12: 83–87.

Kauppinen, T.M., Higashi, Y., Suh, S., Escartin, C., Nagasawa, K. and Swanson, R.A. (2008). Zinc triggers microglial activation. *J. Neurosci.* 28: 5827–5835.

Kettenmann, H., Kirchhoff, F. and Verkhratsky, A. (2013). Microglia: new roles for the synaptic stripper. *Neuron* 77: 10–18.

Khamaysi, Z., Bergman, R. and Weltfriend, S. (2006). Positive patch test reactions to allergens of the dental series and the relation to the clinical presentations. *Contact Dermatitis* 55: 216–218.

Kim, T.W., Kim, W., Mun, J.H. et al. (2015). Patch testing with dental screening series in oral disease. *Ann. Dermatol.* 27: 389–393.

Kimber, I., Hilton, J. and Weisenberger, C. (1989a). The murine local lymph node assay for identification of contact allergens: a preliminary evaluation of in situ measurement of lymphocyte proliferation. *Contact Dermatitis* 21: 215–220.

Kimber, I., Shepherd, C., Mitchell, J., Turk, J. and Baker, D. (1989b). Regulation of lymphocyte proliferation in contact sensitivity: homeostatic mechanisms and a possible explanation of antigenic competition. *Immunology* 66: 577–582.

Klegeris, A., Choi, H., McLarnon, J.and McGeer, P. (2007). Functional ryanodine receptors are expressed by human microglia and THP-1 cells: their possible involvement in modulation of neurotoxicity. *J. Neurosci. Res.* 85: 2207–2215.

Koch, P. and Bahmer, F. (1999). Oral lesions and symptoms related to metals used in dental restorations: a clinical, allergological, and histologic study. *J. Am. Acad. Dermatol.* 41: 422–430.

Kolokitha, O.E. and Chatzistavrou, E. (2009). A severe reaction to ni-containing orthodontic appliances. *Angle Orthod.* 79: 186–192.

Kosten, I.J., Buskermolen, J., Spiekstra, S., de Gruijl, T. and Gibbs, S. (2015). Gingiva equivalents secrete negligible amounts of key chemokines involved in Langerhans cell migration compared to skin equivalents. *J. Immunol. Res.* 2015: 627125.

Laeijendecker, R. and Van, J.T. 1994. Oral manifestations of gold allergy. *J. Am. Acad. Dermatol.* 30: 205–209.

Laeijendecker, R., Dekker, S., Burger, P., Mulder, P., Van, J.T. and Neumann, M.H. (2004). Oral lichen planus and allergy to dental amalgam restorations. *Arch. Dermatol.* 140: 1434–1438.

Langworth, S., Bjorkman, L., Elinder, C., Jarup, L. and Savlin, P. (2002). Multidisciplinary examination of patients with illness attributed to dental fillings. *J. Oral Rehabil.* 29: 705–713.

Lin, H.Y., Bowers, B., Wolan, J., Cai, Z. and Bumgardner, J.D. (2008). Metallurgical, surface, and corrosion analysis of Ni-Cr dental casting alloys before and after porcelain firing. *Dent. Mater.* 24: 378–385.

Lygre, G.B., Gjerdet, N., Gronningsaeter, A. and Bjorkman, L. (2003). Reporting on adverse reactions to dental materials – intraoral observations at a clinical follow-up. *Community Dent. Oral Epidemiol.* 31: 200–206.

Ma, Q. and Wu, F.M. (2011). [Corrosion property and oxide film of dental casting alloys before and after porcelain firing]. *Zhonghua Kou Qiang Yi Xue Za Zhi* 46: 172–176.

Magnusson, B. and Kligman, A. (1969). The identification of contact allergens by animal assay. The guinea pig maximization test. *J. Invest. Dermatol.* 52: 268–276.

Martin, S.F. (2015). Immunological mechanisms in allergic contact dermatitis. *Curr. Opin. Allergy Clin. Immunol.* 15: 124–130.

Matusiewicz, H. (2014). Potential release of in vivo trace metals from metallic medical implants in the human body: from ions to nanoparticles – a systematic analytical review. *Acta Biomater.* 10: 2379–2403.

Maurer, T., Thomann, P., Weirich, E. and Hess, R. (1975). The optimization test in the guinea-pig. A method for the predictive evaluation of the contact allergenicity of chemicals. *Agents Actions* 5: 174–179.

McParland, H. and Warnakulasuriya, S. (2012). Oral lichenoid contact lesions to mercury and dental amalgam – a review. *J. Biomed. Biotechnol.* 2012: 589569.

Mempel, M., Voelcker, V., Kollisch, G. et al. (2003). Toll-like receptor expression in human keratinocytes: nuclear factor kappaB controlled gene activation by Staphylococcus aureus is toll-like receptor 2 but not toll-like receptor 4 or platelet activating factor receptor dependent. *J. Invest. Dermatol.* 121: 1389–1396.

Menne, T. 1981. Nickel allergy – reliability of patch test. Evaluated in female twins. *Derm. Beruf. Umwelt.* 29: 156–160.

Mikulewicz, M., Chojnacka, K. and Wolowiec, P. (2014). Release of metal ions from fixed orthodontic appliance: an in vitro study in continuous flow system. *Angle Orthod.* 84: 140–148.

Mikulewicz, M., Wolowiec, P., Loster, B.W. and Chojnacka, K. (2015). Do soft drinks affect metal ions release from orthodontic appliances? *J. Trace Elem. Med. Biol.* 31: 74–77.

Milheiro, A., J. Muris, C. J. Kleverlaan, and A. J. Feilzer. (2015). Influence of shape and finishing on the corrosion of palladium-based dental alloys. *J. Adv. Prosthodont.* 7: 56–61.

Milheiro, A., Nozaki, K., Kleverlaan, C., Muris, J., Miura, H. and Feilzer, A. (2016). In vitro cytotoxity of metallic ions released from dental alloys. *Odontology* 104: 136–142.

Minang, J.T., Arestrom, I., Troye-Blomberg, M., Lundeberg, L. and Ahlborg, N. (2006). Nickel, cobalt, chromium, palladium and gold induce a mixed Th1- and Th2-type cytokine response in vitro in subjects with contact allergy to the respective metals. *Clin. Exp. Immunol.* 146: 417–426.

Miyazawa, M., Ito, Y., Yoshida, Y., Sakaguchi, H. and Suzuki, H. (2007). Phenotypic alterations and cytokine production in THP-1 cells in response to allergens. *Toxicol. In vitro* 21: 428–437.

Modgil, S., Lahiri, D.K., Sharma, V. and Anand, A. (2014). Role of early life exposure and environment on neurodegeneration: implications on brain disorders. *Transl. Neurodegener.* 3: 9.

Moed, H., von Blomberg, M., Bruynzeel, D., Scheper, R., Gibbs, S. and Rustemeyer, T. (2005). Improved detection of allergen-specific T-cell responses in allergic contact dermatitis through the addition of 'cytokine cocktails'. *Exp. Dermatol.* 14: 634–640.

Moller, H. (2002). Dental gold alloys and contact allergy. *Contact Dermatitis* 47: 63–66.

Mou, Y.H., Yang, J., Cui, N. et al. (2012). Effects of cobalt chloride on nitric oxide and cytokines/chemokines production in microglia. *Int. Immunopharmacol.* 13: 120–125.

Muris, J. and Feilzer, A.J. (2006). Micro analysis of metals in dental restorations as part of a diagnostic approach in metal allergies. *Neuro. Endocrinol. Lett.* 27 (Suppl 1): 49–52.

Muris, J., Kleverlaan, C.J., Rustemeyer, T. et al. (2012). Sodium tetrachloropalladate for diagnosing palladium sensitisation. *Contact Dermatitis* 67: 94–100.

Muris, J., Scheper, R.J., Kleverlaan, C.J. et al. (2014). Palladium-based dental alloys are associated with oral disease and palladium-induced immune responses. *Contact Dermatitis* 71: 82–91.

Muris, J., Goossens, A., Goncalo, M. et al. (2015). Sensitisation to palladium and nickel in Europe and the relationship with oral disease and dental alloys. *Contact Dermatitis* 72: 286–296.

Murphy, K.P. (2012). *Janeway's Immunobiology*. London: Garland Science.

Nelson, S.K., Wataha, J. and Lockwood, P. (1999). Accelerated toxicity testing of casting alloys and reduction of intraoral release of elements. *J. Prosthet. Dent.* 81: 715–720.

Nonaka, H., TNakada, T. and Iijima, M. (2003). Gold allergy in Japan. *Contact Dermatitis* 48: 112–114.

Nonaka, H., Nakada, T., Iijima, M. and Maibach, H. (2011). Metal patch test results from 1990–2009. *J. Dermatol.* 38: 267–271.

Ortiz, A.J., Fernandez, E., Vicente, A., Calvo, J. and Ortiz, C. (2011). Metallic ions released from stainless steel, nickel-free, and titanium orthodontic alloys: toxicity and DNA damage. *Am. J. Orthod. Dentofacial Orthop.* 140: e115–e122.

Oskarsson, A., ASchultz, A., SSkerfving, S. et al. (1996). Total and inorganic mercury in breast milk in relation to fish consumption and amalgam in lactating women. *Arch. Environ. Health* 51: 234–241.

Ouwehand, K., Santegoets, S., Bruynzeel, D.P., Scheper, R., de Gruijl, T. and Gibbs, S. (2008). CXCL12 is essential for migration of activated Langerhans cells from epidermis to dermis. *Eur. J. Immunol.* 38: 3050–3059.

Ouwehand, K., Scheper, R., de Gruijl, T. and Gibbs, S. (2010). Epidermis-to-dermis migration of immature Langerhans cells upon topical irritant exposure is dependent on CCL2 and CCL5. *Eur. J. Immunol.* 40: 2026–2034.

Ouwehand, K., Spiekstra, S., Waaijman, T., Scheper, R., de Gruijl, T. and S. Gibbs. (2011). Technical advance: Langerhans cells derived from a human cell line in a full-thickness skin equivalent undergo allergen-induced maturation and migration. *J. Leukoc. Biol.* 90: 1027–1033.

Oyar, P., Can, G. and Atakol, O. (2014). Effects of environment on the release of Ni, Cr, Fe, and Co from new and recast Ni-Cr alloy. *J. Prosthet. Dent.* 112: 64–69.

Pacini, S., Fiore, M., Magherini, S. et al. (2012). Could cadmium be responsible for some of the neurological signs and symptoms of myalgic encephalomyelitis/chronic fatigue syndrome? *Med. Hypotheses* 79: 403–407.

Penarrocha-Diago, M.A., Cervera-Ballester, J., Maestre-Ferrin, L. and Penarrocha-Oltra, D. (2012). Peripheral giant cell granuloma associated with dental implants: clinical case and literature review. *J. Oral Implantol.* 38 Spec No: 527–532.

Pistoor, F.H., Kapsenberg, M., Bos, J., Meinardi, M., von Blomberg, M. and Scheper, R. (1995). Cross-reactivity of human nickel-reactive T-lymphocyte clones with copper and palladium. *J. Invest. Dermatol.* 105: 92–95.

Qiu, J., Yu, W., Zhang, F., Smales, R., Zhang, Y. and Lu, C. (2011). Corrosion behaviour and surface analysis of a Co-Cr and two Ni-Cr dental alloys before and after simulated porcelain firing. *Eur. J. Oral Sci.* 119: 93–101.

Raghavan, B., Martin, S., Esser, P., Goebeler, M. and Schmidt, M. (2012). Metal allergens nickel and cobalt facilitate TLR4 homodimerization independently of MD2. *EMBO Rep.* 13: 1109–1115.

Rahilly, G. and Price, N. (2003). Nickel allergy and orthodontics. *J. Orthod.* 30: 171–174.

Roach, M.D., Wolan, J., Parsell, D. and Bumgardner, J. (2000). Use of x-ray photoelectron spectroscopy and cyclic polarization to evaluate the corrosion behavior of six nickel-chromium alloys before and after porcelain-fused-to-metal firing. *J. Prosthet. Dent.* 84: 623–634.

Roberts, D.W., Aptula, A. and Patlewicz, G. (2006). Mechanistic applicability domains for non-animal based prediction of toxicological endpoints. QSAR analysis of the schiff base applicability domain for skin sensitisation. *Chem. Res. Toxicol.* 19: 1228–1233.

Roos, P.M., Vesterberg, O., Syversen, T., Flaten, T. and Nordberg, M. (2013). Metal concentrations in cerebrospinal fluid and blood plasma from patients with amyotrophic lateral sclerosis. *Biol. Trace Elem. Res.* 151: 159–170.

Rudolph, M.G., Stanfield, R. and Wilson, I. (2006). How TCRs bind MHCs, peptides, and coreceptors. *Annu. Rev. Immunol.* 24: 419–466.

Rustemeyer, T. and Frosch, P.J. (2000). Occupational contact dermatitis in dental personnel. In: *Handbook of Occupational Dermatology* (eds L. Kanerva, P. Elsner, J.E. Wahlberg and H.I. Maibach), pp.899–905. Berlin: Springer Verlag.

Rustemeyer, T.,. von Blomberg, B.M., van Hoogstraten, I.M., Bruynzeel, D.P. and Scheper, R.J. (2004). Analysis of effector and regulatory immune reactivity to nickel. *Clin. Exp. Allergy* 34: 1458–1466.

Sakaguchi, R.L. and Powers, J. (2012). *Craig's Restorative Materials*, 13e. Philadelphia: Elsevier Mosby.

Schmalz, G. (2002). Materials science: biological aspects. *J. Dent. Res.* 81: 660–663.

Schmalz, G., Garhammer, P. and Reitinger, T. (1999). Metal content of biopsies from the neighborhood of casting alloys. *J. Dent. Res.* 78 (Abstr. No. 1048): 236.

Schmidt, M., Raghavan, B., Muller, V. et al. (2010). Crucial role for human Toll-like receptor 4 in the development of contact allergy to nickel. *Nat. Immunol.* 11: 814–819.

Sicilia, A., Cuesta, S., Coma, G. et al. (2008). Titanium allergy in dental implant patients: a clinical study on 1500 consecutive patients. *Clin. Oral Implants Res.* 19: 823–835.

Sjursen, T.T., Binder, P., Lygre, G., Helland, V., Dalen, K. and Bjorkman, L. (2015). Patients' experiences of changes in health complaints before, during, and after removal of dental amalgam. *Int. J. Qual. Stud. Health Well-being* 10: 28157.

Skoglund, A. (1994). Value of epicutaneous patch testing in patients with oral, mucosal lesions of lichenoid character. *Scand. J. Dent. Res.* 102: 216–222.

Spiekstra, S.W., Toebak, M., Sampat-Sardjoepersad, S. et al. (2005). Induction of cytokine (interleukin-1alpha and tumor necrosis factor-alpha) and chemokine (CCL20, CCL27, and CXCL8) alarm signals after allergen and irritant exposure. *Exp. Dermatol.* 14: 109–116.

Spiewak, R., Moed, H., von Blomberg, B.M. et al. (2007). Allergic contact dermatitis to nickel: modified in vitro test protocols for better detection of allergen-specific response. *Contact Dermatitis* 56: 63–69.

Steele, J.C., Bruce, A., Davis, M., Torgerson, R., Drage, L. and Rogers III, R.S. (2012). Clinically relevant patch test results in patients with burning mouth syndrome. *Dermatitis* 23: 61–70.

Stejskal, V. (2014). Metals as a common trigger of inflammation resulting in non-specific symptoms: diagnosis and treatment. *Isr. Med. Assoc. J.* 16: 753–758.

Sterzl, I., Prochazkova, J., Hrda, P., Bartova, J., Matucha, P. and Stejskal, V. (1999). Mercury and nickel allergy: risk factors in fatigue and autoimmunity. *Neuro. Endocrinol. Lett.* 20: 221–228.

Stockinger, B., Bourgeois, C. and Kassiotis, G. (2006). CD4+ memory T cells: functional differentiation and homeostasis. *Immunol. Rev.* 211: 39–48.

Subramani, K., Jung, R., Molenberg, A. and Hammerle, C. (2009). Biofilm on dental implants: a review of the literature. *Int. J. Oral Maxillofac. Implants* 24: 616–626.

Syed, M., Chopra, R. and Sachdev, V. (2015). Allergic reactions to dental materials – a systematic review. *J. Clin. Diagn. Res.* 9: ZE04–ZE09.

Szameit, S., Vierlinger, K., Farmer, L., Tuschl, H. and Noehammer, C. (2008). Microarray-based in vitro test system for the discrimination of contact allergens and irritants: identification of potential marker genes. *Clin. Chem.* 54: 525–533.

Thornhill, M.H., Pemberton, M., Simmons, R. and Theaker, E.D. 2003. Amalgam-contact hypersensitivity lesions and oral lichen planus. *Oral Surg. Oral Med. Oral Pathol. Oral Radiol. Endod.* 95: 291–299.

Thyssen, J.P. and Menne, T. (2010). Metal allergy – a review on exposures, penetration, genetics, prevalence, and clinical implications. *Chem. Res. Toxicol.* 23: 309–318.

Toebak, M.J., Pohlmann, P.R., Sampat-Sardjoepersad, S.C. et al. (2006). CXCL8 secretion by dendritic cells predicts contact allergens from irritants. *Toxicol. In vitro* 20: 117–124.

Torgerson, R.R., Davis, M.D., Bruce, A.J., Farmer, S.A. and Rogers III, R.S. (2007). Contact allergy in oral disease. *J. Am. Acad. Dermatol.* 57: 315–321.

Upadhyay, D., Panchal, M.A., Dubey, R.S. and Srivastava, V.K. (2006). Corrosion of alloys used in dentistry: a review. *Mater. Sci. Engin. A* 432: 1–11.

van der Meij, E.H., Mast, H. and van der Waal, I. (2007). The possible premalignant character of oral lichen planus and oral lichenoid lesions: a prospective five-year follow-up study of 192 patients. *Oral Oncol.* 43: 742–748.

van Hoogstraten, I.M., Andersen, K.E., von Blomberg, B.M. et al. (1991). Reduced frequency of nickel allergy upon oral nickel contact at an early age. *Clin. Exp. Immunol.* 85: 441–445.

Wataha, J.C. (2000). Biocompatibility of dental casting alloys: a review. *J. Prosthet. Dent.* 83: 223–234.

Wataha, J.C., Lockwood, P.E., Nelson, S.K. and Bouillaguet, S. (1999). Long-term cytotoxicity of dental casting alloys. *Int. J. Prosthodont.* 12: 242–248.

Wataha, J.C., Drury, J.L. and Chung, W.O. (2013). Nickel alloys in the oral environment. *Expert. Rev. Med. Devices* 10: 519–539.

Wohrl, S., Hemmer, W., Focke, M., Gotz, M. and Jarisch, R. (2001). Copper allergy revisited. *J. Am. Acad. Dermatol.* 45: 863–870.

Yoshihisa, Y. and Shimizu, T. (2012). Metal allergy and systemic contact dermatitis: an overview. *Dermatol. Res. Pract.* 2012: 749561.

Yoshihisa, Y., Rehman, M.U., Yamakoshi-Shibutani, T. and Shimizu, T. (2015). In vitro effects of zinc on the cytokine production from peripheral blood mononuclear cells in patients with zinc allergy. *Springerplus* 4: 404.

Yu, F., Addison, O., Baker, S.J. and Davenport, A.J. (2015). Lipopolysaccharide inhibits or accelerates biomedical titanium corrosion depending on environmental acidity. *Int. J. Oral Sci.* 7: 179–186.

13

Inflammation and Immune Response in Arthrogenous Temporomandibular Disorders

Siew Wui Chan[1] and Wei Seong Toh[2]

[1] *Department of Oral and Maxillofacial Clinical Sciences, Faculty of Dentistry, University of Malaya, Kuala Lumpur, Malaysia*
[2] *Faculty of Dentistry, National University of Singapore, Singapore*

13.1   Introduction

The temporomandibular joints are often subject to a variety of pathological conditions that may be myogenous or arthrogenous in origin. Long-term successful management of temporomandibular joint disorders or temporomandibular disorders (TMDs) remains challenging as there is no recognised, unequivocal universal cause for these disorders. The current consensus is that the majority of TMDs have complex and multifactorial or unknown aetiologies. Identifying the precise cause of TMD is challenging because of the intertwining complexity of elements that may upset the dynamic equilibrium among the components of the masticatory system (de Leeuw and Klasser 2018). Despite the multifactorial aetiology of TMDs, trauma remains the most tangible and explicable cause on many occasions.

Reasonable advances have been made to relate immune system plasticity in the pathogenesis of TMDs, particularly atherogenic temporomandibular dysfunctions such as disc displacement disorders, osteoarthritis and rheumatoid arthritis, as well as for the diagnosis and development of novel immunomodulatory therapies. There has been immense advancement in this area due to the development of animal models, including surgical, mechanical, chemical and genetic models that replicate acute and chronic inflammation present in several arthrogenous TMD subtypes (Wang et al. 2012, 2015). In addition, studies using synovial, serum and urinary samples have yielded a plethora of potential diagnostic biomarkers, the majority of which are inflammatory cytokines (Zwiri et al. 2020) that have been recognised as key to the initiation, progression and clinical manifestation of TMD (Kellesarian et al. 2016).

13.2   Anatomy of the Temporomandibular Joint

Temporomandibular joints (TMJs) are a pair of complex joints of the hinge and sliding synovial type. Structurally, the TMJ is composed of the squamous portion of the temporal bone, mandibular condyle and articular disc bounded by collateral ligaments and a capsule. Unlike most synovial joints, the TMJ has an avascular articular surface lined with dense fibrocartilage instead of hyaline cartilage (Norton et al. 2017). The extracellular matrix within the fibrocartilage consists of large aggregates of hyaluronic acid and proteoglycan monomers enmeshed in a primarily type II collagen matrix (Bouloux 2009). The articular disc separates the TMJ into superior and inferior compartments. There are also cells, known as synoviocytes, on the internal surfaces of both compartments which are part of the synovial membrane or synovium (Norton et al. 2017).

The synovium is made up of a connective tissue sublining layer and a synovial lining cell layer (synovial intima) (Figure 13.1). The synoviocytes in the synovial intima consist of morphologically different macrophage-like type A cells and fibroblast-like type B cells. Type A cells have a monocyte lineage and function like a residential macrophage while type B cells are responsible for the production, secretion and resorption of synovial fluid. Type B cells also produce specialised matrix constituents including hyaluronan, collagens and fibronectin for the intimal interstitium and joint cavity (Iwanaga et al. 2000). The possibility of the existence of a third kind of cell, termed intermediate cells, has been suggested, but to date not much is known about the morphology or function of these cells (Carvalho de Moraes et al. 2015).

Immunology for Dentistry, First Edition. Edited by Mohammad Tariqur Rahman, Wim Teughels and Richard J. Lamont.
© 2023 John Wiley & Sons Ltd. Published 2023 by John Wiley & Sons Ltd.

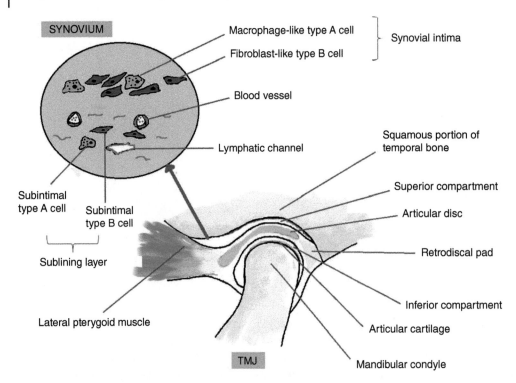

Figure 13.1 Diagrammatic representation of the TMJ components and synovial membrane (synovium).

Synovial fluid in the TMJ functions like a lubricant to enable smooth jaw movements, effectively reducing friction and serving as a shock absorber. In addition, it is the transporting medium for nutrients and waste products to and from the articular surfaces. The synovial fluid contains lipids, cholesterol, phospholipids, hyaluronic acid, glycosaminoglycans, albumin, immunoglobulin, elastase, collagenase, cathepsins, proteinase inhibitors, phospholipase A2 and alpha-2-macroglobulin. Synovial membrane and synovial fluid are considered integral in normal joint function and pathological conditions (Bouloux 2009).

13.3 Temporomandibular Disorders

Disorders of the temporomandibular joint are a group of musculoskeletal disorders affecting the masticatory structures which include the TMJs, muscles of mastication and associated structures such as the coronoid process. Based on the affected components, the majority of TMDs are broadly categorised either into TMJ disorders (arthrogenous) or masticatory muscle disorders (myogenous). Masticatory muscle disorders include pathologies involving muscles and/or their related tendons responsible for jaw movement such as masseter, medial pterygoid, temporalis, digastric and lateral pterygoid muscles. On the same note, TMJ disorders refer to pathologies or abnormalities in relation to the intricate structures of the joint itself. TMDs are recognised as the most common cause of chronic pain in the orofacial region. TMDs demonstrate strong female predilection and peak between 25 and 45 years of age. TMDs have a multifactorial aetiology involving anatomical and pathophysiological factors, as well as psychosocial characteristics and macro- or microtrauma (de Leeuw and Klasser 2018).

The TMD Research Diagnostic Criteria for Temporomandibular Disorders (RDC/TMD) or its revised version, DC-TMD, along with the American Academy of Orofacial Pain (AAOP) are the two most frequently used diagnostic classifications for TMDs. In fact, the latest AAOP classification has also adopted DC-TMD as the basis of its classification outlines (Figure 13.2) (de Leeuw and Klasser 2018).

In the course of continual improvement of the diagnostic classifications, discrepancies for certain terminologies are inevitable in much of the TMD-related literature due to the authors' preference for different classifications, as well as the existing classifications at the time of publication. Notable inconsistencies that are relevant to the discussion here mainly involve the terminologies for certain subtypes of TMJ disorders. For instance, disc derangement (previously known as

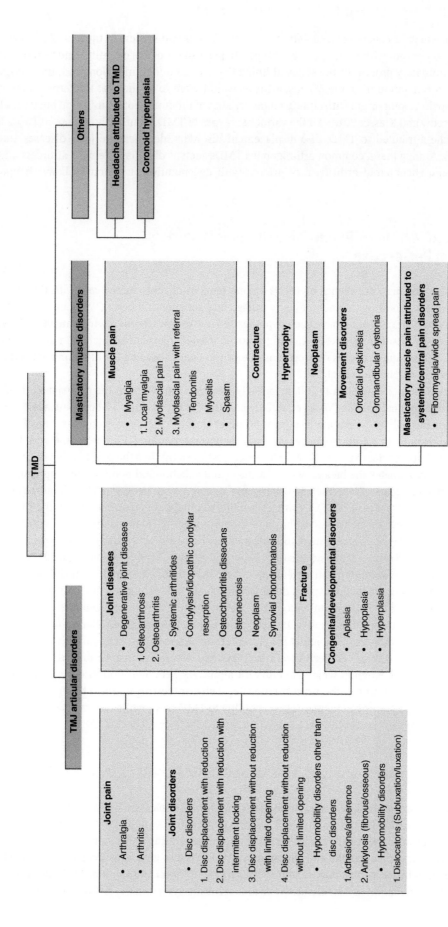

Figure 13.2 Expanded TMD taxonomy. *Source:* Adapted from Peck et al. (2014).

internal derangement), which has been replaced with disc-condyle complex disorders in the new classification, still refers to disc displacement disorders but with more specific subtypes. In place of synovitis, capsulitis and retrodiscitis, 'joint pain' now embodies an inflammatory process of the synovial lining that can be due to infection, an immunological condition secondary to cartilage degeneration or trauma. Thus, arthritis would seem to be the best reinterpretation of synovitis or capsulitis as it refers to pain of joint origin with clinical characteristics of inflammation or infection but with a less restricted nociceptive field (de Leeuw and Klasser 2018). Of the various subtypes of TMD, commonly diagnosed TMDs include myalgia, arthralgia, headache attributed to TMD, disc displacement disorders, degenerative joint diseases and subluxation (Schiffman et al. 2014). Among these, common arthrogenous TMDs such as disc displacement disorders and, to a greater extent, osteoarthritis and rheumatoid arthritis may present with degenerative or structural bony changes (Schiffman et al. 2014).

13.4 Female Predilection in Temporomandibular Disorders: An Immunological Perspective

Many studies have linked the high prevalence of TMDs among females of reproductive age with the negative effects of female hormones, particularly oestrogen, on condylar cartilage and subchondral bone (Wang et al. 2015). The negative effects of oestrogen on condylar resorption have been hypothesised in two ways, both of which are yet to be validated. One hypothesis suggests the role of sex hormones in causing synovial tissue hyperplasia which stimulates the production of destructive substrates. The second proposes oestrogen as one of the factors causing dysfunctional condylar remodelling leading to condylar resorption (Nicolielo et al. 2017).

The proinflammatory effects of oestrogen in inflamed TMJ have been attributed to the conversion of estrone/17-beta-oestradiol to proinflammatory metabolites (Wang et al. 2015). In the TMJ synovium, 17-beta-oestradiol reportedly aggravates acute inflammation through the NF-kappa-B pathway (Wang et al. 2012). Increasing concentration of 17beta-oestradiol also leads to greater expression of proinflammatory cytokines such as interleukin (IL)-1-beta, IL-6 and IL-8 in the culture of mandibular condylar chondrocytes (Yu et al. 2009). Moreover, oestrogen inhibits the proliferation of chondrocytes in the mandibular condyle and exacerbates the breakdown of cartilage and subchondral bone through upregulation of Fas and caspase 3-related proapoptotic genes. Nevertheless, oestrogen also confers protection to TMJ chondrocytes by inhibiting nitric oxide (NO) production (Wang et al. 2015). Oestrogen's ability to modify metabolic activity in the TMJ is theoretically dependent on binding to its receptors such as ER-alpha and ER-beta in the TMJ. However, the very existence of these receptors within the articular disc has been questioned and disputed by the conflicting results from clinical randomised controlled trials, cohort studies and case–control studies (de Leeuw and Klasser 2018; Nicolielo et al. 2017).

Pain neurotransmission and pain modulation systems are different in males and females. The influence of oestrogen on the regulative mechanism of pain might also explain the sex dimorphism in TMDs, given that pain is a common manifestation of TMDs and closely related to TMJ inflammation or synovitis. Oestrogen possibly regulates pain neurotransmission by affecting the expression of neuropeptide Y and NO in sensory neurons. The combined effect of oestrogen and inflammation has been suggested to affect the expression and properties of ion channels in TMJ neurons (Wang et al. 2008). TMD pain modulation is possible via central and peripheral neural systems where oestrogen can affect the nociception of the TMJ by targeting the trigeminal ganglion which contains ER-alpha, ER-beta and a novel oestrogen receptor called the G-protein-coupled receptor 30. However, the exact relationship between oestrogen and TMD pain remains ambiguous since many studies suggest that oestrogen increases susceptibility to TMD pain, while others have shown that low oestrogen or a rapid change in oestrogen concentration results in increased TMD pain (Bi et al. 2015).

13.5 Inflammation in Arthrogenous Temporomandibular Disorders

The element of inflammation is present in many intracapsular TMD conditions, such as disc displacement disorders, synovitis, fibrous adhesions, osteoarthritis and rheumatoid arthritis (Ogura and Kondoh 2015). TMJ tissues may undergo an inflammatory process that can be induced by macro- or microtrauma generating a situation of joint overload exceeding the adaptive capacity of the joint tissues (Poluha and Grossmann 2018). It is also generally accepted that synovitis or synovial inflammation often features in disc derangements and/or osteoarthritis (Ogura and Kondoh 2015). Regardless of the actual aetiology, the resultant inflammation of TMJ tissues leads to most of the symptomatic arthrogenous TMDs.

Clinical symptoms of TMD often include pain and dysfunction during jaw movements, basically a clinical manifestation of inflammation. Inflammation in the TMJ may modify its physical and functional properties reversibly or irreversibly, eventually compromising its function (de Alcântara Camejo et al. 2017). Histologically, inflammation in TMJ is characterised by hyperplastic synovial linings, hyperaemia and infiltration of various inflammatory cells (Ohta et al. 2017), e.g. T cells, monocytes or macrophages, in the synovium of patients with disc displacement and osteoarthritis. In addition, neutrophil and macrophage accumulation in the inflamed TMJ may lead to structural damage to arthritic joints (Ogura and Kondoh 2015).

Temporomandibular joint synoviocytes or fibroblast-like synoviocytes (FLS) are thought to produce and excrete various inflammation mediators into the synovial fluid in response to damage to the synovial membrane. Histamine, serotonin, kinins, eicosanoids, platelet-activating factor, nitric oxide, tumour necrosis factor (TNF) and interleukins are among the major inflammatory mediators in TMDs (Poluha and Grossmann 2018).

The most frequently identified inflammatory mediators are cytokines: IL-1, IL-6, IL-8 and TNF (Zwiri et al. 2020). Under normal circumstances, the communication network of pro- and anti-inflammatory cytokines maintains the homeostasis of the TMJ. However, in the diseased state, inflammatory cytokines secreted into the synovial fluid of the inflamed TMJ may be involved in the enhancement of inflammation, the transition from acute inflammation to chronicity, and clinical manifestation of TMJ pain (Ibi 2019). These molecules have been studied extensively for their roles in the mechanism of synovial cellular infiltration and joint degeneration, with the following sequence of events proposed.

In response to damage to the synovium, FLS releases chemokines which stimulate chemotaxis of neutrophils, macrophages and T lymphocytes. These inflammatory cells will in turn produce inflammatory cytokines such as IL-1-beta, matrix degradative enzymes and various products of oxidative metabolism. The enzymes and oxidative metabolites cause degradation of the extracellular matrix while inflammatory cytokines stimulate FLS to release more chemokines. Some chemokines may promote angiogenesis but also recruit inflammatory cells, leading to joint degeneration (Ogura and Kondoh 2015).

Prolonged inflammation has been associated with disc displacement disorders and osteoarthritis, and contributes to the degradation of cartilage and bone joints through the release of proteinases and other inflammatory factors. Although the underlying molecular mechanisms remain to be fully elucidated, higher levels of proinflammatory cytokines such as IL-1-beta and TNF-alpha in synovial fluids of patients with disc derangement and osteoarthritis, compared to healthy TMJ, are thought to stimulate synoviocytes to produce and secrete inflammatory cytokines or chemokines (Wang et al. 2012; Kellesarian et al. 2016; Ibi 2019). Notably, IL-1-beta and TNF-alpha are pleiotropic cytokines known for their important roles in immune reactions, inflammation and cartilage/bone remodelling, particularly cartilage degradation and bone resorption (Ogura and Kondoh 2015).

13.6 Cytokines in Temporomandibular Disorders

13.6.1 Interleukin-1

At present, the IL-1 family consists of 11 cytokines and 10 receptors, all of which are extremely potent modulators of inflammation. Among them are IL-1-alpha and IL-1-beta, two cytokines of similar molecular weight that bind to the same receptor and induce a similar immunological effect (Dinarella 2018). IL-1-alpha and IL-1-beta are produced by various cell types, such as macrophages, fibroblasts, osteoblasts and synoviocytes. Both cytokines have been detected in synovial fluid from patients with internal derangement and osteoarthritis but IL-1-beta was more frequently reported. IL-1-beta was also predominantly expressed in synoviocytes (Ogura and Kondoh 2015). Increased expression of IL-1 in the synovial fluid at different phases indicates that these cytokines may result in the development and progression of TMD (Zwiri et al. 2020).

While IL-1-alpha is synthesised in its active form, IL-1-beta undergoes posttranslational modification to become an active agonist in IL-1 signalling. Generally, processing of the IL-1-beta precursor may or may not involve caspase-1 (also known as IL-1-converting enzyme, ICE) (Dinarello 2011) that is contained within a specialised intracellular complex termed the inflammasome (Turner et al. 2014). IL-1-beta plays a crucial role in conditions like arthritic joint and following blunt trauma, hypoxia, haemorrhage or exposure to irritants, but ICE may not be necessary. For example, irritant-induced inflammation in muscle tissue, cartilage destruction in joints and urate crystal-induced inflammation are all IL-1-beta dependent but caspase-1 independent (Dinarello 2011). Hence, it may be a caspase-1-independent process in the case of internal derangement and osteoarthritis.

In the IL-1 system, IL-1-alpha and IL-1-beta are activated through binding to the IL-1 receptor – a complex of two chains, namely IL-1 receptor type I (IL-1RI) and IL-1 receptor accessory protein (IL-1RAcP). The assembled complex leads to the induction of intracellular signal transduction, beginning with the recruitment of myeloid differentiation primary response gene 88 (MyD88) adaptor protein (Ogura and Kondoh 2015). MyD88 serves as a scaffold protein on which IL-I receptor-associated kinase 4 (IRAK-4) is presumed to phosphorylate IRAK-1, leading to the autophosphorylation and activation of IRAK-1 itself. MyD88 only binds non-phosphorylated IRAK-1, so IRAK-1 is then released from the receptor complex and binds to TNF-receptor-associated factor 6 (TRAF6), ultimately resulting in activation of the nuclear factor kappa B (NF-kappa-B) and mitogen-activated protein kinase, i.e. MAPK pathways involving p38, JNKs (Janus kinases) and ERKs (extracellular signal-regulated kinases). TRAF6 recruits TGF-beta-activated kinase 1 (TAK1, a MAPK kinase) which then activates the I-kappa-B kinase (IKK) complex, which is essentially made up of two kinases (IKK-alpha and IKK-beta) and a regulatory unit NF-kappa-B essential modifier (NEMO/IKK-gamma). Activated IKK-beta phosphorylates inhibitor of NF-kappa-B (I-kappa-B-alpha), triggering its degradation and thereby freeing NF-kappa-B. Translocation of the active NF-kappa-B dimer (comprising RelA/p65 and NFκB1/p50 subunits in most cells) into the nucleus leads to activation of the NF-kappa-B pathway through which various genes involved in inflammation and other immune responses are activated. On the other hand, TAK1 also phosphorylates MAPK kinases such as MKK3/6 and MKK4/7, which in turn stimulates p38/SAPKs (stress-activated protein kinases) and JNKs (c-Jun N-terminal kinases), respectively (Ogura and Kondoh 2015; Flannery and Bowie 2010).

Chronic inflammation may over time disrupt the homeostatic balance of the extracellular matrix within the cartilaginous tissue of the TMJ, causing its eventual net loss (Morel et al. 2019). Progressive connective tissue loss is a shared characteristic in rheumatoid arthritis and osteoarthritis, that is mediated mainly by chondrocytes, synovial fibroblasts and even osteoclasts (Vincenti and Brinckerhoff 2002). This process is heavily influenced by IL-1-alpha, IL-1-beta and TNF-alpha through the regulation of MMPs (Morel et al. 2019; Aida et al. 2012). MMP and a disintegrin and metalloproteinase with thrombospondin motifs (ADAMTS) are catabolic enzymes with crucial roles in cartilage matrix degradation (Ogura and Kondoh 2015). Aggrecanase-1 (ADAMTS-4) and aggrecanase-2 (ADAMTS-5/11) of the ADAMTS family are responsible for the degradation of proteoglycan in osteoarthritis (Legendre et al. 2005). MMP-1, MMP-8 and MMP-13 degrade type II collagen, also a component of the ECM within the TMJ fibrocartilage. In particular, IL-1-beta and TNF-alpha increase the expression of MMP-1 and MMP-13 (Vincenti and Brinckerhoff 2002). MMP-1 (also known as collagenase-1) is more ubiquitously expressed, but MMP-13 (also known as collagenase-3) degrades type II collagen more efficiently (Vincenti and Brinckerhoff 2002). Transcriptional induction of MMP-1 and MMP-13 is possible via NF-kappa-B and MAPK pathways. On the other hand, MMP transcription involving the MAPK family would also include the ERKs, besides JNK and p38 kinases.

Most promoters of MMP contain a TATA box, the core transcriptional unit, and cis-acting DNA elements like the activating protein-1 (AP-1) binding site (Vincenti and Brinckerhoff 2002; Legendre et al. 2005). JNKs and ERKs phosphorylate and activate the AP-1 family member c-Jun, which dimerises with c-Fos at the AP-1 sites on the MMP promoters, leading to the expression of MMPs. The ERK pathway also regulates the activity of erythroblastosis 26 (ETS) transcription factors, which interact with AP-1 proteins in multiple MMP promoters. Meanwhile, p38 contributes indirectly to MMP transcription by promoting the expression of AP-1 (Vincenti and Brinckerhoff 2002). Incidentally, raised synovial fluid viscosity due to increased cytokine expression by infiltrating chronic inflammatory cells also contributes to the breakdown of joint ultrastructure by impairing nutrition and lubrication of the disc and articular cartilage (Kellesarian et al. 2016).

13.6.2 Tumour Necrosis Factor Alpha

Tumour necrosis factor-alpha is a proinflammatory cytokine mainly produced by activated macrophages and T lymphocytes during inflammation and infection. TNF-alpha is likely to mediate acute and chronic inflammation associated with connective tissue degeneration in TMD. T-cell-induced inflammation reportedly contributes to the pathogenesis of TMD, as T cells and macrophages were found in samples from patients with generalised osteoarthritis and rheumatoid arthritis of TMJ. On the other hand, TNF-alpha is frequently detected in synovial fluid and expressed by synoviocytes in samples taken from patients with disc derangement. TNF-alpha enhances the production of several chemokines, such as IL-8, C-X-C motif ligand 1 (CXCL1) and C-C motif chemokine ligand 20 (CCL20) in synovial fibroblasts. It is also a potent inducer of NF-kappa-B and NF-kappa-B-dependent IL-8, CXCL10 and cyclo-oxygenase-2 expression in synovial fibroblasts of the TMJ. These chemokines may promote and shape the pathological condition of the TMJ by attracting inflammatory cells such as T cells and neutrophils to the inflamed synovium (Ohta et al. 2017).

The TNF-alpha signalling pathway is initiated with the binding of ligand TNF-alpha to its receptors, either TNFR1 or TNFR2. TNFR1 is a strong inducer of proinflammatory activities while TNFR2 possesses both pro- and anti-inflammatory effects. In the TNF-alpha–TNFR1 axis, the TNFR-associated death domain (TRADD) interacts with the intracellular death domain of TNFR1 to recruit TNF receptor-associated factor 2 (TRAF-2) and receptor-interacting protein 1(RIP-1), which are essential for the activation of NF-kappa-B, and Fas-associated death domain (FADD) that regulates the apoptotic pathway. The TNFR1 signalling complex (also known as complex I) undergoes various modifications which in turn allow the recruitment of TAK-1 via the adapter protein TAK1-binding protein-2 (TAB2). TAK1 can then activate the IKK-beta and subsequently trigger the events of the classic NF-kappa-B pathway. In addition, TNF-alpha also triggers the signalling cascades of MAPKs such as p38 and JNK (Ogura and Kondoh 2015; Pobezinskaya and Liu 2012; Wajant and Siegmund 2019).

Tumour necrosis factor-alpha may also bind to TNFR2 on the cell surface to form a signalling complex, which consists of TRAF-2, a cellular inhibitor of apoptosis protein 2 (cIAP2) and cIAP-1. Unlike TNFR1, TNFR2 lacks the death domain but receptors of this subgroup can directly recruit TRAF adapter proteins, especially TRAF2, through a short peptide motif. In contrast to the TNFR2-associated cytotoxic activity, cell signalling associated with TNFR2-induced gene induction is currently poorly understood. However, there is evidence of IKK complex recruitment to the TNFR2 signalling complex which results in activation of the classic NF-kappa-B pathway too, albeit less efficient than in the case of TNFR1 (Wajant and Siegmund 2019; Siegmund et al. 2018).

13.6.3 Interleukin-6

The proinflammatory IL-6 is another cytokine frequently implicated in the pathogenesis of TMJ inflammation and disorders. This pleiotropic cytokine is produced by cells such as FLS, monocytes, macrophages, T cells and B cells and has important roles in immune reactions, inflammation, haematopoiesis, carcinogenesis, osteoclastic activity and differentiation. Elevated levels of IL-6 and soluble IL-6R are regularly detected in correlation with greater severity of disease, in the synovial fluid of patients with rheumatoid arthritis, internal derangement and osteoarthritis of the TMJ (Ogura and Kondoh 2015).

Interleukin-6 exerts its biological activity by forming an IL-6 receptor complex with the cell membrane-bound IL-6R-alpha (gp80 or CD126) and subsequently the signal-transducing protein IL-6R-beta (gp130 or CD130). IL-6R-alpha is only present in limited cells, including hepatocytes and some leucocytes, but IL-6R-beta is expressed in all cells. IL-6R-alpha may also exist in a soluble form as soluble IL-6R (sIL-6R) and bind to IL-6 with similar affinity. The formation of a IL-6/IL-6R/IL-6Rβ complex initiates classic intracellular signalling and activates the JAK/STAT3, P13K/AKT and MAPK/ERK signalling pathways. However, IL-6 trans-signalling is mediated by forming the complex with a soluble rather than the cell-bound IL-6R.

Classic signalling is important for the acute phase of immunological response and promotes anti-inflammatory activities through the synthesis of acute-phase proteins with anti-inflammatory properties. This pathway is indispensable for immune defence. Meanwhile, IL-6 trans-signalling is proinflammatory in various inflammation and autoimmune diseases, as well as inflammation-associated cancer (Ogura and Kondoh 2015; Choy and Rose-John 2017; Su et al. 2017).

The complicated properties of IL-6 in inflammation remain controversial as the pathogenetic roles of IL-6 classic and trans-signalling may be different in different diseases. However, trans-signalling has been described as markedly stronger and used in many cell types and tissues compared to classic signalling. IL-6 initiated pro- and anti-inflammatory responses that are dependent on the expression ratios of the membrane-bound IL-6R-alpha to IL-6R-beta on the cell surface (Reeh et al. 2019). Soluble IL-6R and soluble IL-6R-beta modulate IL-6-induced signalling through a buffer system. In the excess of sIL-6R, trans-signalling is favoured but when sIL-6R-beta is in excess, both IL-6-induced signalling pathways are blocked. This is because sIL-6R-beta at a high concentration forces free IL-6 into IL-6/IL-6R-alpha/sIL-6R-beta complexes (Reeh et al. 2019). The concentrations of sIL-6R and sIL-6R-beta are generally much higher than their effector IL-6 under steady-state conditions. Hence, IL-6R-beta will associate with the IL-6/sIL-6R complex which will then be neutralised. This will change during inflammation, as the concentration of IL-6 will be increased drastically (up to a million fold) in contrast to the relatively small increase (2–5-fold) for sIL-6R and sIL-6R-beta (Rose-John 2012).

Dysregulated IL-6 activity is associated with the acute stage of patients with degenerative joint disease due to its role as a major mediator of the acute-phase response. In rheumatoid arthritis, therapeutic targeting with anti-IL-6R antibody to neutralise the increased levels of IL-6 has been shown to be beneficial, and comparable to the benefits of blocking TNF-alpha activity. Tocilizumab (anti-IL-6R-alpha antibody) and JAK inhibitors (tofacitinib, baricitinib) have been approved for treatment of rheumatoid arthritis but do not differentially block trans- and classic signalling (Reeh et al. 2019). Tocilizumab reduces C-reactive protein (CRP) levels, one of the acute-phase proteins released during inflammation (Choy and Rose-John 2017).

Acute inflammation is an innate and immediate response following tissue injury, characterised by local leucocyte recruitment, death and emigration. IL-6 has been implicated in regulating the transition from neutrophil to monocyte recruitment, a hallmark of acute inflammation. This transition might be related to the release of chemokines, IL-8 and monocyte chemotactic protein-1 (MCP-1) in the inflammatory site. IL-8 predominantly recruits polymorphonuclear leucocytes (PMN) in the first 24 hours before gradually being replaced by MCP-1-recruited monocytes. IL-8 and other chemoattractants induce the shedding of IL-6R from neutrophil membranes to form sIL-6R. Together with locally produced IL-6, sIL-6R stimulates the non-IL-6R-expressing endothelial cells to secrete MCP-1 rather than IL-8, resulting in decreased neutrophil but increased monocyte recruitment. This transition is enhanced by IL-6-induced PMN apoptosis, which also prevents further tissue injury because there is no discharge of the intracellular toxic contents. Moreover, PMN apoptosis indirectly leads to monocyte recruitment as phagocytosis of apoptotic neutrophils induces MCP-1 production by macrophages (Kaplanski et al. 2003). On another note, IL-6-mediated upregulation of macrophage colony-stimulating factor (M-CSF) receptors on monocytes has been shown to switch the differentiation of monocytes to macrophages, instead of dendritic cells (Su et al. 2017).

Interleukin-6 plays important roles in the activation of T cells and B cells, both of which are integral to cellular and humoral immune responses and are usually elevated in sepsis or aseptic inflammation such as rheumatoid arthritis (de Alcântara Camejo et al. 2017). IL-6 is involved in the maturation of B cells into plasma cells and the induction of regulatory B cells. IL-6 causes the differentiation of T cells (CD4$^+$ and CD8$^+$) into subsets that produce IL-21, which in turn stimulates the maturation of B cells (Choy and Rose-John 2017). On the other hand, IL-6 is involved in the regulation of T-cell differentiation between regulatory T (Treg) cells and T helper 17 (Th17) cells. IL-6 in concert with transforming growth factor (TGF)-beta stimulates Th17 helper cell differentiation from naive CD4$^+$ T cells by enhancing the expression of transcription factors, including retinoic acid-related orphan receptor gamma t (ROR-gamma-t). This process is amplified by the presence of sIL-6R, which is produced by naive and memory CD4$^-$ T cells during the activation of T-cell receptors. At the same time. IL-6 also inhibits signal transducer and activator of transcription 3 (STAT3)-mediated generation of Treg cells. Hence, Th17 cells secrete proinflammatory cytokines such as IL-17 and initiate various inflammatory responses, which could intensify due to the lack of mediation by the reduced Treg cells (Su et al. 2017).

Interleukin-6 induces receptor activator of NF-kappa-B ligand (RANKL) expression in osteoblasts and synoviocytes, which in turn stimulates osteoclast formation causing structural changes to the joint, pivotal in the pathogenesis of intracapsular TMD, particularly rheumatoid arthritis. A positive correlation between increased levels of IL-6 and other cytokines such as IL-1-beta and TNF-alpha in the synovial fluid and the extent of TMJ destruction has been suggested (Kellesarian et al. 2016). However, IL-1-beta, TNF-alpha and IL-6 can trigger a cytokine amplification loop via IL-6–STAT3 that promotes sustained inflammation and joint destruction in rheumatoid arthritis. These cytokines activate STAT3 which then induces the expression of IL-6, thus further activating STAT3 in osteoblastic and fibroblastic cells. Membrane-bound IL-6Rs are expressed at low levels on osteoblasts and fibroblasts. STAT3 activation is also involved in the induction of RANKL expression which is essential for osteoclastogenesis (Mori et al. 2011).

In rheumatoid arthritis and osteoarthritis, IL-6 may inhibit the synthesis of type II collagen and aggrecan, and induce expression of MMP-1, MMP-3, MMP-13, ADAMTS-4 and ADAMTS-5/11. IL-6 also amplifies IL-1-induced MMP synthesis and proteoglycan depletion (Legendre et al. 2005). Likewise, IL-1-beta may promote the autocrine action of IL-6 in chondrocytes by increasing IL-6 receptor expression (Aida et al. 2012). MMP-3 (or stromelysin) is an aggrecan-degrading enzyme that also activates MMP-1, which is a collagen-degrading enzyme (Vincenti and Brinckerhoff 2002; Legendre et al. 2005). IL-6, in the presence of sIL-6R, greatly enhances MMP production. This is because FLS constitutively expresses gp130, but not IL-6R. Formation of the IL-6/sIL-6R/IL-6R-beta complex is increased since sIL-6R exists in synovial fluids and IL-6 is produced by FLS in the presence of IL-1-beta and/or TNF-alpha (Ogura and Kondoh 2015). IL-6/sIL-6R stimulates both JAK-STAT and MAPK signalling cascades, which co-operate to maximise induction of MMP and ADAMTS gene transcription in the chondrocytes (Legendre et al. 2005). Janus kinases (JAK) are tyrosine kinase effectors that can activate the cytoplasmic transcription factor STAT, which then translocates to the nucleus and acts on target gene transcription.

The presence of IL-6 and sIL-6R also induces the synthesis of tissue inhibitors of metalloproteinase-1 (TIMP-1). TIMP-1 is an endogenous MMP inhibitor that can bind activated forms of MMP-1, -3 and -13. Therefore, IL-6 and sIL-6r activate the turnover of cartilage matrix proteins through the increased production of MMP-1, -13 and TIMP-1 via the ERK signalling cascade (Aida et al. 2012).

13.6.4 Interleukin-8

Interleukin-8 belongs to the C-X-C subfamily of chemokines that is significantly upregulated following IL-1-beta- and TNF-alpha-induced signalling cascades, so is frequently analysed in TMD research in conjunction with IL-1 and/or TNF (Zwiri et al. 2020). IL-8 (also known as CXCL-8) is similarly increased in the synovial fluid of rheumatoid arthritis, osteoarthritis and internal derangement. It is also expressed by chondrocytes and synoviocytes of patients with osteoarthritis and rheumatoid arthritis (Bouloux 2009; Ogura and Kondoh 2015). Transcription of IL-8, a proinflammatory chemokine, is possible via the NF-kappa-B and MAPK pathways. This could be attributed to the presence of two NF-kappa-B binding sites and one AP-1 binding site in the CXCL8 promoter. Stimuli such as TNF and IL-1 are capable of simultaneously triggering NF-kappa-B and SAPK/JNK cascades to produce synergistic activation of IL-8 transcription and secretion. In addition, activation of the p38 MAP kinase cascade stabilises IL-8 mRNA to further complement IL-8 synthesis (Holtmann et al. 1999).

Functionally, IL-8 is largely associated with neutrophil chemotaxis and activation. It is also implicated in the recruitment of monocytes, lymphocytes, basophils and eosinophils at sites of inflammation, as well as being an angiogenic factor (Turner et al. 2014). Regulation of chemokines such as IL-8 is important to control the intensity of inflammation as excessive amounts can result in destruction of host tissue (Holtmann et al. 1999). IL-8 may reversibly exist as monomers or dimers, an ability that is essential in the regulation of neutrophil recruitment (Turner et al. 2014). Either form is capable of binding, with differential affinity, to glycosaminoglycans (GAGs) on endothelial cells and ECM (Das et al. 2010). GAG-binding may induce a conformational change that facilitates the consequent binding to G-protein-coupled receptors, CXC chemokine receptors (CXCR) 1 or 2 on neutrophils (Schlorke et al. 2012). GAG-binding also creates a chemotactic gradient crucial in enhancing the binding of IL-8 to the receptors (Schlorke et al. 2012). Following that, intracellular signalling cascades are initiated through the activation of intracellular G proteins to induce chemotaxis and degranulation. The G proteins are subunits (G-alpha, -beta, -gamma) that dissociate from the receptor. The G-alpha subunit activates the membrane-bound adenylate cyclase (AC), generating cyclic AMP (cAMP) which then activates protein kinase A (PKA). The dissociated G-beta-gamma heterodimer stimulates phospholipase beta (PLC-beta), which catalyses phospholipids to produce inositol 3,4,5-triphosphate (IP3) and diacylglycerol (DAG). IP3 triggers neutrophil degranulation by stimulating the release of intracellular calcium stores. Meanwhile, DAG activates protein kinase C (PKC), which then induces MAPK activation. IL-8-mediated MAPK and phosphatidylinositol-3 kinase (PI3K) signalling induce the expression of adhesion molecules responsible for chemotaxis (Turner et al. 2014).

13.7 Pain and Inflammation in the Temporomandibular Joint

The joint capsule, synovial membrane and articular disc are innervated by myelinated and unmyelinated nerve fibres with free nerve endings. Many of these nerve fibres are mechanical and chemical nociceptors that are part of the peripheral mechanism generally associated with TMJ pain. However, the pathophysiology of TMJ pain is unclear. The multiple aetiologies of TMD, poor correlation between pain severity and actual tissue damage, as well as concomitant pain in other areas of the body, are unresolved issues that cannot be satisfactorily explained by a common pain mechanism.

Mechanical nociceptors may be triggered by excessive jaw movements or overloading of the joints that can be exacerbated by the presence of pathological changes to the joint structures. Chemically induced nociception is possible via the release of neuropeptides, inflammatory mediators and/or local hypoxia. Sustained peripherally induced nociceptive stimuli could result in prolonged sensitisation of the central nervous system (Cairns 2010).

Neuroradiological studies offer further insights into structural and functional brain alterations in TMD patients with chronic pain (Yin et al. 2020). Central sensitisation may reduce pain thresholds and tolerance, hence better explaining phenomena such as pain–tissue damage discrepancies, referred pain and generalised pain sensitivity or co-existing chronic pain in other body areas. Another less proven proposed consequence of chronic TMJ pain is the reflex masticatory muscle spasm which could also contribute to pain in TMDs, especially since myogenous and arthrogenous TMDs are not mutually exclusive.

Other pathophysiological factors contributing to TMJ pain that have been proposed are generalised hyperexcitability of the central nociceptive neurons, decreased endogenous pain control mechanisms and psychosocial stressors. Stress is implicated since many of the mediators for stress responses and pain modulation are similar. Furthermore, stress can promote parafunctional habits and affect the muscles through sympathetic nervous system activation. In lesser roles, genetic predisposition to chronic pain and oestrogen effect on pain transduction and endogenous analgesia have also been described (Cairns 2010).

Inflammatory responses in TMD are associated with neural changes involving the peripheral and central nervous systems. A number of inflammatory mediators within the synovium and synovial fluid contribute to peripheral sensitisation, possibly via mediation by nerve growth factors released during inflammation. In addition, raised levels of angiogenic factors such as vascular endothelial growth factor (VEGF) and fibroblast growth factor (FGF) during inflammation have been identified in patients with internal derangement, with neurite extension and arborisation occurring post angiogenesis thought to contribute to pain (Bouloux 2009).

Detection of proinflammatory cytokines such as TNF-alpha, IL-1-beta, IL-6 and interferon (IFN)-gamma correlate with TMJ pain in samples that include disc derangements and osteoarthritis (Bouloux 2009). These cytokines promote the release of pronociceptive compounds including potassium chloride, leukotriene B4 (LTB4), prostaglandin (PG) E2, bradykinin, serotonin, histamine, glutamate and adenosine triphosphate (ATP) (Cairns 2020). Bradykinin, leukotriene B4, PGE2 and substance P have been associated with pain in patients with internal derangement and osteoarthritis. Patients with higher pain scores post arthrocentesis correspond to greater detection of these mediators (Bouloux 2009). The concentration of PGE2, leukotriene B4, malondialdehyde, NO and myeloperoxidase also correlates with the Wilkes criteria, a five-stage classification describing the severity of internal derangement including presence/absence of pain (Bouloux 2009).

Histamine is positively correlated with pain-related TMD as it induces nociception indirectly via a mechanism stimulating serotonin (5-hydroxytryptamine, 5-HT) release. Serotonin induces nociception through activation of beta-1 and beta-2 adrenoreceptors in the TMJ, and local release of adrenergic amines and prostaglandins. It was found to be significantly increased in the synovial fluid of temporomandibular arthralgias (Poluha and Grossmann 2018). Serotonin has a lesser role in vasodilation and increased vascular permeability in inflammation of the TMJ, but it has a conversely significant role in inflammatory pain of the region (Poluha and Grossmann 2018). Kinins (bradykinin, lysyl-bradykinin, methionyl-lysyl-bradykinin) are implicated in TMDs due to their proinflammatory properties. They interact with beta-1 and beta-2 receptors on inflammatory cells to promote the synthesis of IL-1 and TNF, and to activate phospholipases A2 and C. This has been demonstrated to correlate with the degree of synovitis (Poluha and Grossmann 2018).

In turn, these pronociceptive compounds trigger spontaneous discharge within nociceptive neurons in the TMJ and subnucleus caudalis. Stimulation of TMJ nociceptors results in the release of neuropeptides such as calcitonin gene-related peptide (CGRP) and substance P, leading to neurogenic inflammation (Cairns 2010). CGRP, neuropeptide Y (NPY), serotonin and the capsaicin receptor transient receptor potential vanilloid-1 (TRPV1) are some specific pain mediators that have been found to be correlated with the degree of pain or synovitis (Bouloux 2009). Expression of CGRP and substance P may be increased in patients with painful disc displacements, but only CGRP shows a weak correlation with pain intensity. These pain-related neuropeptides may be expressed due to progressive joint injury or subsequent to local hypoxia induced by injury to the joint (Cairns 2010).

Inflammation may also stimulate the mechanical nociceptors through increased intra-articular pressure from joint oedema (Cairns 2010). Joint effusion or swollen joint is one of the signs seen in inflammatory conditions such as osteoarthritis and rheumatoid arthritis. More importantly, joint effusion correlates with increased protein content and pain. Increased IL-6 expression has been associated with joint effusion, and demonstrated an indirect connection with pain. High IL-6 and TIMP-1 levels have both been detected in synovial fluids of painful chronic TMJ disorders (Bouloux 2009).

The concentration of free radicals such as NO levels was significantly higher in painful joints compared to pain-free joints, especially in osteoarthritis. Incidentally, proinflammatory cytokines like TNF-alpha, IL-1-beta and IFN-gamma may induce NO production in many cells, including articular chondrocytes and synoviocytes. NO is a potent vasodilator that could culminate in hyperaemia, a feature that is consistent with synovitis. With the association between pain and synovitis previously demonstrated, NO-mediated TMJ pain is therefore plausible. The painful joints could also be explained by increased sensitivity of peripheral nociceptors caused by the elevated NO levels (Takahashi et al. 1999).

Furthermore, cyclo-oxygenase-2 (COX-2) was found to be expressed in synovial lining, infiltrating mononuclear cells, fibroblast-like cells and endothelial cells in the synovium of patients with internal derangement and osteoarthritis. COX-2 is an inducible isoform of COX, which is an enzyme involved in the production of various prostaglandins, including PGE2 which is essential in pain signalling (Seki et al. 2004). Various cytokines, growth factors and free radicals may induce COX-2 production via activation of transcriptional regulatory proteins such as NF-kappa-B, AP1 and CCAAT/enhancer binding protein (C/EBP) that act on promoter sites (Ogura and Kondoh 2015; Seki et al. 2004). For instance, IL-1-beta, TNF-alpha, NO donor S-nitros-N-acetyl-D and L-penicillamine have all been demonstrated to increase the production of COX-2 in synovial cells of osteoarthritis or rheumatoid arthritis. Upregulation of COX-2, stimulated directly by proinflammatory cytokines or indirectly by NO, correlates with synovitis and joint pain. Prostaglandins are also capable of sensitising nociceptors to other mediators (Seki et al. 2004).

13.8 Other Inflammation-related Biomarkers in Temporomandibular Disorders

Extensive research in TMD has identified a great number of molecules, particularly inflammatory mediators including but not limited to the following: histamine, serotonin, eicosanoids, platelet-activating factor, nitric oxide, interferon, tumour necrosis factor and interleukins. Figure 13.3 provides an overview of the commonly studied markers in TMD, expressly those using samples from synovial fluid or tissues from the TMJ.

In the event of tissue insult, mast cells found in the retrodiscal zone of the TMJ may degranulate and release histamine. Histamine contributes to TMJ inflammation by promoting vasodilation and increasing vascular permeability and

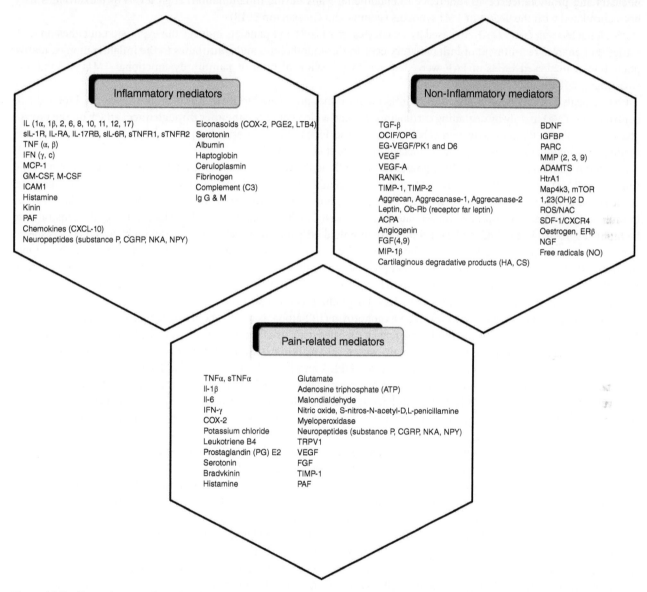

Figure 13.3 Expansive overview of molecules investigated in relation to TMD. Some of these molecules are not mutually exclusive and may interact with each other in inflammation, non-inflammation and pain-related functions. ICAM, intercellular adhesion molecules; NKA, neurokinin A; MCP-1, monocyte chemotactic protein-1; GM-CSF, granulocyte-macrophage colony-stimulating factor; TGF, transforming growth factor; OCIF, osteoclastogenesis inhibitory factor; OPG, osteoprotegerin; EG-VEGF/PK1, endocrine gland-derived vascular endothelial growth factor/prokineticin-1; VEGF, vascular endothelial growth factor; TIMP, tissue inhibitors of metalloproteinases; ACPA, anti-citrullinated peptide antibodies; FGF, fibroblast growth factors; MIP, macrophage inflammatory protein; HA, hyaluronic acid; CS, chondroitin sulfate; BDNF, brain-derived neurotrophic factor; IGFBP, insulin-like growth factor-binding protein; PARC, pulmonary and activation-regulated protein; HtrA1, high-temperature requirement serine protease A1; MAP4K3, mitogen-activated protein kinase kinase kinase kinase 3; mTOR, mammalian target of rapamycin; ROS, reactive oxygen species; NAC, N-acetyl cysteine; SDF, stromal cell-derived factor; NGF, nerve growth factor.

endothelial activation. Histamine concentration tends to be higher in osteoarthritis than in other TMDs and has been implicated in TMD pain (Poluha and Grossmann 2018).

Eicosanoids are a group of molecules derived from 20-carbon polyunsaturated fatty acids, usually arachidonic acid. Arachidonic acids are generated through hydrolysis of phospholipids on the cell membrane by the enzymes phospholipase A2 and C. Arachidonic acid subsequently follows COX or lipoxygenase pathways to produce eicosanoids such as prostaglandins, thromboxanes and leukotrienes. Prostaglandins and prostacyclins enhance the effects of histamine and kinins during late inflammation by increasing the sensitivity of specific receptors. Prostaglandins, especially PGE2, have an additional role in TMJ nociception. Leukotrienes are implicated in chemotaxis, aggregation and degranulation of polymorphonuclears and promote leucocyte adherence to endothelial walls during inflammation. High levels of leukotrienes have been correlated with the degree of TMJ synovitis (Poluha and Grossmann 2018).

Platelet-activating factor (PAF) released by leucocytes, mast cells and platelets induces the expression of adhesion molecules that enables recruitment of inflammatory cells to the endothelium and contributes to the inflammation exudative phenomena. Increased levels of PAF were detected in the synovial fluid of painful, dysfunctional TMJs (Poluha and Grossmann 2018).

Free radicals like NO have minor roles in inflammation that are related to their effects on blood vessels. Free radicals contribute to TMD mainly by degrading cartilaginous tissue which could occur either through direct attack on the proteoglycan and collagen fibres or activation of latent collagenase. Free radicals generated in proximity to bone surfaces may also incite the formation of bone-resorbing osteoclasts (Tomida et al. 2003).

Interferon-gamma is another cytokine produced by T cells and natural killer cells that can be found in the synovial fluid samples of TMD patients. IFN-gamma possesses both proinflammatory and anti-inflammatory properties. IFN-gamma, alone or particularly in combination with TNF-alpha, promotes the expression of CXCR3 chemokines like CXCL-10 by binding to CXCR3 receptors present on activated T cells. With CXCR3 chemokines and T cells previously demonstrated to be highly expressed in the inflamed synovium of rheumatoid arthritis, the synergistic effect of both cytokines was speculated to recruit numerous T cells to the inflammation site. Conversely, IFN-gamma has inhibitive effects on TNF-alpha-mediated IL-8 and CXCL-1 production, TNF-alpha-induced collagenase expression in chondrocytes and induction of osteoclastogenesis in bone marrow macrophages. IFN-gamma may differentially regulate TNF-alpha-induced chemokines in the synovial fibroblasts of the TMJ via JAK/STAT1 signalling (Ohta et al. 2017).

Tumour necrosis factor-beta, also known as lymphotoxin (LT)-alpha, is a close homologue to TNF-alpha that was also found to be elevated in the synovial fluid of patients with osteoarthritis of the TMJ. However, due to the relative scarcity of literature on this molecule, less is known especially with regard to its role in the pathogenesis of TMD. TNF-beta is expressed by T cells, B cells and natural killer cells, and binds to TNFR-1 and TNFR-2 like TNR-alpha. There is in vitro evidence that TNF-beta induces proliferation and production of proinflammatory cytokines in FLS. A study of chondrocyte cultures of unspecified origin showed that TNF-beta stimulates activation of the NF-kappa-B pathway and consequent proinflammatory activity. Within an inflammatory microenvironment, TNF-beta also increases the adhesiveness of T cells to chondrocytes.

These results indicate that TNF-beta exerts similar effects to TNR-alpha in inflamed chondrocytes. This observation is supported by additional findings from several studies on biological therapy. Anti-TNF-beta treatment was comparable to anti-TNF-alpha, significantly improving clinical symptoms of rheumatoid arthritis in animal studies. While anti-TNF-alpha has been used in the treatment of rheumatoid arthritis with promising results, a TNF-beta antibody, pateclizumab, also received a favourable evaluation in a phase I clinical trial (Buhrmann et al. 2013).

Besides IL-1, IL-6 and IL-8, other interleukins have also been investigated in association with TMD. IL-2, -10, -11, -12 and -17 have all been correlated with TMD (Kellesarian et al. 2016). IL-2, IL-12 and IL-17 were upregulated while IL-10 was downregulated in osteoarthritis of the TMJ. However, little else was discussed on IL-2, a cytokine with a primary function in the proliferation and activation of T and B cells (Turner et al. 2014). In contrast, although IL-12 showed no significant difference in a study examining cytokine levels following irrigation of TMJ with chronic closed lock, previous studies have implicated elevated IL-12 in disease activity in rheumatoid arthritis patients.

Interleukin-10, on the other hand, is recognised for its anti-inflammatory properties. IL-10 has been shown to inhibit the synthesis of IL-1-alpha, IL-1-beta, IL-6, IL-8, IL-12, TNF-alpha in monocyte/macrophage, IL-2 and IL-12 in T helper cell 1(Th-1), IFN-gamma in dendritic cell and NK, as well as reactive oxygen and nitrogen intermediates. IL-10 also induces the production of anti-inflammatory cytokines like IL-1RA. In addition, the presence of IL-10 in healthy TMJ contributes to the speculation that it has a protective role in the pathophysiology of TMD.

Interleukin-17 has been detected in the synovial fluid of rheumatoid arthritis and reportedly promotes bone degradation through the induction of RANKL. Relevant IL-17 activities also include inducing synovitis and cartilage degradation, inhibiting the proliferation of chondrocytes, and enhancing the production of NO and osteoclastogenic cytokines like IL-1-beta and IL-6. TNF-alpha and IFN-gamma may augment IL-17-induced effects (Vernal et al. 2008). IL-11 is another scarcely discussed interleukin that was found to be significantly increased together with IL-6 in TMJs exhibiting osseous changes in the condyle (Kellesarian et al. 2016).

Recently, there has been some interest in the activation of inflammasomes as a new mechanism of inflammation induction in TMD. The inflammasome is a multiprotein complex comprising a sensor protein, an adapter protein and the inflammatory protease caspase-1. Activated caspase-1 converts inactive precursors of IL-1-beta and IL-18 into their active counterparts. Secreted IL-1-beta and IL-18 then proceed to evoke an inflammatory response. Internal derangement and osteoarthritis of TMJ were considered comparable to diseases like atherosclerosis and Alzheimer disease that have been investigated in relation to inflammasomes because all these diseases are characterised by sterile inflammation. Since IL-1-beta is a major proinflammatory cytokine in TMJ inflammation, inflammasome involvement is thought highly possible. NLRP3, as one of the sensor proteins of the inflammasome, has been investigated for possible involvement in osteoarthritis pathology (Ibi 2019).

13.9 Conclusion

The fact that inflammation and its associated biological factors are pivotal in the pathogenesis of arthrogenous TMD is undeniable. However, full disclosure of the mechanisms underlying the pathogenesis has yet to be achieved despite the abundance of related research. This chapter discusses arthrogenous TMD from an immunological point of view based on the current understanding of associated inflammatory mediators. Most of the commonly identified molecules have been discussed in depth or in passing while others were not discussed because they are not primarily inflammation-related molecules. Unfortunately, potential inadequacies of sampling techniques in synovial fluid collection, differences in the precision and sensitivity level of methods employed in cytokine profiling, and inconsistent patient recruitment criteria of an already diagnostically challenging group of diseases remain concerning issues that prevent clear interpretation of many research findings.

References

Aida, Y., Honda, K., Tanigawa, S. et al. (2012). IL-6 and soluble IL-6 receptor stimulate the production of MMPs and their inhibitors via JAK-STAT and ERK-MAPK signalling in human chondrocytes. *Cell Biol. Int.* 36 (4): 367–376.

Bi, R.Y., Ding, Y. and Gan, Y.H. (2015). A new hypothesis of sex-differences in temporomandibular disorders: estrogen enhances hyperalgesia of inflamed TMJ through modulating voltage-gated sodium channel 1.7 in trigeminal ganglion. *Med. Hypoth.* 84: 100–103.

Bouloux, G.F. (2009). Temporomandibular joint pain and synovial fluid analysis: a review of the literature. *J. Oral Maxillofac. Surg.* 67: 2497–2504.

Buhrmann, C., Shayan, P., Aggarwal, B.B. and Shakibaei, M. (2013). Evidence that TNF-β (lymphotoxin α) can activate the inflammatory environment in human chondrocytes. *Arthritis Res. Ther.* 15: R202.

Cairns, B.E. (2010). Pathophysiology of TMD pain – basic mechanisms and their implications for pharmacotherapy. *J. Oral Rehabil.* 37: 391–410.

Carvalho de Moraes, L.O., Tedesco, R.C., Arraez-Aybar, L.A., Klein, O., Merida-Velasco, J.R. and Alonso, L.G. (2015). Development of synovial membrane in the temporomandibular joint of the human fetus. *Eur. J. Histochem.* 59: 2569.

Choy, E. and Rose-John, S. (2017). Interleukin-6 as a multifunctional regulator: inflammation, immune response, and fibrosis. *J. Scleroderma Relat. Disord.* 2: S1–S5.

Das, S.T., Rajagopalan, L., Guerrero-Plata, A. et al. (2010). Monomeric and dimeric CXCL8 are both essential for in vivo neutrophil recruitment. *PLoS One* 5 (7): e11754.

de Alcântara Camejo, F., Azevedo, M., Ambros, V. et al. (2017). Interleukin-6 expression in disc derangement of human temporomandibular joint and association with osteoarthrosis. *J. Cranio-Maxillofac. Surg.* 45 (5): 768–774.

de Leeuw, R. and Klasser, G.D. (2018). *Orofacial Pain: Guidelines for Assessment, Diagnosis, and Management*. 6e. Hanover Park, IL: Quintessence Publishing.

Dinarello, C.A. (2011). Interleukin-1 in the pathogenesis and treatment of inflammatory diseases. *Blood* 117: 3720–3732.

Dinarello, C.A. (2018). Overview of the IL-1 family in innate inflammation and acquired immunity. *Immunol. Rev.* 281: 8–27.

Flannery, S. and Bowie, A.G. (2010). The interleukin-1 receptor-associated kinases: critical regulators of innate immune signalling. *Biochem. Pharmacol.* 80: 1981–1991.

Holtmann, H., Winzen, R., Holland, P. et al. (1999). Induction of interleukin-8 synthesis integrates effects on transcription and mRNA degradation from at least three different cytokine-or stress-activated signal transduction pathways. *Mol. Cell. Biol.* 19 (10): 6742–6753.

Ibi, M. (2019). Inflammation and temporomandibular joint derangement. *Biol. Pharmaceut. Bull.* 42: 538–42.

Iwanaga, T., Shikichi, M., Kitamura, H., Yanase, H. and Nozawa-Inoue, K. (2000). Morphology and functional roles of synoviocytes in the joint. *Arch. Histol. Cytol.* 63: 17–31.

Kaplanski, G., Marin, V., Montero-Julian, F., Mantovani, A. and Farnarier, C. (2003). IL-6: a regulator of the transition from neutrophil to monocyte recruitment during inflammation. *Trends Immunol.* 24: 25–29.

Kellesarian, S.V., Al-Kheraif, A.A., Vohra, F. et al. (2016). Cytokine profile in the synovial fluid of patients with temporomandibular joint disorders: a systematic review. *Cytokine* 77: 98–106.

Legendre, F., Bogdanowicz, P., Boumediene, K. and Pujol, JP. (2005). Role of interleukin 6 (IL-6)/IL-6R-induced signal tranducers and activators of transcription and mitogen-activated protein kinase/extracellular. *J. Rheumatol.* 32: 1307–1316.

Morel, M., Ruscitto, A., Pylawka, S., Reeve, G. and Embree, M.C. (2019). Extracellular matrix turnover and inflammation in chemically-induced TMJ arthritis mouse models. *PLoS One* 14: e0223244.

Mori, T., Miyamoto, T., Yoshida, H. et al. (2011). IL-1β and TNFα-initiated IL-6–STAT3 pathway is critical in mediating inflammatory cytokines and RANKL expression in inflammatory arthritis. *Int. Immunol.* 23 (11): 701–712.

Nicolielo, L.F.P., Jacobs, R., Albdour, E.A. et al. (2017). Is oestrogen associated with mandibular condylar resorption? A systematic review. *Int. J. Oral Maxillofac. Surg.* 46 (11): 1394–1402.

Norton, N.S., Netter, F.H. and Machado, C.A.G. (2017). *Netter's Head and Neck Anatomy for Dentistry*. Philadelphia: Elsevier.

Ogura, N. and Kondoh, T. (2015). Molecular aspects in inflammatory events of temporomandibular joint: microarray-based identification of mediators. *Japan. Dent. Sci. Rev.* 51: 10–24.

Ohta, K., Naruse, T., Kato, H. et al. (2017). Differential regulation by IFN-γ on TNF-α-induced chemokine expression in synovial fibroblasts from temporomandibular joint. *Mol. Med. Rep.* 16 (5): 6850–6857.

Peck, C.C., Goulet, J.P., Lobbezoo, F. et al. (2014). Expanding the taxonomy of the diagnostic criteria for temporomandibular disorders. *J. Oral Rehabil.* 41 (1): 2–23.

Pobezinskaya, Y.L. and Liu, Z. (2012). The role of TRADD in death receptor signaling. *Cell Cycle* 11 (5): 871–876.

Poluha, R.L. and Grossmann, E. (2018). Inflammatory mediators related to arthrogenic temporomandibular dysfunctions. *Braz. J. Pain* 1: 60–65.

Reeh, H., Rudolph, N., Billing, U. et al. (2019). Response to IL-6 trans-and IL-6 classic signalling is determined by the ratio of the IL-6 receptor α to gp130 expression: fusing experimental insights and dynamic modelling. *Cell Commun. Signal.* 17 (1): 1–21.

Rose-John, S. (2012). IL-6 trans-signaling via the soluble IL-6 receptor: importance for the pro-inflammatory activities of IL-6. *Int. J. Biol. Sci.* 8: 1237–1247.

Schiffman, E., Ohrbach, R., Truelove, E. et al. (2014). Diagnostic criteria for temporomandibular disorders (DC/TMD) for clinical and research applications: recommendations of the International RDC/TMD Consortium Network and Orofacial Pain Special Interest Group. *J. Oral Fac. Pain Headache* 28 (1): 6.

Schlorke, D., Thomas, L., Samsonov, S., Huster, D., Arnhold, J. and Pichert, A. (2012). The influence of glycosaminoglycans on IL-8-mediated functions of neutrophils. *Carbohydrate Res.* 356: 196–203.

Seki, H., Fukuda, M., Iino, M., Takahashi, T. and Yoshioka, N. (2004). Immunohistochemical localization of cyclooxygenase-1 and -2 in synovial tissues from patients with internal derangement or osteoarthritis of the temporomandibular joint. *Int. J. Oral Maxillofac. Surg.* 33: 687–692.

Siegmund, D., Ehrenschwender, M. and Wajant, H. (2018). TNFR2 unlocks a RIPK1 kinase activity-dependent mode of proinflammatory TNFR1 signaling. *Cell Death Dis.* 9: 921.

Su, H., Lei, C.T. and Zhang, C. (2017). Interleukin-6 signaling pathway and its role in kidney disease: an update. *Front. Immunol.* 8: 405.

Takahashi, T., Kondoh, T., Ohtani, M., Homma, H. and Fukuda, M. (1999). Association between arthroscopic diagnosis of temporomandibular joint osteoarthritis and synovial fluid nitric oxide levels. *Oral Surg. Oral Med. Oral Pathol. Oral Radiol. Endodont.* 88: 129–136.

Tomida, M., Ishimaru, J.I., Miyamoto, K. et al. (2003). Biochemical aspects of the pathogenesis of temporomandibular joint disorders. *Asian J. Oral Maxillofac. Surg.* 15 (2): 118–127.

Turner, M.D., Nedjai, B., Hurst, T. and Pennington, D.J. (2014). Cytokines and chemokines: at the crossroads of cell signalling and inflammatory disease. *Biochim. Biophys. Acta* 1843: 2563–2582.

Vernal, R., Velásquez, E., Gamonal, J., Garcia-Sanz, J.A., Silva, A. and Sanz, M. (2008). Expression of proinflammatory cytokines in osteoarthritis of the temporomandibular joint. *Arch. Oral Biol.* 53: 910–915.

Vincenti, M.P. and Brinckerhoff, C.E. (2002). Transcriptional regulation of collagenase (MMP-1, MMP-13) genes in arthritis: integration of complex signaling pathways for the recruitment of gene-specific transcription factors. *Arthritis Res.* 4: 157–164.

Wajant, H. and Siegmund, D. (2019). TNFR1 and TNFR2 in the control of the life and death balance of macrophages. *Front. Cell Dev. Biol.* 7: 91.

Wang, J., Chao, Y., Wan, Q. and Zhu, Z. (2008). The possible role of estrogen in the incidence of temporomandibular disorders. *Med. Hypoth.* 71: 564–567.

Wang, X.D., Kou, X.X., Mao, J.J., Gan, Y.H. and Zhou, Y.H. (2012). Sustained inflammation induces degeneration of the temporomandibular joint. *J. Dent. Res.* 91: 499–505.

Wang, X.D., Zhang, J.N., Gan, Y.H. and Zhou, Y.H. (2015). Current understanding of pathogenesis and treatment of TMJ osteoarthritis. *J. Dent. Res.* 94: 666–673.

Yin, Y., He, S., Xu, J. et al. (2020). The neuro-pathophysiology of temporomandibular disorders-related pain: a systematic review of structural and functional MRI studies. *J. Headache Pain* 21 (1): 1–20.

Yu, S., Xing, X., Liang, S. et al. (2009). Locally synthesized estrogen plays an important role in the development of TMD. *Med. Hypoth.* 72 (6): 720–722.

Zwiri, A., Al-Hatamleh, M.A.I., Ahmad, W.M.A. et al. (2020). Biomarkers for temporomandibular disorders: current status and future directions. *Diagnostics* 10 (5): 303.

14

Prospects of Passive Immunotherapy to Treat Pulpal Inflammation

Shelly Arora[1], Srinivas Sulugodu Ramachandra[2], Paul R. Cooper[1] and Haizal M. Hussaini[1]

[1] Faculty of Dentistry, Sir John Walsh Research Institute, University of Otago, Dunedin, New Zealand
[2] Department of Preventive Dental Sciences, College of Dentistry, Gulf Medical University, Ajman, United Arab Emirates

14.1 Introduction

Dental caries is the microbial invasion of the tooth structures including enamel, dentin and finally the pulp, resulting in pulpitis (Moss et al. 2021). It is one of the major dental diseases afflicting the general population in both developed and especially in developing countries (Wen et al. 2021). Dental caries results in significant morbidity, affecting the quality of life of the individual, and if left untreated may result in tooth loss (Moss et al. 2021). Pulpitis is characterised by chronic inflammation and elevated cytokine levels and if untreated, it can lead to irreversible pulpitis, tissue necrosis and periapical pathology (Cooper et al. 2014). Increased amounts of cytokines, such as tumour necrosis factor (TNF)-alpha, interleukin (IL)-1-alpha, IL-1-beta, IL-4, IL-6 and IL-8, are found in the inflamed pulp which amplify the immune response and cause exacerbation of pulpal inflammation (Cooper et al. 2014).

Chronic pulpal inflammation delays reparative events, and pulp healing can only occur after removal of pathogenic bacteria with subsequent reduction in the intensity of the pulpal inflammation (Baumgardner and Sulfaro 2001). This premise is based on findings from classic animal studies which demonstrated that dental tissue repair was found in germ-free mice with artificial cavities but was significantly impeded in mice with infected and inflamed pulps (Inoue and Shimono 1992). In vitro studies suggested the effect of inflammation on regeneration and showed the biphasic effects of proinflammatory mediators (Lara et al. 2003; Simon et al. 2010).

The inflammatory response can be a double-edged sword, beneficial in certain instances and harmful in others. At relatively low levels, proinflammatory mediators, such as TNF-alpha, transforming growth factor (TGF)-beta, reactive oxygen species (ROS) and lipopolysaccharides (LPS), can stimulate repair-associated events in dental pulp cells. However, at higher levels, during persistent inflammation they can cause cell death (He et al. 2005; Wang et al. 2015; Cooper et al. 2017). Although disinfection and removal of bacteria is key to enabling dental tissue repair, an in-depth understanding of the pulp's cellular inflammatory response is required for the possible development of immunomodulatory approaches for future regenerative endodontics based on immunotherapy.

With a fuller description of both active and passive immunotherapy, this chapter deals with the potential role of passive immunomodulatory and anti-inflammatory therapies in the treatment of oral diseases, specifically dental caries. The advantages of passive immunotherapies locally delivered to the carious lesions are also highlighted.

14.2 Current Status of Immunotherapy in Periodontitis

Immunotherapy has been explored in oral diseases including periodontitis (Pers et al. 2008) and pulpal inflammation (Arora et al. 2021). Periodontitis is an oral disease caused by association of subgingival plaque on the periodontium, which results in destruction of the hard and soft tissues of the periodontium (Ramachandra et al. 2017b). Currently, the pathogenesis of periodontitis is explained by the host–bacteria interaction model (Page and Kornman 1997; Ramachandra et al. 2017a). In a susceptible host, bacterial antigens, lipopolysaccharides and endotoxins interact with antibodies, local tissue cells and polymorphonuclear leucocytes, resulting in the excessive production of cytokines and matrix metalloproteinases (MMPs), which contribute to hard and soft tissue destruction respectively (Page and Kornman 1997). Even though microbial plaque has an initiating role in the aetiology of periodontitis, current evidence suggests that the host's immuno-inflammatory system has a major role in the pathogenesis of periodontitis (Hajishengallis and Lamont 2021).

Defects in the immuno-inflammatory system have been demonstrated in diabetics (Das et al. 2011) and smokers (Zhang et al. 2021), resulting in increased risk of advanced periodontitis in these individuals (Zhang et al. 2021; Das et al. 2011). Existing treatment approaches, including hard (Singh and Ramachandra 2016; Kocak Oztug et al. 2021; Majid et al. 2022) and soft tissue regeneration (Ramachandra et al. 2014; Rana et al. 2013), are, on the whole, regarded as being successful but are considered to be tertiary levels of treatment wherein regeneration and repair of lost structures are attempted (Ramachandra et al. 2014; Kocak Oztug et al. 2021).

The pivotal role played by inflammation in the aetiopathogenesis of periodontitis allows therapeutic approaches based on blocking the inflammatory cascade at various levels to be considered. Disease-modifying antirheumatic drugs (DMARDs) have been shown to be effective in the treatment of rheumatoid arthritis (RA) (Cantini et al. 2021). Since periodontitis and RA share similar aetiopathogenesis, Coat et al. (2015) studied the reduction in pocket depths and clinical attachment. Interestingly, data indicated that periodontitis patients who were on rituximab (anti-B lymphocyte therapy for the treatment of RA) continued to show significant disease improvement up to the two-year time-point. Another disease-modifying drug, infliximab, blocks TNF-alpha used in the treatment of RA, resulting in increased gingival inflammation, whereas clinical attachment loss decreased (Pers et al. 2008). Encouragingly, blocking cytokines like TNF-alpha and anti-B lymphocyte therapy has shown improvement in periodontal parameters (Yang et al. 2021).

Use of these agents in periodontitis can be justified owing to the generalised extent of the disease and consequently the application of a more systemic therapy. However, pulpitis is localised, although in rare instances could involve multiple teeth. Consequently, the use of immune therapy which utilises an appropriate localised delivery vehicle for the therapeutic agents would be preferred (Liang et al. 2020).

14.3 Immunotherapies for Dental Caries

Immunotherapies are broadly classified into two types: (i) active immunotherapy, which essentially utilises vaccines to develop immunity within the body (Arora et al. 2021), and (ii) passive immunotherapy which delivers laboratory-synthesised immune system components, antibodies or anticytokine molecules to enable the individual to resist infection or progression of the disease (Farhangnia et al. 2022). Active immunotherapy in the prevention of caries has explored the potential use of a caries vaccine (Cherukuri et al. 2020). The causation of caries is known to be through microbial dysbiosis supported by frequent carbohydrate intake with increases in acid-producing bacteria resulting in demineralisation of the hard tissues of the teeth (Tanner et al. 2018).

Historically, classic microbiological studies have associated dental caries with specific bacteria including *Streptococcus mutans* and *Streptococcus sobrinus* (smooth surface caries) (Costalonga and Herzberg 2014) and *Lactobacillus acidophilus* (proximal caries) (Caufield et al. 2015). However, next-generation sequencing technologies have highlighted the possible role of other cariogenic bacteria and an entirely dysbiotic microbial community in the causation of caries (Tanner et al. 2018).

The discovery of other bacteria, including *Scardovia wiggsiae*, in the aetiopathogenesis of dental caries indicates that a caries vaccine targeting *Streptococcus mutans* alone may not be the solution in the fight against dental caries (Kressirer et al. 2017; Cherukuri 2020). While several major research groups have made substantial efforts to develop a caries vaccine over the past four decades, a significant breakthrough is still awaited, especially in terms of clinical translation (Patel 2020). Worryingly, human heart tissue vaccine reactivity has been shown by immunofluorescence, raising concerns over the safety of caries vaccines in humans. This aspect has limited the potential of clinical translation of dental caries vaccine candidates, i.e. active immunotherapy in man (Russell and Wu 1990).

Passive immunotherapy, including the delivery of anticytokine molecules to the inflamed area, is yet to be explored in the caries model. Hypothetically, this approach would deliver anticytokine molecules in a suitable delivery vehicle, such as micro/nanoparticle, dendrimer or hydrogel mixed with hydraulic calcium silicate cement molecules and applied locally on the exposed pulp (Arora et al. 2021). Notably, compared with an active immunotherapy approach, systemic side-effects would be minimised in this approach due to localised application (Cherukuri et al. 2020). Figure 14.1 summarises the main differences between active and passive immunotherapies in potentially preventing or treating dental caries.

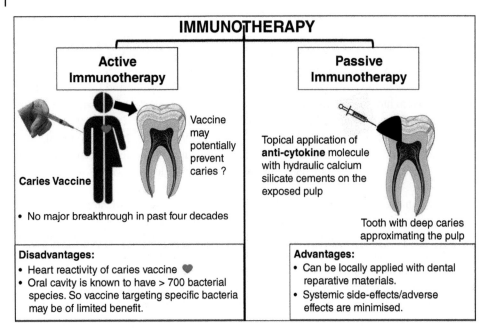

Figure 14.1 Key features of active and passive immunotherapies with potential for preventing or treating dental caries.

14.4 Inflammatory Responses in Dental Pulp

In order to develop better therapeutic approaches for dental caries, it is necessary to understand the molecular and cellular reactions that occur in the dental pulp as the disease progresses. Odontoblasts form the first line of defence against bacterial invasion and activate innate and adaptive dental pulp immunity (Durand et al. 2006). Pathogen-associated molecular patterns (PAMPs) on bacterial pathogens responsible for dental caries can be detected by odontoblasts using their pattern recognition receptors (PRRs), including members of the Toll-like receptor (TLR), nucleotide-binding oligomerisation domain (NOD) receptor and nod-like receptor (NLR) families. Members of these receptor families are present not only on odontoblasts but also on fibroblasts, neurons, endothelial and stem cells (Beutler 2009; Kumar et al. 2011).

Binding of the bacterial component to the receptor results in stimulation of downstream intracellular signalling molecules, including TRIF (TIR-domain-containing adapter-inducing interferon-b) and MyD88 (myeloid differentiation primary response gene 88). This further leads to the activation of IRF (IFN regulatory factor), NF-kappa-B and MAPK signalling pathways, resulting in nuclear translocation and transcription factor activation. Activation of these pathways leads to activation and production of proinflammatory cytokines (Beutler 2009; Durand et al. 2006). Subsequently, the release of these signalling molecules invokes and modulates the cellular immune response within the dental pulp (Figure 14.2).

Bacterial infection in the pulp, i.e. pulpitis, triggers an early immune response as part of immunosurveillance which results in the recruitment of dendritic cells (DCs), mast cells and T lymphocytes to the involved site (Farges et al. 2003). As part of the initial response, a large number of polymorphonuclear leucocytes surround the microbes in the infected pulp. Even though pulpitis is considered an immuno-inflammatory response to bacteria invading the pulp, initiation of the entire process starts with ingress of bacteria and their components into the pulp. Bacterial translation and protein synthesis result in the formation of N-formylmethionine-leucyl-phenylalanine (fMLP), which is a potent chemoattractant, especially for polymorphonuclear leucocytes, with each cell expressing ~50 000 fMLP receptors. The initial recruitment of neutrophils is followed by monocytes which later differentiate into macrophages (Jontell et al. 1998; Hahn and Liewehr 2007a; Cooper et al. 2011, 2014, 2017). DCs and macrophages engulf the invading bacteria, resulting in the activation of T lymphocytes which activate both innate and adaptive immune responses (Jontell et al. 1998; Hahn and Liewehr 2007a;

Figure 14.2 The molecular and cellular inflammatory responses involved in the activation of expression of cytokines and recruitment of immune cells during pulpal inflammation.

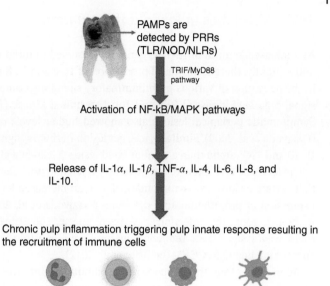

PAMPs are detected by PRRs (TLR/NOD/NLRs)

TRIF/MyD88 pathway

Activation of NF-kB/MAPK pathways

Release of IL-1α, IL-1β, TNF-α, IL-4, IL-6, IL-8, and IL-10.

Chronic pulp inflammation triggering pulp innate response resulting in the recruitment of immune cells

Neutrophils   T lymphocytes   Macrophages   Dendritic cells

Durand et al. 2006). The uptake of bacterial antigens results in the maturation of DCs, which subsequently migrate to the lymph nodes, thereby presenting the bacterial antigens to the T-helper (Th) or CD4 lymphocytes. This results in the activation of Th cells to effector Th cells or induced T regulatory cells (Tregs) (Onoé et al. 2007).

The generation of Tregs results in the production of cytokines which subsequently leads to a cascade of IL-2, interferon (IFN)-gamma and other cytokines. Subsequently, the activated macrophages express IL-1, platelet-activating factor, prostaglandins and leukotrienes (Hahn and Liewehr 2007b). The differentiation of Th2 cells also results in secretion of IL-4, IL-5, IL-6, IL-10, IL-13 and IL-14 which initiate the humoral immune response. The release of IL-6 and TGF-beta leads to differentiation of Th17. The secreted inflammatory cytokines and recruited neutrophils consequently aim to combat the microbial challenge (Hahn and Liewehr 2007b) (Figure 14.3).

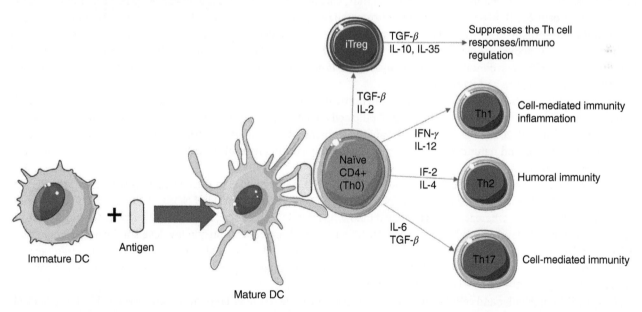

Figure 14.3 The complexity of the immune cell response and cytokines involved in an inflamed pulp. The role of DCs and the stimulated differentiation of naive T cells into iTreg, Th1, Th2 and Th17 subtypes are shown. *Source:* Adapted from Arora et al. (2021) with permission of John Wiley & Sons.

14.5   Cytokines in Pulpal Inflammation

An increased amount of IL-17 is generally observed in inflamed pulp compared to healthy pulp tissue (Xiong et al. 2015). Subsequently, there is increased production of IL-6 and IL-8 in a dose-dependent manner (Xiong et al. 2015). This results in the activation of various proinflammatory signalling components, including involvement of NF-kappa-B, extracellular signal-regulated kinase (ERK) and Jun N-terminal kinase (JNK), in human dental pulp fibroblasts (Xiong et al. 2015). Symptomatic periapical lesions also showed higher levels of IL-1, IL-6 and IL-8 compared with asymptomatic lesions (Gazivoda et al. 2009). Similarly, a larger lesion harbours higher percentages of CD8 cells and secretes higher levels of IL-6, IL-10 and TNF-alpha than a smaller sized lesion (Gazivoda et al. 2009).

The levels of TGF-beta are also inversely related to proinflammatory cytokine levels and this probably highlights the fact that certain lesions are asymptomatic due to an increased level of anti-inflammatory TGF-beta, which downregulates the expression of proinflammatory cytokines (Gazivoda et al. 2009). Significantly higher levels of CD4, CD28 and CD8 cell markers in root canal infections have been reported (de Brito et al. 2012). Seven days following initial root canal treatment, there was a significant reduction in the levels of proinflammatory cytokines, including IFN-gamma, IL-1-beta and chemokine ligand 5 (CCL5) (de Brito et al. 2012).

Much earlier than these reports, the formation of immune complexes in immunised monkeys following the application of bovine serum albumin on the exposed dentin confirmed the immune-inflammatory reactions occurring in the pulp (Bergenholtz et al. 1977). Indeed, the experimental approach taken then still serves as an appropriate model for studying pulpal inflammation in animals.

14.6   Antimicrobial Peptides in Pulpal Defence

Generally speaking, antimicrobial peptides (AMPs) are a class of small peptides that are an important part of the innate immune system of different organisms, including humans. AMPs have a wide range of inhibitory effects against pathogens. Upon TLR stimulation by the bacterial pathogen, odontoblasts will simultaneously produce antibacterial agents (beta-defensins [BDs] and nitric oxide [NO]). BDs are cationic, broad-spectrum antimicrobial peptides that cause microbial cell lysis by forming channel-like micropores that disrupt cell membranes and cause leakage of cellular contents (Semple and Dorin 2012). BD-1 is constitutively expressed, whereas BD-2, BD-3 and BD-4 are expressed when host cells encounter micro-organisms. In vitro studies have found the specific defensive protection of BDs in pulp against caries pathogens. BD-2 is active against *Streptococcus mutans* and *Lactobacillus casei* whereas BD-3 has shown antibacterial activity against biofilms containing *Actinomyces naeslundii*, *Lactobacillus salivarius*, *Streptococcus mutans* and *Enterococcus faecalis* (Lee and Baek 2012).

Interestingly, it has also been shown that BD-2 can upregulate in vitro synthesis of IL-6 and IL-8 in odontoblast-like cells (Dommisch et al. 2007). In cultured human dental pulp cells (HDPCs), IL-1-alpha and TNF-alpha can stimulate the secretion of BD-2 (Kim et al. 2010). BD-2 also has the ability to chemoattract immature antigen-presenting DCs, macrophages, CD4$^+$ memory T cells and natural killer (NK) cells, thus demonstrating its multifaceted proinflammatory characteristics (Semple and Dorin 2012).

Another antibacterial molecule secreted by odontoblasts is NO, a free radical produced by NO synthases which exists in three isoforms: NOS1 (neuronal NOS), NOS2 (inducible NOS) and NOS3 (endothelial NOS). NOS1 and NOS3 are present mostly in healthy tissues whereas NOS2 is secreted following microbial challenge; hence NOS2 participates mostly in host defence (Arthur and Steven 2013; Bogdan 2015). NOS2 has been observed at relatively low levels in healthy human pulp while high levels were found in inflamed pulps (Di Nardo Di Maio et al. 2004). Odontoblasts secrete NO to fight against *Streptococcus mutans* and in inflamed pulp the secretion of NO is facilitated by the stimulation of NOS2 aimed at combatting the later stages of the disease (Korkmaz et al. 2011).

The described molecular and cellular immune responses contribute to the inflammatory response and if left unchecked, associated processes may lead to irreversible pulpal tissue damage. Consequently, regulation of the immune response would be key to limiting the damage to the pulp and, notably, the pulp tissue is well equipped to undertake this challenge with the help of in situ regulatory cells.

14.7 Potential for Immunotherapy to Treat Pulpal Inflammation

Pulp has a natural tendency to heal (Bjørndal et al. 2014) and therefore, vital pulp therapy (VPT) is recommended for the management of deep caries and in some cases of teeth with signs and symptoms indicative of partial irreversible pulpitis, in order to preserve the remaining pulp (Duncan et al. 2019).

Deep caries lesions not extending to the pulp are usually treated with direct and indirect pulp capping techniques using different medicaments, including mineral trioxide aggregate (MTA), hydraulic calcium silicate cements and calcium hydroxide (Duncan 2022). However, these medicaments have certain drawbacks. MTA is known to contain some cytotoxic elements, has a prolonged setting time, is difficult to handle and expensive, and may result in tooth discoloration (Shahi et al. 2022). Additionally, once MTA is set, it is difficult to remove and does not dissolve in any available solvents (Shahi et al. 2022). Calcium hydroxide-based medicaments create a reparative hard tissue barrier in direct pulp capping procedures and their outcomes following placement are not always predictable (Duncan 2022). Furthermore, treatment with calcium hydroxide requires multiple appointments and the formation of a hard tissue barrier may take from three months up to 18 months. Susceptibility to fracture and coronal microleakage are additional disadvantages in the use of calcium hydroxide (Duncan 2022).

Caries lesions extending to the pulp or in clinically diagnosed irreversible pulpitis are treated with endodontic therapy. Endodontic therapy is usually considered as tertiary stage dental treatment and is expensive in many countries. The procedures involved in an endodontic treatment include opening of the pulp and biomechanical preparation which involves removal of the tooth structure and unfortunately causes the remaining tooth structure to be weak. Endodontically treated posterior teeth usually require further coverage with a metallic or porcelain crown to sustain the heavy occlusal forces.

As the afore-mentioned approaches exhibit several disadvantages, there is a need to develop improved treatment options for use in regenerative endodontics (Arora et al. 2021).

14.8 Immunoregulation/Immunomodulation for Dental Pulp Therapy

Many therapeutic strategies for pulp treatment aim to function as anti-inflammatory immunomodulators, and are based on molecular, cellular, anticytokine, modified dental biomaterial, epigenetic and microRNA technologies (Table 14.1). These strategies alleviate pulpal inflammation by modulating the ongoing inflammatory processes within the pulp and consequently decrease the production of excessive cytokines. This will lead to a more conducive environment for the pulp to heal and reparative events could be initiated in the treated pulp. Furthermore, as our understanding of immunomodulation therapy increases, it is expected that molecular targeted approaches can be developed to facilitate dentine–pulp complex healing. Therefore, more research is needed to investigate these anti-inflammatory approaches in the dentin–pulp complex and determine if these therapeutic molecules may be used as adjunct treatments with established VPT protocols.

14.8.1 Molecular Therapy Candidates

Molecular therapy involves the utilisation of novel molecule mediators such as adrenomedullin (ADM), resolvins, etc. which have immunomodulatory properties. ADM has been identified to be upregulated during reversible pulpitis (McLachlan et al. 2003). ADM belongs to the neuropeptide family, and is a pleiotropic molecule able to undertake various contextual activities, such as antibacterial, immunomodulation, initiation of differentiation of hard tissue and promotion of angiogenesis in bone (Delgado and Ganea 2008; Zudaire et al. 2006). Further studies on ADM have demonstrated that it shows similar activities within the dental hard tissues, and it is deposited within the dentin during primary dentinogenesis (Musson et al. 2010).

Resolvins, which are derived from fatty acids, exhibit great potential as a pulp therapeutic agent. They have anti-inflammatory properties, including reduction of the migration and stimulation of neutrophils, inhibition of DCs to produce IL-12 and intensifying the differentiation of the M2 phenotype of pro-resolving macrophages (Bannenberg et al. 2005; Winkler et al. 2013; Arita et al. 2005). A dentally related resolvin, resolvin E1 (RvE1), binds to the ligand specific receptor, Chem R23, that is present on macrophages, neutrophils, DCs and T cells and in turn downregulates NF-kappa-B signalling and thus modulates the inflammatory response (Arita et al. 2005; Ariel and Serhan 2007).

Table 14.1 Summary of the various types of immunoregulatory/immune modulation therapies with potential in chronic pulpal diseases.

No.	Type of pulp therapy	Mode of action	Potential advantages and disadvantages
1	Molecular therapies, e.g. adrenomedullin (ADM) and resolvin E1 (RvE1)	Molecules stimulate cellular responses, e.g. ADM acts as a growth factor/cytokine, and stimulates mineralised tissue differentiation, secretion and angiogenic processes (Delgado and Ganea 2008; Zudaire et al. 2006). RvE1 binds to Chem R23 present on macrophages, neutrophils, dendritic cells and T cells, causing downregulation of NF-kappa-B signalling (Arita et al. 2005)	Molecules should elicit healing and/or other beneficial host responses but ensuring correct dosage and most appropriate delivery mode may be problematic, e.g. ADM has antibacterial properties and potential to be used as a biological therapeutic molecule for pulp repair (McLachlan et al. 2003) RvE1 works better to reduce inflammation in the early stages and is not effective at later stages of inflammation (Scarparo et al. 2014)
2	Cell therapies, e.g. mesenchymal stem cells (MSCs)	MSCs modulate the inflammatory response via interaction with immune system cells. Subsequently, this leads to the production of TGF-beta and indolamine-2,3-dioxygenase-1 which attenuates the inflammatory activity and can enable the healing response (Leprince et al. 2012)	Dental pulp stem cells are known to have low immunogenic potential, which is a major advantage. Potential disadvantages include the secretion of proangiogenic factors and hypoxia may potentially result in tumorigenesis (Suzuki et al. 2011). Clinical application may also be costly
3	Antibody therapies, e.g. anticytokines (anti-IL-17, anti-IL-23)	Anticytokine antibodies directly bind to a specific proinflammatory cytokine, thereby neutralising it and preventing its binding to its receptor (Arora et al. 2021)	Topical application of anticytokine molecules may allow lower systemic adverse effects unlike systemically administered anticytokine drugs. Potential side-effects include increased susceptibility to infections, such as candida (Arora et al. 2021)
4	Modified dental biomaterials, e.g. dental resins supplemented with antioxidant N-acetyl cysteine, peroxisome proliferator-activated receptor gamma, ascorbic acid and 2-hydroxyethylmethacrylate	Their ability to neutralise reactive oxygen species, such as superoxide anions, hydrogen peroxide and hydroxyl radicals and thus restrict NF-kappa-B inflammatory pathway activation (Yamada et al. 2008)	Incorporation of anti-inflammatory agents into dental materials creates a new set of bioactive dental materials with associated advantages. However, the materials' restorative properties may be adversely affected and they may be expensive for clinical use
5	Epigenetic regulating molecules, e.g. histone deacetylase inhibitors and suberoylanilide hydroxamic acid	Regulate the DNA-associated histone acetylation process which results in accumulation of acetylated proteins causing transcriptional and cellular changes (Duncan et al. 2012, 2013)	Proposed to be used as a topical, low-cost epigenetic-based drug for pulp repair (Kearney et al. 2018). Although the concept looks promising, the use of these materials is in the early stages. Research is still ongoing to demonstrate their clinical efficacy
6	MicroRNA technologies, e.g. miR-21	These microRNAs may re-establish equilibrium by tipping the balance from a chronic inflammatory environment to more conducive conditions which favour pulp repair (Cooper and Smith 2013)	Can be targeted to specific molecules but currently may be costly to translate this technology into clinical practice

14.8.2 Cell Therapy Involving Mesenchymal Stem Cells

Novel therapeutics in the form of cell therapy which involve the use of mesenchymal stem cells (MSCs) are also emerging. MSCs are a type of adult stem cells which were first identified by Friedenstein et al. (1970) in bone marrow and are hence called bone marrow stem cells (BMSCs) or bone marrow mesenchymal stem cells (BMMSCs). MSCs have the ability to modulate inflammatory processes and promote tissue repair (Friedenstein et al. 1970). Their immunomodulatory action occurs through inhibition of immune cell proliferation, cytokine and/or antibody secretion, immune cell maturation and antigen presentation by T cells, B cells, NK cells and DCs. MSC regulatory actions include directing cell-to-cell contact with immune cells resulting in the release of TGF-beta-1 and IDO, which attenuate the inflammatory response (Wang et al. 2012; de Miguel et al. 2012; Leprince et al. 2012; Li et al. 2014; Tomic et al. 2011).

Dental pulp stem cells (DPSCs) are a type of MSC which are multipotent in nature. Recently, it has been shown that these cells can exert anti-inflammatory effects (Xu et al. 2018). Current knowledge about DPSCs and their interaction with their surrounding tissues along with their low immunogenic potential and immunomodulation makes them a promising therapeutic target for use in disease treatment and tissue regeneration.

14.8.3 Anticytokine and Antibody Molecules

Teeth with signs and symptoms indicative of irreversible pulpitis most frequently arise in response to microbial insult from dental caries, are characterised by chronic inflammation with high cytokine expression levels, and if left untreated progress to irreversible pulpitis, tissue necrosis and periapical disease (Cooper et al. 2014). Interestingly, the pathogenesis of inflammatory bowel diseases (IBD) such as Crohn's disease (CD), ulcerative colitis and psoriasis includes a bacterial component (Wlodarska et al. 2015), which is consistent with dental caries and teeth with signs and symptoms indicative of irreversible pulpitis. Moreover, RA is characterised by chronic inflammation affecting both soft and hard tissues, and is also reported to have an associated microbial component, which may be responsible for initiating and perpetuating disease activity (Manasson et al. 2020).

These findings suggest that chronic inflammatory diseases and teeth with signs and symptoms indicative of irreversible pulpitis share common pathological mechanisms (Arora et al. 2021). Therefore, anticytokine therapies have been successfully applied in the treatment of chronic inflammatory diseases and antibody therapies already exist for many cytokines, including TNF-alpha, IL-1-beta, IL-6, IL-8, IL-17 and IL-23; their application may be translatable into VPT and other regenerative endodontic procedures (Arora et al. 2021; Smith 2020).

As discussed earlier, relatively high levels of cytokines, including TNF-alpha, IL-1-beta, IL-6, IL-8, IL-17 and IL-23, have been identified in inflamed pulp tissue (Huang et al. 1999; Guo et al. 2000; Barkhordar et al. 2002; Pezelj-Ribaric et al. 2002; Farges et al. 2011; Nibali et al. 2012; Xiong et al. 2015), so it can be envisaged that anticytokine therapy might have application in chronic pulpal diseases (Wlodarska et al. 2015; Arora et al. 2021).

Currently, we are studying the effects of using an anti-IL-23 antibody on inflamed dental pulp tissue in in vitro and in vivo models. Our preliminary findings indicate that blockade of the IL-23 cytokine signalling pathway in the dental pulp modulates inflammation and enables tissue healing (unpublished data). Consequently, this research will contribute to our understanding of IL-23-mediated inflammation in pulpal diseases and will identify new avenues in both experimental modelling and therapeutic treatments.

14.8.4 Modified Dental Biomaterials for Immunomodulation

This category includes dental resins supplemented with antioxidant N-acetyl cysteine (NAC), peroxisome proliferator-activated receptor gamma (PPAR-gamma), ascorbic acid along with 2-hydroxyethylmethacrylate (HEMA), etc. In vitro studies performed using these molecules have indicated their potential to limit the activation of the NF-kappa-B pathway (Yamada et al. 2008; Kim et al. 2012; Diomede et al. 2019). A dental resin supplemented with NAC has been shown to be capable of neutralising ROS, such as superoxide anions, hydrogen peroxide and hydroxyl radicals, and this may limit stimulation of the NF-kappa-B inflammatory pathway followed by a diminished production of cytokines (Yamada et al. 2008). This modification may protect pulp cells and provide a more conducive environment for repair. Similarly, it has also been shown that exogenous application of PPAR-gamma in HDPCs exhibits anti-inflammatory properties by removing nitric oxide and ROS, which leads to suppression of ERK1/2 and NF-kappa-B inflammatory signal (Kim et al. 2012). Recent work has shown that use of ascorbic acid with HEMA downregulates ROS production and the NF-kappa-B/pERK/ERK signalling pathway and could be used as a therapeutic agent to promote pulp regeneration (Diomede et al. 2019).

14.8.5 Epigenetic Regulating Molecules

Epigenetic regulating molecules, such as histone deacetylase inhibitors (HDACi) and suberoylanilide hydroxamic acid (SAHA), exhibit anti-inflammatory properties and have the ability to facilitate hard tissue regeneration-associated processes, such as cell differentiation and mineralisation (Duncan et al. 2016). HDACis regulate DNA-associated histone acetylation process which results in the accumulation of acetylated proteins causing transcriptional and cellular changes (Duncan et al. 2012, 2013). These molecules also show potential to be used as a therapeutic tool within the pulp. Indeed, proof-of-principle studies have shown their capacity to promote primary pulp cell differentiation and mineralisation-related processes in vivo (Duncan et al. 2011, 2012, 2013). However, further exploration of these inhibitors is required to determine their suitability for dental tissue restoration in humans.

14.8.6 MicroRNA Technologies

Work using regulatory microRNA (miRNA) technologies indicated their application within the pulp. Healthy and diseased pulps have shown the presence of different types of miRNAs with immunomodulatory capabilities (Zhong et al. 2012). Hypothetically, if these molecules are delivered to the pupal tissue, they have the potential to re-establish an equilibrium in the local environment and tip the balance from chronic inflammation to one that favours tissue repair and regeneration (Cooper and Smith 2013). Thus, modulating the expression of miRNA molecules may have potential benefit for addressing pulpal inflammation and subsequent application in clinical VPT protocols (Cooper et al. 2010, 2011; Cooper and Smith 2013).

14.8.7 Miscellaneous Therapies with Potential for Pulpal Regeneration

Apart from the above-mentioned potential therapies for pulpal regeneration, other therapies could also have potential benefits for pulpal lesions. Glutamine has been shown to exert an anti-inflammatory effect on HDPCs in vitro by blocking MAPK pathways and this may contribute to inhibition of pulp inflammatory responses, which may favour pulp healing (Kim et al. 2015). The application of low-level light has been shown to modulate inflammation which has prompted its potential use in dental tissue repair (Milward et al. 2014). Furthermore, naturally derived compounds, such as pachymic acid derived from the mushroom variety *Formitopsis niagara*, have also demonstrated anti-inflammatory properties as well as the ability to activate the haem oxygenase-1 pathway in increasing odontoblast differentiation and activity (Lee et al. 2013). These studies, which highlight the relationship between inflammation and repair, further indicate opportunities to develop novel therapeutics for VPT.

14.9 Conclusion

Inflammatory and immune responses are complex cascades, which are triggered by antigens arising from pathogens. The blocking of a particular pathway may result in the activation of alternative pathways to continue the inflammatory process. Additionally, the literature is currently unclear on the potential of different anticytokine blockers under different disease conditions and for different individuals. Consequently, research regarding immunotherapy for dental caries and pulpitis is in the nascent stages and more research is essential before definitive conclusions can be arrived at. Nonetheless, the application of immunoregulation or immunomodulation for VPT is an exciting area with significant potential to identify novel therapeutic approaches which regulate inflammation and hence favour pulp repair.

References

Ariel, A. and Serhan, C.N. (2007). Resolvins and protectins in the termination program of acute inflammation. *Trends Immunol.* 28: 176–183.

Arita, M., Bianchini, F., Aliberti, J. et al. (2005). Stereochemical assignment, antiinflammatory properties, and receptor for the omega-3 lipid mediator resolvin E1. *J. Exp. Med.* 201: 713–722.

Arora, S., Cooper, P.R., Friedlander, L.T. et al. (2021). Potential application of immunotherapy for modulation of pulp inflammation: opportunities for vital pulp treatment. *Int. Endod. J.* 54: 1263–1274.

Arthur, J.S.C. and Steven, C.L. (2013). Mitogen-activated protein kinases in innate immunity. *Nat. Rev. Immunol.* 13: 679.

Bannenberg, G.L., Chiang, N., Ariel, A. et al. (2005). Molecular circuits of resolution: formation and actions of resolvins and protectins. *J. Immunol.* 174: 4345–4355.

Barkhordar, R.A., Ghani, Q.P., Russell, T.R. and Hussain, M.Z. (2002). Interleukin-1beta activity and collagen synthesis in human dental pulp fibroblasts. *J. Endod.* 28: 157–159.

Baumgardner, K.R. and Sulfaro, M.A. (2001). The anti-inflammatory effects of human recombinant copper-zinc superoxide dismutase on pulp inflammation. *J. Endod.* 27: 190–195.

Bergenholtz, G., Ahlstedt, S. and Lindhe, J. (1977). Experimental pulpitis in immunized monkeys. *Scand. J. Dent. Res.* 85: 396–406.

Beutler, B. (2009). Microbe sensing, positive feedback loops, and the pathogenesis of inflammatory diseases. *Immunol. Rev.* 227: 248.

Bjørndal, L., Demant, S. and Dabelsteen, S. (2014). Depth and activity of carious lesions as indicators for the regenerative potential of dental pulp after intervention. *J. Endod.* 40: S76–S81.

Bogdan, C. (2015). Nitric oxide synthase in innate and adaptive immunity: an update. *Trends Immunol.* 36: 161–178.

Cantini, F., Goletti, D., Benucci, M., Foti, R., Damiani, A. and Niccoli, L. (2021). Tailored first-line biologic and targeted synthetic disease modifying anti-rheumatic drugs therapy in patients with rheumatoid arthritis: 2021 updated ITABIO statements. *Expert Opin. Drug Saf.* 1–11.

Caufield, P.W., Schön, C.N., Saraithong, P., Li, Y. and Argimón, S. (2015). Oral lactobacilli and dental caries: a model for niche adaptation in humans. *J. Dent. Res.* 94: 110s–118s.

Cherukuri, G., Veeramachaneni, C., Rao, G.V., Pacha, V.B. and Balla, S.B. (2020). Insight into status of dental caries vaccination: a review. *J. Conserv. Dent.* 23: 544–549.

Coat, J., Demoersman, J., Beuzit, S. et al. (2015). Anti-B lymphocyte immunotherapy is associated with improvement of periodontal status in subjects with rheumatoid arthritis. *J. Clin. Periodontol.* 42: 817–823.

Cooper, P.R. and Smith, A.J. (2013). Molecular mediators of pulp inflammation and regeneration. *Endod. Topics* 28: 90–105.

Cooper, P.R., Takahashi, Y., Graham, L.W., Simon, S., Imazato, S. and Smith, A.J. (2010). Inflammation-regeneration interplay in the dentine-pulp complex. *J. Dent.* 38: 687–697.

Cooper, P.R., McLachlan, J.L., Simon, S., Graham, L.W. and Smith, A.J. (2011). Mediators of inflammation and regeneration. *Adv. Dent. Res.* 23: 290–295.

Cooper, P.R., Holder, M.J. and Smith, A.J. (2014). Inflammation and regeneration in the dentin-pulp complex: a double-edged sword. *J. Endod.* 40: S46–S51.

Cooper, P.R., Chicca, I.J., Holder, M.J. and Milward, M.R. (2017). Inflammation and regeneration in the dentin-pulp complex: net gain or net loss? *J. Endod.* 43: S87–S94.

Costalonga, M. and Herzberg, M.C. (2014). The oral microbiome and the immunobiology of periodontal disease and caries. *Immunol. Lett.* 162: 22–38.

Das, M., Upadhyaya, V., Ramachandra, S.S. and Jithendra, K.D. (2011). Periodontal treatment needs in diabetic and non-diabetic individuals: a case-control study. *Indian J. Dent. Res.* 22: 291–294.

De Brito, L.C., Teles, F.R., Teles, R.P., Totola, A.H., Vieira, L.Q. and Sobrinho, A.P. (2012). T-lymphocyte and cytokine expression in human inflammatory periapical lesions. *J. Endod.* 38: 481–485.

Delgado, M. and Ganea, D. (2008). Anti-inflammatory neuropeptides: a new class of endogenous immunoregulatory agents. *Brain Behav. Immun.* 22: 1146–1151.

De Miguel, M.P., Fuentes-Julián, S., Blázquez-Martínez, A. et al. (2012). Immunosuppressive properties of mesenchymal stem cells: advances and applications. *Curr. Mol. Med.* 12: 574–591.

Di Nardo di Maio, F., Lohinai, Z., D'Arcangelo, C. et al. (2004). Nitric oxide synthase in healthy and inflamed human dental pulp. *J. Dent. Res.* 83: 312–316.

Diomede, F., Marconi, G.D., Guarnieri, S. et al. (2019). A novel role of ascorbic acid in anti-inflammatory pathway and ROS generation in HEMA treated dental pulp stem cells. *Materials* 13: 130.

Dommisch, H., Winter, J., Willebrand, C., Eberhard, J. and Jepsen, S. (2007). Immune regulatory functions of human beta-defensin-2 in odontoblast-like cells. *Int. Endod. J.* 40: 300–307.

Duncan, H.F. (2022). Present status and future directions – vital pulp treatment and pulp preservation strategies. *Int. Endod. J.* 55: 497–511.

Duncan, H.F., Smith, A.J., Fleming, G.J. and Cooper, P.R. (2011). HDACi: cellular effects, opportunities for restorative dentistry. *J. Dent. Res.* 90: 1377–1388.

Duncan, H.F., Smith, A.J., Fleming, G.J. and Cooper, P.R. (2012). Histone deacetylase inhibitors induced differentiation and accelerated mineralization of pulp-derived cells. *J. Endod.* 38: 339–345.

Duncan, H.F., Smith, A.J., Fleming, G.J. and Cooper, P.R. (2013). Histone deacetylase inhibitors epigenetically promote reparative events in primary dental pulp cells. *Exp. Cell Res.* 319: 1534–1543.

Duncan, H.F., Smith, A.J., Fleming, G.J. et al. (2016). The histone-deacetylase-inhibitor suberoylanilide hydroxamic acid promotes dental pulp repair mechanisms through modulation of matrix metalloproteinase-13 activity. *J. Cell Physiol.* 231: 798–816.

Duncan, H.F., Galler, K.M., Tomson, P.L. et al. (2019). European Society of Endodontology position statement: management of deep caries and the exposed pulp. *Int. Endod. J.* 52: 923–934.

Durand, S.H., Flacher, V., Roméas, A. et al. (2006). Lipoteichoic acid increases TLR and functional chemokine expression while reducing dentin formation in in vitro differentiated human odontoblasts. *J. Immunol.* 176: 2880–2887.

Farges, J.C., Romeas, A., Melin, M. et al. (2003). TGF-beta1 induces accumulation of dendritic cells in the odontoblast layer. *J. Dent. Res.* 82: 652–656.

Farges, J.C., Carrouel, F., Keller, J.F. et al. (2011). Cytokine production by human odontoblast-like cells upon Toll-like receptor-2 engagement. *Immunobiology* 216: 513–517.

Farhangnia, P., Dehrouyeh, S., Safdarian, A.R. et al. (2022). Recent advances in passive immunotherapies for COVID-19: the evidence-based approaches and clinical trials. *Int. Immunopharmacol.* 109: 108786.

Friedenstein, A.J., Chailakhjan, R.K. and Lalykina, K.S. (1970). The development of fibroblast colonies in monolayer cultures of guinea-pig bone marrow and spleen cells. *Cell Tissue Kinet.* 3: 393–403.

Gazivoda, D., Dzopalic, T., Bozic, B., Tatomirovic, Z., Brkic, Z. and Colic, M. (2009). Production of proinflammatory and immunoregulatory cytokines by inflammatory cells from periapical lesions in culture. *J. Oral Pathol. Med.* 38: 605–611.

Guo, X., Niu, Z., Xiao, M., Yue, L. and Lu, H. (2000). Detection of interleukin-8 in exudates from normal and inflamed human dental pulp tissues. *Chin. J. Dent. Res.* 3: 63–66.

Hahn, C.-L. and Liewehr, F.R. (2007a). Innate immune responses of the dental pulp to caries. *J. Endod.* 33: 643–651.

Hahn, C.-L. and Liewehr, F.R. (2007b). Update on the adaptive immune responses of the dental pulp. *J. Endod.* 33: 773–781.

Hajishengallis, G. and Lamont, R.J. (2021). Polymicrobial communities in periodontal disease: their quasi-organismal nature and dialogue with the host. *Periodont. 2000* 86: 210–230.

He, W.X., Niu, Z.Y., Zhao, S.L. and Smith, A.J. (2005). Smad protein mediated transforming growth factor beta1 induction of apoptosis in the MDPC-23 odontoblast-like cell line. *Arch. Oral Biol.* 50: 929–936.

Huang, G.T., Potente, A.P., Kim, J.W., Chugal, N. and Zhang, X. (1999). Increased interleukin-8 expression in inflamed human dental pulps. *Oral Surg. Oral Med. Oral Pathol. Oral Radiol. Endod.* 88: 214–220.

Inoue, T. and Shimono, M. (1992). Repair dentinogenesis following transplantation into normal and germ-free animals. *Proc. Finn. Dent. Soc.* 88 Suppl 1: 183–194.

Jontell, M., Okiji, T., Dahlgren, U. and Bergenholtz, G. (1998). Immune defense mechanisms of the dental pulp. *Crit. Rev. Oral Biol. Med.* 9: 179–200.

Kearney, M., Cooper, P.R., Smith, A.J. and Duncan, H.F. (2018). Epigenetic approaches to the treatment of dental pulp inflammation and repair: opportunities and obstacles. *Front. Genet.* 9: 1–18.

Kim, D.S., Shin, M.R., Kim, Y.S. et al. (2015). Anti-inflammatory effects of glutamine on LPS-stimulated human dental pulp cells correlate with activation of MKP-1 and attenuation of the MAPK and NF-κB pathways. *Int. Endod. J.* 48: 220–228.

Kim, J.C., Lee, Y.H., Yu, M.K. et al. (2012). Anti-inflammatory mechanism of PPARγ on LPS-induced pulp cells: role of the ROS removal activity. *Arch. Oral Biol.* 57: 392–400.

Kim, Y.-S., Min, K.-S., Lee, S.-I., Shin, S.-J., Shin, K.-S. and Kim, E.-C. (2010). Effect of proinflammatory cytokines on the expression and regulation of human beta-defensin 2 in human dental pulp cells. *J. Endod.* 36: 64–69.

Kocak Oztug, N.A., Ramachandra, S.S., Lacin, C.C., Alali, A. and Carr, A. (2021). Regenerative approaches in periodontics. In: *Regenerative Approaches in Dentistry: An Evidence-Based Perspective* (eds S. Hosseinpour, L.J. Walsh and K. Moharamzadeh). Cham: Springer International Publishing.

Korkmaz, Y., Lang, H., Beikler, T. et al. (2011). Irreversible inflammation is associated with decreased levels of the α1-, β1-, and α2-subunits of sGC in human odontoblasts. *J. Dent. Res.* 90: 517–522.

Kressirer, C.A., Smith, D.J., King, W.F., Dobeck, J.M., Starr, J.R. and Tanner, A.C.R. (2017). Scardovia wiggsiae and its potential role as a caries pathogen. *J. Oral Biosci.* 59: 135–141.

Kumar, H., Kawai, T. and Akira, S. (2011). Pathogen recognition by the innate immune system. *Int. Rev. Immunol.* 30: 16–34.

Lara, V.S., Figueiredo, F., Da Silva, T.A. and Cunha, F.Q. (2003). Dentin-induced in vivo inflammatory response and in vitro activation of murine macrophages. *J. Dent. Res.* 82: 460–465.

Lee, S.-H. and Baek, D.-H. (2012). Antibacterial and neutralizing effect of human β-defensins on enterococcus faecalis and enterococcus faecalis lipoteichoic acid. *J. Endod.* 38: 351–356.

Lee, Y.H., Lee, N.H., Bhattarai, G. et al. (2013). Anti-inflammatory effect of pachymic acid promotes odontoblastic differentiation via HO-1 in dental pulp cells. *Oral Dis.* 19: 193–199.

Leprince, J.G., Zeitlin, B.D., Tolar, M. and Peters, O.A. (2012). Interactions between immune system and mesenchymal stem cells in dental pulp and periapical tissues. *Int. Endod. J.* 45: 689–701.

Li, Z., Jiang, C.M., An, S. et al. (2014). Immunomodulatory properties of dental tissue-derived mesenchymal stem cells. *Oral Dis.* 20: 25–34.

Liang, J., Peng, X., Zhou, X., Zou, J. and Cheng, L. (2020). Emerging applications of drug delivery systems in oral infectious diseases prevention and treatment. *Molecules* 25: 516.

Majid, H., Ramachandra, S.S., Kumar, S., Wei, M. and Gundavarapu, K.C. (2022). Influence of grafting on pocket depth and dentin hypersensitivity around third molar extraction sites: a split-mouth randomized controlled trial. *Compend. Contin. Educ. Dent.* 43: e5–e8.

Manasson, J., Blank, R.B. and Scher, J.U. (2020). The microbiome in rheumatology: where are we and where should we go? *Ann. Rheum. Dis.* 79: 727–733.

McLachlan, J.L., Smith, A.J., Sloan, A.J. and Cooper, P.R. (2003). Gene expression analysis in cells of the dentine-pulp complex in healthy and carious teeth. *Arch. Oral Biol.* 48: 273–283.

Milward, M.R., Holder, M.J., Palin, W.M., Hadis, M.A., Carroll, J.D. and Cooper, P.R. (2014). Low level light therapy (LLLT) for the treatment and management of dental and oral diseases. *Dent. Update* 41: 763–772.

Moss, M.E., Luo, H., Rosinger, A.Y., Jacobs, M.M. and Kaur, R. (2021). High sugar intake from sugar-sweetened beverages is associated with prevalence of untreated decay in US adults: NHANES 2013–2016. *Commun. Dent. Oral Epidemiol.* 50: 579–588.

Musson, D.S., McLachlan, J.L., Sloan, A.J., Smith, A.J. and Cooper, P.R. (2010). Adrenomedullin is expressed during rodent dental tissue development and promotes cell growth and mineralization. *Biol. Cell* 102: 145–157.

Nibali, L., Fedele, S., D'Aiuto, F. and Donos, N. (2012). Interleukin-6 in oral diseases: a review. *Oral Dis.* 18: 236–243.

Onoé, K., Yanagawa, Y., Minami, K., Iijima, N. and Iwabuchi, K. (2007). Th1 or Th2 balance regulated by interaction between dendritic cells and NKT cells. *Immunol. Res.* 38: 319–332.

Page, R.C. and Kornman, K.S. (1997). The pathogenesis of human periodontitis: an introduction. *Periodontology 2000* 14: 9–11.

Patel, M. (2020). Dental caries vaccine: are we there yet? *Lett. Appl. Microbiol.* 70: 2–12.

Pers, J.O., Saraux, A., Pierre, R. and Youinou, P. (2008). Anti-TNF-alpha immunotherapy is associated with increased gingival inflammation without clinical attachment loss in subjects with rheumatoid arthritis. *J. Periodontol.* 79: 1645–1651.

Pezelj-Ribaric, S., Anic, I., Brekalo, I., Miletic, I., Hasan, M. and Simunovic-Soskic, M. (2002). Detection of tumor necrosis factor alpha in normal and inflamed human dental pulps. *Arch. Med. Res.* 33: 482–484.

Ramachandra, S.S., Rana, R., Reetika, S. and Jithendra, K.D. (2014). Options to avoid the second surgical site: a review of literature. *Cell Tissue Bank.* 15: 297–305.

Ramachandra, S.S., Dopico, J., Donos, N. and Nibali, L. (2017a). Disease staging index for aggressive periodontitis. *Oral Health Prev. Dent.* 15: 371–378.

Ramachandra, S.S., Gupta, V.V., Mehta, D.S., Gundavarapu, K.C. and Luigi, N. (2017b). Differential diagnosis between chronic versus aggressive periodontitis and staging of aggressive periodontitis: a cross-sectional study. *Contemp. Clin. Dent.* 8: 594–603.

Rana, R., Ramachandra, S.S., Lahori, M., Singhal, R. and Jithendra, K.D. (2013). Combined soft and hard tissue augmentation for a localized alveolar ridge defect. *Contemp. Clin. Dent.* 4: 556–558.

Russell, M.W. and Wu, H.Y. (1990). Streptococcus mutans and the problem of heart cross-reactivity. *Crit. Rev. Oral Biol. Med.* 1: 191–205.

Scarparo, R.K., Dondoni, L., Böttcher, D.E. et al. (2014). Intracanal delivery of Resolvin E1 controls inflammation in necrotic immature rat teeth. *J. Endod.* 40: 678–682.

Semple, F. and Dorin, J.R. (2012). β-defensins: multifunctional modulators of infection, inflammation and more? *J. Innate Immun.* 4: 337–348.

Shahi, S., Fakhri, E., Yavari, H., Maleki Dizaj, S., Salatin, S. and Khezri, K. (2022). Portland cement: an overview as a root repair material. *Biomed. Res. Int.* 2022: 3314912.

Simon, S., Smith, A.J., Berdal, A., Lumley, P.J. and Cooper, P.R. (2010). The MAP kinase pathway is involved in odontoblast stimulation via p38 phosphorylation. *J. Endod.* 36: 256–259.

Singh, R. and Ramachandra, S.S. (2016). Resective or regenerative periodontal therapy: considerations during treatment planning: a case report. *N.Y. State Dent. J.* 82: 46–49.

Smith, A.J. (2020). Reflections and future visions for pulp biology research. *J. Endod.* 46: S42–S45.

Suzuki, K., Sun, R., Origuchi, M. et al. (2011). Mesenchymal stromal cells promote tumor growth through the enhancement of neovascularization. *Mol. Med.* 17: 579–587.

Tanner, A.C.R., Kressirer, C.A., Rothmiller, S., Johansson, I. and Chalmers, N.I. (2018). The caries microbiome: implications for reversing dysbiosis. *Adv. Dent. Res.* 29: 78–85.

Tomic, S., Djokic, J., Vasilijic, S. et al. (2011). Immunomodulatory properties of mesenchymal stem cells derived from dental pulp and dental follicle are susceptible to activation by toll-like receptor agonists. *Stem Cells Dev.* 20: 695–708.

Wang, L., Zhao, Y. and Shi, S. (2012). Interplay between mesenchymal stem cells and lymphocytes: implications for immunotherapy and tissue regeneration. *J. Dent. Res.* 91: 1003–1010.

Wang, Z., Ma, F., Wang, J. et al. (2015). Extracellular signal-regulated kinase mitogen-activated protein kinase and phosphatidylinositol 3-kinase/akt signaling are required for lipopolysaccharide-mediated mineralization in murine odontoblast-like cells. *J. Endod.* 41: 871–876.

Wen, P.Y.F., Chen, M.X., Zhong, Y.J., Dong, Q.Q. and Wong, H.M. (2021). Global burden and inequality of dental caries, 1990 to 2019. *J. Dent. Res.* 101: 392–399.

Winkler, J.W., Uddin, J., Serhan, C.N. and Petasis, N.A. (2013). Stereocontrolled total synthesis of the potent anti-inflammatory and pro-resolving lipid mediator resolvin D3 and its aspirin-triggered 17R-epimer. *Org. Lett.* 15: 1424–1427.

Wlodarska, M., Kostic, A.D. and Xavier, R.J. (2015). An integrative view of microbiome-host interactions in inflammatory bowel diseases. *Cell Host Microbe* 17: 577–591.

Xiong, H., Wei, L. and Peng, B. (2015). IL-17 stimulates the production of the inflammatory chemokines IL-6 and IL-8 in human dental pulp fibroblasts. *Int. Endod. J.* 48: 505–511.

Xu, K., Xiao, J., Zheng, K. et al. (2018). MiR-21/STAT3 signal is involved in odontoblast differentiation of human dental pulp stem cells mediated by TNF-α. *Cell Reprogram.* 20: 107–116.

Yamada, M., Kojima, N., Paranjpe, A. et al. (2008). N-acetyl cysteine (NAC)-assisted detoxification of PMMA resin. *J. Dent. Res.* 87: 372–377.

Yang, B., Pang, X., Li, Z., Chen, Z. and Wang, Y. (2021). Immunomodulation in the treatment of periodontitis: progress and perspectives. *Front. Immunol.* 12: 781378.

Zhang, J., Yu, J., Dou, J., Hu, P. and Guo, Q. (2021). The impact of smoking on subgingival plaque and the development of periodontitis: a literature review. *Front. Oral Health* 2: 751099.

Zhong, S., Zhang, S., Bair, E., Nares, S. and Khan, A.A. (2012). Differential expression of microRNAs in normal and inflamed human pulps. *J. Endod.* 38: 746–752.

Zudaire, E., Portal-Núñez, S. and Cuttitta, F. (2006). The central role of adrenomedullin in host defense. *J. Leukoc. Biol.* 80: 237–244.

15

Techniques in Immunology

Mohammad Tariqur Rahman[1] and Muhammad Manjurul Karim[2]

[1] *University of Malaya, Kuala Lumpur, Malaysia*
[2] *Department of Microbiology, University of Dhaka, Dhaka, Bangladesh*

15.1 Principles of Immunoassays

15.1.1 Interaction between Antigen and Antibody

Laboratory techniques of immunology are mostly based on antigen–antibody interactions. An antibody (Ab) uses its fragment antigen binding (Fab) arms to bind with the specific site of an antigen (Ag), called an epitope. The formation of the Ag–Ab complex can be detected if the Ab is conjugated with a marker (also known as a reporter) to generate detectable or visible signals.

Immunological techniques are used to identify, quantify or purify a target biomolecule which is usually protein in nature, which is referred to as Ag, one of the most common terms in the field of immunology. The principle is applied to detect, quantify or separate cells having the target Ag. The target Ag could be present on the cell membrane, in the cytoplasm or even inside cellular organs. Therefore, the distribution and localisation of specific cellular components that are attached to the cells, either on their cell membrane or inside the cells, can be visualised using immunological techniques (Figure 15.1).

In certain techniques such as enzyme-linked immunosorbent assay (ELISA) and Western blotting, the Ab is conjugated with an enzyme that eventually can be detected by the visible signals generated from the enzyme–substrate reaction. In other techniques, such as immunofluorescence-based techniques, the Ab is conjugated with a fluorescent marker that can be detected using fluorescent microscopy. The detection marker such as the enzyme or fluorescent marker is generally conjugated or attached to the Ab through covalent bonding.

The Ag–Ab interactions are also used for the separation of a target biomolecule or even cells. For instance, when a mixture of biomolecules such as proteins is present in a solution, an immobilised (inert) surface coated with Ab can selectively retain the target protein through Ag–Ab interactions. The remaining unbound proteins can be washed off the inert surface, thus allowing selective separation of a target protein. This principle is used to separate proteins using immune affinity chromatography.

Similarly, a specific cell type can be attached to an inert surface through Ag–Ab interactions. Practically, this is possible as each cell type has its unique surface or membrane-bound proteins (or glycol-proteins) that can be used as the target for binding with a specific Ab. Binding of a fluorescent conjugated Ab (Ab*) on a cell surface protein (commonly known as a marker) is also used to separate and often quantify the cell–Ab* complex, a technique known as fluorescent activated cell sorting (FACS). When the Ab is conjugated with a magnetic bead (●), then the cell–Ab● complex can be separated using a magnetic field, also known as magnetic assisted cell sorting (MACS).

15.1.2 Direct and Indirect Immunoassays

Depending on the approaches applied to bind the target Ag by the detecting Ab, immunological techniques can be *direct* or *indirect assays* (Figure 15.2). In the direct approach, the Ab, i.e. the 1°Ab against the target Ag, is conjugated to a reporter (visualisation marker). In the indirect method of detection, a 2°Ab is applied which is conjugated with the visualisation

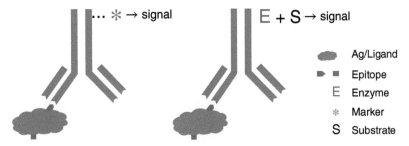

Figure 15.1 Basic principles of immunological techniques based on Ag–Ab interactions. The F_{ab} site ( ) of an Ab ( ) binds to an epitope (or) of an Ag (ligand). The Ab molecule carries a fluorescent marker (*) or is conjugated with an enzyme (E).

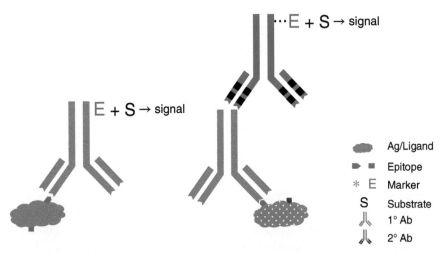

Figure 15.2 Direct and indirect immunoassays. In the direct assay, the detection marker is conjugated with the 1°Ab. In the indirect assay, the detection marker is conjugated with the 2°Ab which generally binds at the fragment crystallisable (Fc) site of the 1°Ab. The Fab site ( ) of an Ab ( ) binds to an epitope (or) of an Ag (ligand). The Ab molecule carries a fluorescent marker (*) or an enzyme (E).

marker. The 2°Ab can bind the 1°Ab which is not conjugated with the visualisation marker but binds the target Ag. Conjugated visualisation markers could be either an enzyme, mostly horseradish peroxidase (HRP) or alkaline phosphatase (AP), or a fluorophore.

While direct detection does not require an additional step of adding a 2°Ab, signal amplification is not possible by applying this method, therefore detection might be difficult for a small quantity of the target Ag. Additionally, the conjugation process may in some cases interfere with the binding of the 1°Ab with the target Ag.

15.1.3 Samples Suitable for Immunoassays

Different kinds of samples are used to evaluate the presence or absence of the target Ag. Specific protocols are applicable to collect the respective samples which may vary depending on the types of cells or tissues, as well as the amount, nature (soluble or bound) and location (membrane, cellular organelle, cytoplasm) of the target Ag.

Generally, after collection, samples are stored before proceeding with the immunoassays. In whichever conditions the samples are stored, repeated freeze-thaw cycles must be avoided for all sample types.

15.1.3.1 Serum

Blood serum is a common source of sample used to analyse cytokines or secreted proteins, including enzymes. Serum is separated from blood and collected in a serum separator tube. To separate the serum, blood is allowed to clot for 30 minutes at room temperature followed by centrifugation for 15 minutes at 1000 g. Serum often looks yellowish in colour unless there is haemolysis (which might turn the colour of the serum more red). The serum is separated as the supernatant. Serum can be stored in aliquots at ≤ –20 °C.

15.1.3.2 Plasma

Plasma is also separated from the blood and collected with anticoagulant agents such as EDTA, heparin or citrate. Once the blood is collected with the anticoagulant agent, it is centrifuged for 15 minutes at 1000 g (within 30 minutes of collection). The plasma is separated as supernatant, aliquoted and stored at ≤ -20 °C.

15.1.3.3 Platelet-poor (Platelet-free) Plasma

To obtain platelet-poor or platelet-free plasma, an additional centrifugation step at 10 000 g for 10 minutes at 2–8 °C is required for platelet removal. After centrifugation, the pellet will contain the platelets and the supernatant will contain the platelet-poor (-free) plasma.

15.1.3.4 Cell Culture Supernatant

If a cell population is cultured in a given medium, the culture supernatant also works as a source of samples for immunoassays, especially to analyse the proteins secreted by the cells. To collect the culture supernatant, a centrifugation step at 500 g for 5 minutes is required to remove cell debris. The supernatant is aliquoted and stored at ≤ 20 °C.

15.1.3.5 Tissue Lysate/Homogenate

The preparation of tissue homogenates varies depending upon tissue type. Generally, a step of tissue homogenisation is required. Tissue can be homogenised by a number of means such as sonication, repeated cycles of freezing and thawing, and by crushing using a mortar and pestle where tissue is soaked in liquid nitrogen before the crushing step. After homogenisation, the homogenates are mixed with the desired buffer such as PBS and centrifuged for 5 minutes at 5000 g. A number of commercially available kits provide the buffer and reagents to prepare tissue lysates or homogenates depending on the target use of the samples.

15.1.3.6 Saliva

Saliva is an easy and non-invasive source of sample for immunoassays. Unlike other samples, saliva collection is generally simpler and involves a step of centrifugation for 5 minutes at 10 000 g. The supernatant is collected in aliquots for storage (at ≤ -20 °C) or immediate analysis.

15.1.3.7 Urine

Collection of urine is also simple and straightforward involving a centrifugation step for 5 minutes at 10 000 g to remove particulate matter.

15.1.3.8 Human Milk

Human milk is also a non-invasive source of samples for immunoassay. It involves centrifugation for 15 minutes at 1000 g at 2–8 °C to collect the aqueous supernatant fraction.

15.1.4 Antibodies for Immunoassays

In immunological assays, Abs are classified as primary (1°) or secondary (2°). The source of the 1°Ab must be an animal which is different from the animal the target Ag of interest belongs to. For example, if the target Ag is a human cytokine IL-6, then the 1°Ab must be raised in another animal such as rat, rabbit or horse. Therefore, the 1°Ab could be rat anti-human IL-6.

If a 2°Ab is used for detection, then it must be raised in an animal different from the animal where the 1°Ab was raised. Notably, the target Ag for the 2°Ab is the 1°Ab, i.e. an immunoglobulin of the species in which the 1°Ab is raised, for example, horse anti-rat IgG.

The antibodies used for specific detection can be polyclonal or monoclonal. Monoclonal antibodies show specificity for a single epitope.

15.1.5 Use of Polyclonal or Monoclonal Antibodies

15.1.5.1 Polyclonal Antibodies

Polyclonal antibodies (pAbs) are a heterogeneous mix of antibodies in which each antibody recognises a specific epitope, i.e. Ab binding site on the Ag, on the same antigen. Each of the antibodies is produced by a specific plasma cell (Figure 15.3).

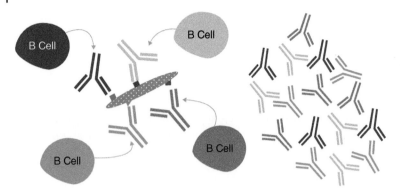

Figure 15.3 Polyclonal antibodies. Polyclonal antibodies (pAbs) are a mixture of heterogeneous antibodies that are usually produced by different B-cell clones in the body. They can recognise and bind to many different epitopes of a single Ag.

In the natural course of immune response, a number of plasma cells are programmed to produce antibodies against the same antigen, albeit targeting different epitopes. Therefore, it is possible that the mixture of polyclonal antibodies from one batch will vary from the mixture of polyclonal antibodies from another batch, although they are all capable of targeting and binding the same antigen.

Polyclonal antibodies are produced by injecting the target Ag into an animal, which could be rat, rabbit, horse, chicken or goat. Choosing the animal is important as an Ag originating from a given animal species will not elicit an immune response in another animal of the same species. Phylogenetically, the greater the distance between the source animal of the target Ag and the host animal to be used for Ab production, the better will be the immune response. After injecting the target Ag, polyclonal antibodies can be obtained from the serum.

The major advantages of using pAbs in immunoassays are (i) higher Ab affinity that results in quicker binding to the target Ag, (ii) superior for use in detecting a native protein, and (iii) easy to conjugate with Ab labels and rather unlikely to affect binding capability. However, use of pAbs might result in false-positive results as they offer a high chance of cross-reactivity due to recognition of multiple epitopes.

15.1.5.2 Monoclonal Antibodies

Monoclonal antibodies (mAbs) are antibodies which can recognise one epitope on an Ag. Hence, they come from plasma cells that originated from one B cell. In other words, monoclonal antibodies producing plasma cells are all clones of the same B cell. To produce a large amount of monoclonal antibodies, the target B cells are immortalised by fusion with hybridoma cells in a technique called hybridoma technology (Figure 15.4).

Monoclonal antibodies are produced ex vivo in tissue culture media. However, the target Ag needs to be injected into an animal. Once the animal develops an immune response, the B lymphocytes are isolated from the animal's spleen, separated and fused with a myeloma cell line. This is important to generate a large number of the same plasma cells producing the same Ab. The hybridoma of the B cells and the immortal myeloma cells can grow continuously in culture while producing the target antibodies.

Among the major advantages of using mAb are (i) high specificity to a single epitope reflected in low cross-reactivity, (ii) greater sensitivity in assays requiring quantification of protein levels, and (iii) low background noise. However, binding of conjugates for detection (labelling) may change the affinity of an mAb.

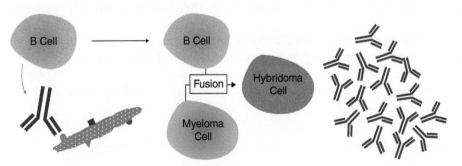

Figure 15.4 Monoclonal antibodies (mAbs) are generated by identical B cells which are clones from a single parent cell. This means that the mAbs only recognise the same epitope of an Ag.

Currently, recombinant mAbs are available which are developed by in vitro synthetic genes. The gene expression from the encoding sequences can be controlled to allow optimised binding and improved reproducibility over mAbs produced naturally, such as using hybridoma.

For applications such as therapeutic drug development that require large volumes of identical antibodies specific to a single epitope, mAbs are a better solution. For general research applications, however, the advantages of polyclonal antibodies typically outweigh the few advantages that monoclonal antibodies provide. With affinity purification of serum against small antigen targets, the advantages of polyclonal antibodies are further extended.

15.1.6 Specificity and Sensitivity of Ag–Ab Binding

In living cells, antibodies bind with high specificity to antigens which were used to trigger the immune system. However, Abs may also show cross-reactivity by binding to other antigens that share structural, conformational and biochemical properties with the original antigen.

Injection of an antigen into an animal results in a polyclonal antibody response in which different antibodies are produced that react with the various epitopes on the antigen.

Since monoclonal antibodies specifically detect a particular epitope on the antigen, they are less likely than polyclonal antibodies to cross-react with other proteins.

15.1.7 Reporter (Visualisation Marker) and Linker

If an enzyme is used, then it is either HRP or alkaline phosphatase (AP) that is conjugated with the detecting Ab. Upon reacting with the given substrate, a coloured product is produced which is then visualised and the intensity of which is also used for the quantification. Notably, the activity of HRP and AP depends on enzyme and substrate concentration, buffer, pH and temperature, all of which need to be optimised accordingly.

Fluorescein molecules such as fluorescein isothiocyanate (FITC) are often used as reporters. Generally, fluorescein reporters are conjugated with primary Abs but secondary Abs can also be conjugated with these reporters.

FITC

15.1.7.1 Fluorescein Isothiocyanate

Fluorescein isothiocyanate is a derivative of fluorescein which has an isothiocyanate reactive group (–N=C=S). This derivative is reactive towards nucleophiles, including amine and sulfhydryl groups on proteins.

Several modifications have been adopted to amplify the signal from the E–S complex during immunological assays. For visualisation purposes, Abs are conjugated with a linker (such as biotin) which ultimately binds to an avidin-, streptavidin- or neutravidin-bound enzyme. This modification allows a higher ratio of E–S complex compared to Ag–Ab complex, and so results in more colour development.

15.1.7.2 Enzyme: Horseradish Peroxidase

Horseradish peroxidase (M_r 40 kDa) catalyses the oxidation of substrates in the presence of hydrogen peroxide (H_2O_2), resulting in a coloured product or the release of light as a byproduct of the reaction. Its high turnover rate, good stability, low cost and wide availability of substrates make HRP the enzyme of choice for most applications.

15.1.7.3 Enzyme: Alkaline Phosphatase

Alkaline phosphatase is a heat-stable enzyme, also known as basic phosphatase, which consists of two similar monomers, hence it is a homodimeric enzyme (M_r 86 kDa). Five cysteine residues, two Zn and one Mg play crucial roles in its catalytic function. The enzyme is present in both prokaryotes and eukaryotes having the same catalytic function. AP is a nonspecific enzyme which catalyses the hydrolysis of a wide range of phosphate esters.

Alkaline phosphatase hydrolyses a colourless substrate called 5-bromo-4-chloro-3-indolyl phosphate (BCIP) and reduces p-nitroblue tetrazolium chloride (NBT) to produce a deep purple reaction product.

In the presence of H_2O_2, 3-amino-9-ethyl carbazole and 4-chlorine naphthol will be oxidised to a brown substance and a blue product respectively under the catalysation of HRP. Enhanced chemiluminescence is another method employed in HRP detection.

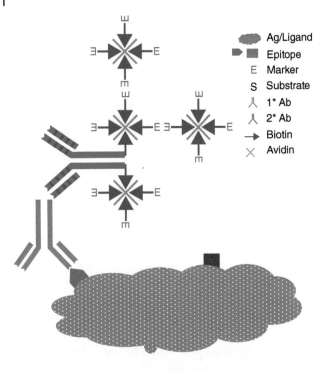

	Ag/Ligand
	Epitope
E	Marker
S	Substrate
人	1* Ab
人	2* Ab
→	Biotin
×	Avidin

signal amplifiction

15.1.7.4 Streptavidin–Biotin Complex

Streptavidin, originally isolated from *Streptomyces avidinii*, can bind biotin. Each subunit of streptavidin binds one molecule of biotin with affinity similar to that of avidin.

15.1.7.5 Common Substrates

The compatible substrate that reacts with HRP in the presence of peroxide is 3,3'-diaminobenzidine tetrahydrochloride (DAB; M_r 214.1). The HRP–DAB reactions yield an insoluble brown-coloured product at locations where peroxidase-conjugated antibodies are bound to samples. The brown precipitate is insoluble in alcohol and other organic solvents, making it an excellent substrate for immunohistochemical staining that requires the use of traditional counterstains and mounting media.

There are a number of other substrates that are used for different immunoassays.

- O-phenylenediamine dihydrochloride (OPD) turns amber to detect HRP (which is often used as a conjugated protein).
- 3,3',5,5'-Tetramethylbenzidine (TMB) turns blue when detecting HRP and turns yellow after the addition of sulfuric or phosphoric acid.
- 2,2'-Azinobis [3-ethylbenzothiazoline-6-sulfonic acid]-diammonium salt (ABTS) turns green when detecting HRP.
- p-Nitrophenyl phosphate, disodium salt (PNPP) turns yellow when detecting alkaline phosphatase.

DAB

HRP + H_2O_2 → Quinone iminium cation → brown precipitate

15.1.8 Different Types of Immunoassays and Their Applications

Different types of immunoassays are being used for research purposes and clinical investigations. A few of the most common techniques, namely ELISA, IHC/ICC, Western blotting and FACS, are discussed in detail in the following sections. In relation to their applications, different techniques are used for different purposes.

- IHC/ICC and FACS can be used for the diagnosis and identification of cells during the course of disease, such as cells from cancerous tissue and cells or tissue infected with infectious agents.
- ELISA, IHC/ICC and Western blotting can be used to identify specific molecular markers that are characteristic of particular cellular events such as proliferation and cell death (apoptosis), as well as pathological and inflammatory status.
- IHC/ICC is widely used in basic research to understand the distribution, localisation and expression pattern of specific proteins related to specific cellular responses and events.
- ELISA, IHC/ICC and Western blotting can be used to detect the presence of a pathogenic micro-organism in an infected cell or tissue.
- Western blotting is mainly applied for the simultaneous detection of a specific protein by means of its antigenicity and its molecular mass.

- Western blotting can also be used to elute specific antibodies from specific proteins resolved out of a complex mixture, many of whose components react with a given antiserum. One can electrophorese a mixture of proteins, cut out a specific band from a gel or membrane, and use this to fish out specific antibodies from a serum.

15.2 Enzyme-linked Immunosorbent Assay

15.2.1 Basic Concept and Steps

The most common and simplest form of ELISA is based on attaching the target antigens (or ligand), generally present in a liquid sample such as serum or cell culture supernatant, to solid surfaces (solid phase) in wells of a microtitre plate. A specific Ab that can bind the target Ag, more specifically an epitope of an antigen, is added. The Ab is conjugated to an enzyme, which can react with a specific substrate that is generally added at the final step. The subsequent reaction produces a detectable signal, most commonly a change in colour of the substrate.

An ELISA-based detection or quantification of target Ag can involve 1–3 types of Abs.

The sample to be tested to detect the target Ag, its presence and/or quantity is dispensed into wells of a polystyrene microtitre plate to immobilise or attach the Ag on the surface of the well. Attachment of the target Ag in the well can be performed non-specifically which involves adsorption of the Ag directly on the polystyrene surface. Alternatively, a pre-coated microtitre plate, i.e. the plate surface of its well is coated with a specific Ab, can be used in which the target Ag will bind (such binding is also called 'immunosorbed') the attached Ab.

The attached Ag is then targeted for binding with a detection Ab which is covalently linked to an enzyme or can itself be detected by a 2°Ab that is linked to an enzyme. At the final step, a substrate is added into the plate which then reacts with the enzyme to produce a visible coloured signal. The intensity of the colour indicates the quantity of Ag remaining attached in the well of the plate. Between each step, the plate is washed with a buffer containing mild detergent solution to remove any proteins or antibodies that are non-specifically bound or were unbound.

15.2.2 Types of ELISA

ELISA-based assays are classified based on whether the target Ag is detected by the 1°Ab conjugated with the detection marker (called *direct ELISA*) or by a 2°Ab conjugated with the detection marker (called *indirect ELISA*). However, the use and meaning of the names indirect or direct ELISA differ in the literature and on websites depending on the context of the experiment. A third type of ELISA, 'sandwich ELISA', is clearly distinct from an indirect ELISA (Figure 15.5).

In a sandwich ELISA, the microtitre plate is coated with an Ab called the 'capture Ab'. The capture Ab is expected to bind the target Ag. A second Ab, called the 'detecting Ab', is then used to bind the same Ag but at a different site from that of the capture Ab. A third Ab (also called anti-antibody) is then used that can bind at the Fc site of the detecting Ab. This third Ab conjugates with the detection marker such as an enzyme.

A sandwich ELISA used for research often needs validation because of the risk of false-positive results.

15.2.3 General Steps in Direct or Indirect ELISA

Like any other immunoassays, the simplest form of ELISA involves three major stages: (i) immobilisation of the Ag in wells of a microtitre plate, (ii) addition of the 1°Ab to bind the target Ag at the corresponding epitope, (iii) detection of the target Ag, through the Ag–1°Ab* complex in direct ELISA and Ag–1°Ab–2°Ab* complex in indirect ELISA using the detection marker (*) conjugated to the 1°Ab and 2°Ab respectively. In a sandwich ELISA, a microtitre plate precoated with a capture Ab is used to trap the target Ag on the surface of the well.

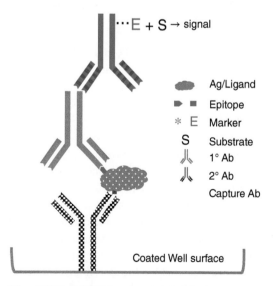

Figure 15.5 Molecular arrangements in sandwich ELISA.

Therefore, the protocol generally involves the following steps.

1) Addition of a sample solution, generally prepared in a prescribed buffer, containing the target Ag to each well of a 96-well plate and allowing adhesion to the polystyrene surface of the plate through charge interactions. The sample solutions are discarded after a given time before proceeding to the next step.

2) In case of a sandwich ELISA, a precoated microtitre plate is used. The coating is performed using a known quantity of capture Ab which can bind the target Ag. After allowing the sample containing the target Ag to bind the capture Ab, solutions are discarded before proceeding to the next step.

3) A solution of non-reacting protein, also known as blocking solution, such as bovine serum albumin (BSA) or casein or skimmed milk, is added to the well in order to cover or block any part of the surface which might remain unbound by the target Ag (or Ag–capture Ab complex in case of sandwich ELISA) or any other antigens present in the sample solution. Once again, the blocking solutions are discarded and often washed with a prescribed buffer before the next step.

4) Next, the 1°Ab with a conjugated enzyme (in case of a direct ELISA) is added which binds specifically to the target Ag coated in the well.

5) In the case of indirect ELISA, a 1°Ab is added and washed before adding the 2°Ab conjugated with enzyme.

6) The plate is washed to remove the unbound Ab conjugates to avoid any false-positive results.

7) A substrate for the enzyme is then added. Often, this substrate changes colour upon reaction with the enzyme. The higher the concentration of the antibody conjugate present in the solution, the stronger the colour development through the enzyme–substrate reactions. Often, a spectrometer is used to give quantitative values for colour strength.

8) If the detecting Ab is conjugated with a fluorescent marker (reporter), then the results can be directly recorded without the addition of any other reagents such as substrate.

9) A chemical is added to be converted by the enzyme into a colour or fluorescent or electrochemical signal. The absorbance or fluorescence or electrochemical signal (e.g. current) of the plate wells is measured to determine the presence and quantity of antigen.

10) However, the use of a 2°Ab conjugated with a detection marker is helpful to reduce the cost of purchasing enzyme-linked 1°Ab for every target Ag one might want to detect. It is possible to use the same enzyme-linked 2°Ab that binds the Fc region of other antibodies.

15.2.4 Variations and Advances in ELISA

15.2.4.1 Competitive ELISA

In a competitive ELISA, unlabelled Ab that can bind the target Ag is preincubated in the presence of its antigen (sample) before being added into a well of a microtitre plate. These bound Ag–Ab complexes (immune complexes) are then added to an antigen-coated well. The plate is washed, so unbound antibodies are removed. The more Ag in the sample, the more Ag–Ab complexes are formed and so there are fewer unbound antibodies available to bind to the antigen in the well, hence the name 'competitive'.

Some competitive ELISA kits include enzyme-linked Ag rather than enzyme-linked Ab. The labelled Ag competes for 1°Ab binding sites with the sample Ag (unlabelled). The less Ag in the sample, the more labelled Ag is retained in the well and the stronger the signal.

15.2.4.2 Reverse ELISA

In reverse ELISA, an unlabelled Ab is added with the target Ag suspended in the sample or buffer in a vial or a tube and allowed to form an Ag–Ab complex. Here the Ag is often tagged (*) with a detection molecule.

Reverse ELISA allows multiple Ags to be tagged and counted at the same time. In addition, this technique allows specific strains of bacteria to be identified by two (or more) different tags with different colours. When both tags are expected to be present in a cell, then the target strain can be detected or identified using the combination of the tags.

After mixture, the sample will contain the free *Ag and Ab as well as the *Ag–Ab complex and is then passed through a test tube or a specifically designed flow-through channel called a scavenger container. The surface of the scavenger container has identical or sufficiently similar to the target Ag (without the tag) also called 'scavenger Ag' bound to it. The scavenger Ag can bind the free Ab present in the sample.

If the sample is passed through a detector such as a flow cytometer, when a fluorescence tag is used, the presence of the target Ag can be detected by the fluorescence signal.

15.2.5 Analysis of Results of ELISA

Primarily, ELISA data are obtained in the form of absorbance of the samples. The absorbance data can be used to evaluate the sample in three different ways.

15.2.5.1 Qualitative Analysis
By comparing the developed colour of the negative control, positive control and samples, one can determine if the target protein is present or absent in the sample.

15.2.5.2 Semiquantitative Analysis
Using the absorbance data, i.e. signal intensities, one can infer if the amount of the target protein in the sample is higher or lower than that of the negative and/or positive control. This merely gives an idea on the relative levels of the target protein in the samples since signal intensity is directly related to antigen concentration.

15.2.5.3 Quantitative Analysis
For a more precise calculation of the concentration of the target protein, the signal intensity, i.e. the absorbance data of the target protein, can be converted to a unit of concentration such as µg/ml, ng/ml and mg/l. This is done by plotting a *standard curve* using different concentrations (usually serially diluted) of a positive sample (a known protein).

15.2.5.4 Important Points in Results Analysis
- Using triplicates of each sample in order to determine an average (or mean) absorbance is often critical. Please see Chapter 16 on statistical analysis to determine if mean or average should be used. This provides statistical validation of the results. When a sample is measured in duplicate/triplicate, the absorbance should not vary more than 15–20% of the mean/average.
- Evaluating a blank sample is vital to read the background absorbance.
- The range of absorbance, i.e. reading from the microplate/ELISA reader, should be within 0.2–2.0 for the evaluation or calculation. If necessary, a more diluted sample should be used.
- If the absorbance is below 0.2 then it can be reasonably concluded that the target protein is either absent or below the detection limit. If the absorbance is above 2.0, a diluted sample needs to be analysed for the original calculation.
- Often a cut-off value is used to determine the actual concentration of a sample; this is based on the range of the target protein that is present in a natural or normal condition. For example, if one wants to analyse the change (increase or decrease) in the concentration of a cytokine in a given condition, the normal range of the given cytokine can be used as a cut-off value.

15.2.5.5 Preparing a Standard Curve
A standard curve is prepared by plotting the mean absorbance on the y-axis against the protein concentration on the x-axis of a known protein such as bovine serum albumin (BSA) (Figure 15.6).

Figure 15.6   Standard curve for ELISA.

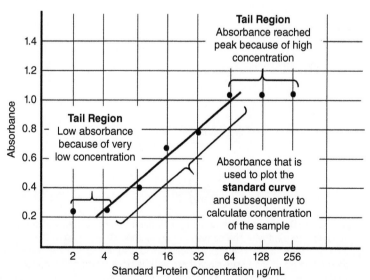

Absorbance of a serial dilution (of its concentration) of the known protein such as BSA is used to plot a standard curve. It is possible the standard curve might have tails at both ends. Only the region of the plot showing progression, i.e. without the tail regions, is acceptable to measure the concentration of the target protein in the unknown sample.

15.3 Immunohisto-(cyto-)-chemical Staining

15.3.1 Basic Concept of IHC/ICC

Primarily, immunohistochemical (IHC) or immunocytochemical (ICC) staining is used to detect the presence of a protein and/or its relative quantity in a given section of a tissue sample or smear of cells that is attached, fixed and stained on a glass slide (Figure 15.7). This technique also reveals the in situ location of the target protein. When combined with detection of an additional protein, the double IHC/ICC staining can also reveal the co-localisation of the target proteins.

In principle, IHC and ICC staining serve the same purposes and are performed in a similar way. The main difference lies with the sample investigated. If the sample is taken from a tissue, the technique is referred to as immunohistochemical staining. If the sample is composed of isolated cells from cell culture, blood or disintegrated tissue, then the technique is called immunocytochemical staining. While the prefix 'immuno' refers to antibodies used in the procedure to detect the target protein, the prefixes 'histo' and 'cyto' refer to tissue and cell respectively.

The simplest form of IHC involves three major steps: (i) immobilisation of the tissue section onto a glass slide, (ii) allowing the binding of the 1°Ab with the target protein (serves as an Ag for the Ab) at the corresponding epitope, and (iii) detection of the target protein, more particularly the Ag–1°Ab* complex, through the detection marker (*) conjugated to the 1°Ab. This approach is called direct IHC staining. To increase the specificity and sensitivity of the staining, a second Ab is often used.

The 2°Ab is chosen so it can bind the 1°Ab, generally on its Fc domain of one of the heavy chains. In this approach, the detection marker (*) is conjugated with the 2°Ab. This approach is called indirect IHC. Therefore, in indirect IHC, the detection marker basically represents the presence of the Ag–1°Ab–2°Ab* complex.

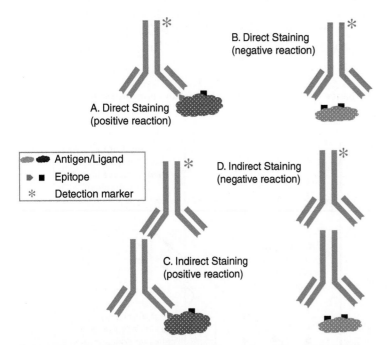

Figure 15.7 Detection of the target Ag using immunohistochemical staining. In cases where the target Ag is present in the sample, 1°Ab is able to bind with the corresponding epitope(s), resulting in the formation of the Ag–1°Ab* complex as in direct IHC staining (a) or a Ag–1°Ab–2°Ab* complex in indirect IHC staining (c). In cases where the target Ag is absent in the sample, 1°Ab is not able to remain attached to the tissue since there will be no corresponding epitopes for its binding; hence, there will be no Ag–1°Ab* complex as in direct IHC staining (b) or Ag–1°Ab–2°Ab* complex in indirect IHC staining (d).

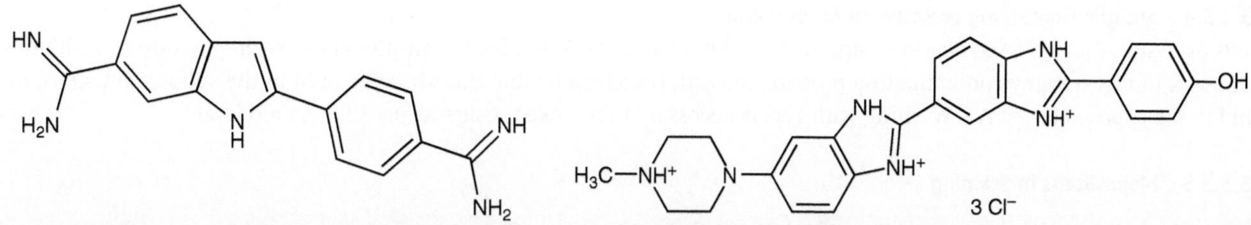

Figure 15.8 (Left) DAPI (4',6-diamidino-2-phenylindole) is a fluorescent stain that binds to A-T-rich regions in DNA and once bound, shows absorption maximum at 358 nm (ultraviolet) and emission maximum 461 nm (blue). (Right) Hoechst 33258 stains are part of a family of blue fluorescent dyes used to stain DNA. There are three related Hoechst stains: Hoechst 33258, Hoechst 33342 and Hoechst 34580.

15.3.2 Basic Requirements for IHC/ICC Staining

- *Sample*: fixed target cell or tissue on an appropriate surface such as on silica or lysine-coated glass slide and chamber slide.
- *Antibodies*: binding of the target protein with a reporter with or without a linker enzyme or fluorescent conjugated Ab. Depending on the design of the experiment, either conjugated 1°Ab* or conjugated 2°Ab* specific for 1°Ab is required.
- *Detection markers*: visualisation of the Ag–Ab interaction which depends on the type of conjugated Ab used. In the most common instance, the detecting Ab is enzyme conjugated. Alternatively, the antibody can also be tagged to a fluorophore, such as fluorescein or rhodamine.
- *Counterstaining*: after IHC/ICC staining of the target Ag, a second stain is applied to provide contrast and show the anatomical location, i.e. the discrete cellular compartments where the target Ag is located.
- Both chromogenic and fluorescent dyes are available for ICC/IHC to provide a vast array of reagents to fit every experimental design. Haematoxylin and eosin, Hoechst stain and 4',6-diamidino-2-phenylindole (DAPI) are commonly used (Figure 15.8).

15.3.3 Basic Steps in ICC/IHC

15.3.3.1 Pretreatment of Slides
Pretreatment to clean the slides is often helpful to avoid any artifacts or false-positive reaction after staining. Generally, the slides are dipped into a 0.1N HCl solution overnight at room temperature. HCl is removed by washing in deionised water (preferably MQ H_2O). The air-dried slides can be autoclaved or flamed before use.

15.3.3.2 Precoating of Slides (Optional)
Glass slides work better for IHC/ICC if coated with poly-L-lysine (PLL). This can be done by using a very low concentration of PLL, such as 1 mg PLL in 10 ml in MQ H_2O. Slides are covered with the PPL solution for about 5 minutes and air dried after draining the solution. Pretreated and precoated slides are currently available commercially.

Poly-L-lysine enhances electrostatic interaction between negatively charged ions of the cell membrane and positively charged surface ions provided by lysine. When adsorbed to the slide surface, PLL increases the number of positively charged sites available for binding by the negatively charged ions of the cell membrane.

15.3.3.3 Preparation of Tissue Sections or Cells
Cells that are separated from cell culture or blood or those suspended in liquid media are generally used for ICC staining. These cells, when ready for staining, are washed in PBS and then resuspended in PBS containing 5% BSA at a density of about 5×10^5 cells/ml which are then spread over the glass slides either by using cytocentrifuge or manually using another slide. The cells can be air dried overnight at room temperature before the next step.

Generally, a tissue section, either fresh frozen or paraffin embedded, is used for IHC. The tissue section of an appropriate thickness, usually 5–10 μM, is placed on the glass slide and allowed to air dry.

15.3.3.4 Antigen Unmasking or Retrieval for Staining

Cells or tissues that are fixed on a slide are treated with 0.1% Triton X-100 for 15 minutes at room temperature or with proteinase K to digest many contaminating proteins present, thereby allowing the Ab, to be used in the subsequent steps, to bind to the exposed target Ag. Washing with PBS is necessary to remove the agents used for Ag retrieval.

15.3.3.5 Major Steps in Staining

1) *Peroxidase blocking*: incubation of the slides in 3% H_2O_2 for 10 minutes. This step is not necessary for immunofluorescence detection.
2) *Serum blocking*: slides are incubated in blocking buffer (such as 1–2% BSA prepared in PBS) for 20 minutes at room temperature. This is useful to block/mask the spaces where the Ab could bind non-specifically, hence preventing false-positive reactions.

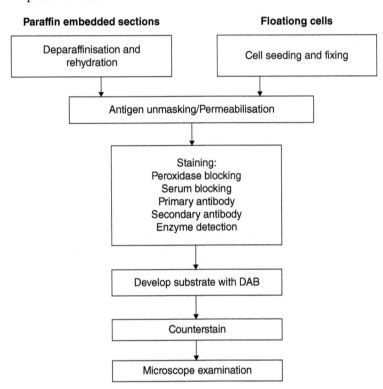

3) *Incubation with Ab*: after removing the blocking buffer, 1°Ab is added at a prescribed dilution and incubated for one hour at room temperature or overnight at 4 °C. Remove the 1°Ab and wash sections in PBS (better to do three times, each for three minutes). In the following step, 2°Ab is added and incubated for 30 minutes at room temperature.
4) *Detection*: detection is performed based on the markers used. If an enzyme-conjugated detection Ab is used, detection is performed using the colour development related to the substrate–enzyme complex. Fluorescent markers are also used for detection where detection is based on emission of fluorescent light.
5) *Counterstain and mounting of cover slips*: counterstaining is often used in IHC/ICC. Slides can be counterstained with haematoxylin, Hoechst stain or DAPI. Before mounting the cover slip, slides need to washed in dH_2O and dehydrated in ascending series of ethanol solutions such as 80%, 95% and finally 100% ethanol. Slides are also cleaned using xylene for 2 × 5 minutes. Finally, cover slips are mounted on the cells/tissue section using a mounting medium such as Permount® (Fisher Scientific) or DPX.

15.3.4 Troubleshooting in IHC/ICC

ICC/IHC may experience either strong or weak background staining. The reasons and solutions linked to such outcomes are as follows.

- *Interference from endogenous peroxidases or phosphatases.*
  Solution: quench endogenous peroxidases with 3% H_2O_2 in H_2O or methanol or use a commercial peroxidase suppressor. Endogenous phosphatases can be inhibited with levamisole.
- *High background:* high background can occur when endogenous biotin and lectins are not blocked prior to adding the avidin–biotin–enzyme complex. If the ABC complex is made with avidin, the highly glycosylated protein can bind to lectins in the tissue sample.
  Solution: block endogenous lectins with 0.2 M alpha-methyl mannoside in dilution buffer. Alternatively, use streptavidin or NeutrAvidin® protein instead of avidin, because they are not glycosylated and therefore will not bind to lectins.
- *The 2°Ab may show a strong or moderate affinity for identical or similar epitopes on non-target antigens.*

Solution: if normal serum from the same species as the 2°Ab is used to block the tissue, then increase the serum concentration by 2% or more. If blocking with another reagent (BSA, skim milk), then add 2% or more normal serum from the species of the 2°Ab. Alternatively, reduce the concentration of the biotinylated 2°Ab.

- *Non-specific interactions between the 1°Ab and non-target epitopes*: the 1°Ab can bind a non-specific site on the tissue sample that occurs regularly during incubation but at a level that does not influence background staining. A high 1°Ab concentration will increase these interactions and thus increase non-specific binding and background staining.
  Solution: reduce the concentration of the 1°Ab.
- The 1°Ab may also show a strong or moderate affinity for identical or similar epitopes on non-target antigens.
  Solution: increase the blocking buffer concentration or use a different 1°Ab.
- *The 1°Ab diluent may contain little or no NaCl, thus reducing ionic interactions.*
  Solution: add NaCl diluents usually containing 0.15 M to 0.6 M NaCl.
- *Absence of enzyme-substrate reactivity*: deionized H_2O can sometimes contain peroxidase inhibitors that can significantly impair enzyme activity. Also, the pH of the substrate buffer must be appropriate for that specific substrate.
  Solution: change the enzyme diluent and/or prepare substrate at the proper pH and repeat the test.
- *Absence of binding of the 1°Ab*: the 1°Ab may lose affinity for the target epitope over time, due to protein degradation or denaturation due to long-term storage, altered pH or harsh treatments (i.e. freeze-thaw cycles).
  Solution: ensure optimum pH (7.0–8.2) of Ab diluent for optimum Ab binding; store the Ab according to the manufacturer's instructions and avoid repeated freezing-thawing.
- *High background colour*: while high concentrations of the 2°Ab can increase background staining, extremely high concentrations can cause the opposite effect and reduce antigen detection.
  Solution: reduce the concentration of the 2°Ab. If the diluent contains antigen-neutralising antibodies, such as those found in serum, then the antibodies will block 2°Ab binding.

15.3.5 Reducing High Background in IHC/ICC Staining

- Carefully prepare tissue samples. Damage to the tissue can cause diffuse staining.
- Prepare thinner sections if the tissue is not being penetrated well.
- Optimise fixation. Each tissue antigen will react differently with different fixatives. Optimise the pH, incubation time and temperature.
- Blocking may be improved by simply draining the excess buffer instead of washing the tissue sample prior to the addition of antibodies.
- Use a monoclonal instead of a polyclonal primary antibody to reduce cross-reactivity.
- Use cross-adsorbed polyclonal antibodies to reduce cross-reactivity.
- Decrease the incubation times with the primary and secondary antibodies to reduce non-specific binding.
- Choose an improved substrate that will produce a higher signal:noise ratio for the system, such as metal enhanced DAB rather than DAB.

15.3.6 Increasing Staining Intensity

- Optimise fixation. The immune reactivity can be affected by the fixative step and the processing step. Avoid freeze-thaw cycles and high temperatures if the antigen is susceptible to heat.
- Use clean slides for mounting of tissue, and use appropriate conditions to prevent tissue from being removed during processing.
- Do not inhibit the enzyme. If an AP system is being used, do not use phosphate buffer. If an HRP system is being used, do not use sodium azide. Both will inhibit enzyme activity.
- Do not overblock the tissue, since antigenic sites may be masked.
- Remember that neutralising antibodies may be in the blocking serum.
- Increase antibody penetration of the tissue by using unmasking agents such as trypsin, pepsin, chymotrypsin and Pronase.
- Increase the detection efficiency, and possibly the sensitivity, by using signal amplification systems such as ABC.
- Properly prepare the enzyme complex. Carefully mix all components of the enzyme–substrate complex in the correct proportions.

- Avoid potential sources of biotin, such as non-fat dry milk or Fraction V-grade BSA (use only IHC grade).
- Increase incubation times or concentrations of the primary or secondary reagents.
- Use a more sensitive substrate system such as the metal enhanced DAB substrate.
- Always run a positive control to determine if the system is working.
- Use the correct counterstain and mountant. Some enzymatic products are soluble in alcohol, xylene or other solvents. Consider aqueous mounting.

15.4 Western Blotting

15.4.1 Basic Concept

Western blotting, also known as immune-blotting or electro-blotting, is a technique used to transfer proteins transversely from polyacrylamide gel to a nitrocellulose membrane and eventually detect a target protein based on its property to specifically bind to an Ab. The name of the technique, 'Western blot', is a play on 'Southern blot', a technique for DNA detection named after its inventor, Edwin Southern. The term 'Western blot' was coined by W. Neal Burnette in 1981, and the method was first introduced by Harry Towbin at the Friedrich Miescher Institute (Basel, Switzerland) in 1979.

This technique uses the binding specificity of Ab to its target Ag which is immobilised on a nitrocellulose membrane. Proteins which are resolved or separated based on molecular mass (more appropriately, this is called relative molecular mass or M_r) by electrophoresis on a polyacrylamide gel are transferred (or blotted) on a nitrocellulose membrane and eventually detected by Ag–Ab interactions.

The attachment of specific Ab to specific immobilised Ag onto the membrane is visualised by indirect enzyme immunoassay techniques, usually using a chromogenic substrate which produces an insoluble coloured product.

While transferring from gel to membrane, the proteins are trapped and remain attached on the membrane as the polyacrylamide gel allows the protein to diffuse towards the membrane based on the flow of the current (from cathode to anode).

The Western blotting technique detects a target protein in a mixture of proteins separated from a cell lysate and cell culture supernatant. Compared to other immunoassays, it offers an additional feature to the result. In other techniques, such as ELISA, the presence of a target protein is detected by visualisation of the detection Ab. In Western blotting, in addition to its presence, the M_r of the target protein can also be revealed (Figure 15.9).

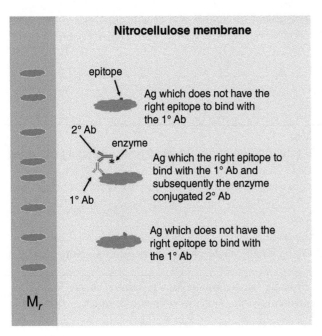

Nitrocellulose membrane

epitope

Ag which does not have the right epitope to bind with the 1° Ab

2° Ab

enzyme

Ag which the right epitope to bind with the 1° Ab and subsequently the enzyme conjugated 2° Ab

1° Ab

Ag which does not have the right epitope to bind with the 1° Ab

M_r

Figure 15.9 Basic concept of Western blotting. The separated target protein along with the other proteins (Ag/Ligand) are transferred onto a nitrocellulose membrane. Once the membrane is incubated with the 1°Ab, it is expected to bind the correct epitope on the target Ag, while the other antigens remain unbound. The 2°Ab will bind only the 1°Ab and so will give a signal depending on the detection marker it carries. The spot (more specifically, the 'band') revealed by the coloured signal can be compared with the proteins with known M_r separated in the same gel and transferred onto the same membrane yet stained separately using Coomassie brilliant blue.

15.4.2 Major Steps in Western Blotting

Western blotting is an experiment in itself. It requires (i) preparation of the sample, i.e. protein, (ii) separation of the proteins into a polyacrylamide gel, (iii) blotting of the separated proteins from the gel to a membrane, and finally (iv) immune detection of the target protein on the membrane, hence the name immunoblotting (Figure 15.10).

Samples are prepared in a denaturing buffer to aid electrophoretic mobility in the polyacrylamide gel, i.e. polyacrylamide gel electrophoresis. Details of polyacrylamide gel electrophoresis are given in a subsequent section of this chapter. Then proteins are moved from within the gel onto a membrane made of nitrocellulose (NC) or polyvinylidene difluoride (PVDF).

The transfer of proteins is conducted in a sandwich-like arrangement of gel-membrane-NC/PVDF filter in between soaked filter papers. A high-intensity electric current is applied for the transfer. Prolonging the time to an appropriate extent will transfer proteins more effectively.

Like any other immunoassay, immune blotting requires the blocking of sites which are not attached with the target or any other proteins. This is again meant to prevent any non-specific false-positive signal through binding of the detection Ab to those sites.

Again, similar to other immunoassays, this technique also requires incubation with the 1°Ab followed by incubation with the 2°Ab (in case of indirect immunoassays). A substrate reacts with the enzyme that is bound to the 2°Ab to generate visible coloured protein bands.

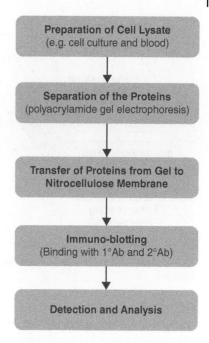

Figure 15.10 Major steps in Western blotting.

15.4.3 Basic Requirements for Western Blotting

- *Reagents and apparatus* to run SDS-PAGE.
- *Membrane to blot the protein*: generally, a nitrocellulose membrane (0.2–0.45 µm pore size) which gives low staining backgrounds with India ink, Amido black, Coomassie brilliant blue, colloidal gold and HRP or AP substrates. Other kinds of membranes include PVDF which can be stained with colloidal gold. Nitrocellulose membranes with 0.45 µm pore size are used to bind proteins with M_r over 20 kDa while pore size of 0.2 µm is used for those below 20 kDa. PVDF membranes provide better resolution of low molecular weight proteins due to their higher sensitivity, resolution and affinity.
- *Filter paper* (Whatman® 3MM) or preferably blotting paper. Filter papers are used for soaking of buffers. The size of the papers must fit the gel to minimise the surface area exposed to the electrode. Bigger papers increase current flow and generate more heat which affects efficient transfer of the proteins from the gel to the membranes.
- *Blotting electrodes*: generally, carbon slabs ($1 \times 20 \times 15$ cm^3) with heavy insulated leads are used as blotting electrodes.
- *Power supply unit*: a high-amperage low-voltage apparatus, capable of supplying 500 mA–1 A current at voltages as low as 5 V is required for optimum transfer.
- *Blotting buffer*: depending on the purpose and the sample, a number of buffers can be used for blotting.
  - 50 mM Tris-HCl/0.196 M glycine pH 8.3 with 20% methanol
  - Laemmli electrophoresis buffer
  - 25 mM Tris-Cl pH 8.3/20% methanol (or pH 7.0–8.8)
  - 25–50 mM phosphate/methanol pH 7.0–8.0.
  - Anodal buffer 1 (for pad nearest anode): 0.3 M Tris/20% MeOH pH 10.4
  - Anodal buffer 2(for other gel pad assemblies): 25 mM Tris/20% MeOH pH 10.4
  - Cathodal buffer (for all pads nearest cathode): 25 mM Tris/40 mM aminocaproic acid/20% MeOH, pH 9.4

15.4.4 Transferring (Blotting) Proteins from Gel to Membrane (Figure 15.11)

1) Dip a freshly electrophoresed SDS-polyacrylamide gel into transfer buffer (0.025 M Tris-HCl/20% (v/v) methanol, pH 8.3).
2) Place 2–3 layers of filter paper soaked in transfer buffer on the ANODE (+) and place the prewetted nitrocellulose membrane on the filter papers. On top of the membrane, place the freshly electrophoresed SDS-polyacrylamide gel. On top of the gel, place another 2–3 layers of filter paper soaked in transfer buffer.

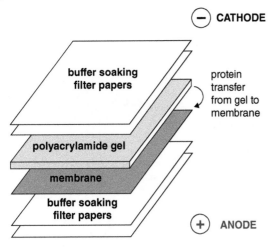

○ **CATHODE**

buffer soaking
filter papers

protein
transfer
from gel to
membrane

polyacrylamide gel

membrane

buffer soaking
filter papers

⊕ **ANODE**

Figure 15.11 Arrangement of components in Western blotting.

3) Care should be taken to exclude bubbles between gel and nitrocellulose, and between nitrocellulose and paper.
4) Place the CATHODE (-) on top of the top layers of filter paper.
5) Apply a current of 500 mA for 20–30 minutes to perform the transfer.

15.4.5 Buffers for Western Blotting

- *Incubation/blocking buffer*: 10 mM Tris-Cl/150 mM NaCl containing 1–5% Protea non-fat milk powder and 0.05% Tween-20 or Triton X-100 (= Nonidet P-40), pH 7.4.
- *Washing buffer*: PBS or 10 mM Tris-Cl/150 mM NaCl pH 7.4 containing 0.05% Tween-20 or Triton™ X-100.
- *Substrate buffer*: 100 mM Tris-Cl/100 mM NaCl/5 mM MgCl2 pH 9.5.
- *Substrate stocks*: Nitroblue tetrazolium (NBT), 75 mg/ml in 70% dimethyl formamide; 5-bromo-4-chloro-3-indolyl phosphate (BCIP), 50 mg/ml in formamide (100%).

It is important to make fresh NBT-BCIP substrate before use.

15.4.6 Protocol for Immunostaining of Proteins on Membranes

Generally, an indirect immunoassay approach is followed for immunostaining of the membrane. In this approach, the membrane is initially incubated in the blocking buffer followed by incubation with 1°Ab and then the marker is conjugated with the 2°Ab. Briefly, the steps would be as follows.

1) Rinse the nitrocellulose blots in transfer buffer then soak for one hour at 37 °C or two hours at room temperature in blocking buffer. This procedure allows blocking of all non-specific protein binding sites on the blots.
2) Incubate the membrane by shaking/rocking in sealed boxes in a buffer containing the 1°Ab for one hour at room temperature (22 °C), followed by washing to eliminate the unbound 1°Ab.
3) Incubate the washed membrane with the 2°Ab at a suitable dilution. Incubation conditions and washing are the same as before.
4) Visualisation of the Ag–Ab complex on the membrane is done by the reaction of NBT and BCIP substrate mixture. The reaction occurs in the dark. Once a visible band is produced, the reaction is terminated by washing with water. Blots are dried under weighted filter paper and stored in the dark. Results may be recorded photographically.

15.4.7 Trouble Shooting in Immunoblotting

15.4.7.1 Blocking of the Non-specific Binding Site of the Membrane

The nitrocellulose membrane used for blotting of the electrophoresed proteins can bind antibodies which are subsequently used for detection purposes. Therefore, non-specific binding of antibodies must be eliminated by incubating with inert protein or non-ionic detergent diluted in blocking buffers. It is important to note that the blocking buffers should not replace target protein on the membrane, bind epitope on the target protein or cross-react with any of the primary or secondary Abs to be used or detection reagents.

The most typical blocking proteins include BSA, non-fat dry milk, casein, gelatin and Tween-20 which are diluted in TBS and/or PBS buffers.

It is best to avoid using non-fat dry milk as a blocking protein if a biotin-conjugated Ab is used for detection purposes, because glycoprotein and biotin present in the milk can give a dark background which obscures the proteins that are present in small amounts.

Generally, BSA is a more appropriate blocking protein for blots if a phosphorylated protein is targeted for detection. Non-fat dry milk should not be used for blots which rely on the alkaline phosphatase system.

Casein is recommended for blots with alkaline phosphatase conjugated secondary antibody. TBS instead of PBS buffer should be chosen because PBS interferes with alkaline phosphatase.

Avoid adding sodium azide (NaN$_3$) to the blocking reagent for blots based on the HRP system because NaN$_3$ can inactivate HRP.

15.4.7.2 Reducing False-positive or False-negative Results

Both polyclonal and monoclonal antibodies work well for Western blots. However, a validated or proven 1°Ab should be used. As discussed earlier, mAbs recognise a single specific antigenic epitope with higher specificity, resulting in lower background. However, during preparation and blotting, if the target epitope is denatured (or destroyed), monoclonal 1°Ab might produce false-negative results.

Polyclonal antibodies recognise more epitopes and often have higher affinity. Blot results will be stable even though a few epitopes are destroyed.

15.4.7.3 Choose the Right Secondary Ab

The choice of secondary antibody depends upon the species of animal in which the primary antibody was raised. For example, if the primary antibody is a mouse monoclonal antibody, the secondary antibody must be an anti-mouse antibody. If the primary antibody is a rabbit polyclonal antibody, the secondary antibody must be an anti-rabbit antibody.

The most popular secondary antibodies are anti-mouse and anti-rabbit immune globulin since the host species for primary antibodies are mainly mouse and rabbit. Goat is used widely to raise anti-mouse and anti-rabbit polyclonal antibodies. Thus, goat anti-mouse and goat anti-rabbit immune globulin are the most commonly used secondary antibodies.

15.5 Polyacrylamide Gel Electrophoresis

Polyacrylamide gel electrophoresis (PAGE) is a technique which separates biomolecules, such as proteins, in a polyacrylamide gel according to the charge carried by the proteins. The migration or separation of the proteins is aided by the electric current running through the gel. The speed of migration of the proteins depends on the pores of the gel through which the proteins run.

The rate of migration of the proteins in the gel depends on the strength of the electric field that is applied, the net charge carried by the proteins, and the size and shape of the protein. The ionic strength, viscosity and temperature of the gel in which the molecules move also greatly influence the speed of migration.

15.5.1 Principles of PAGE

Proteins are amphoteric compounds; their net charge therefore is determined by the pH. In a solution with a pH above its isoelectric point, a protein has a net negative charge and migrates towards the anode in an electrical field. Below its isoelectric point, the protein is positively charged and migrates towards the cathode. The net charge carried by a protein is independent of its size, i.e. the charge carried per unit mass (or length, given proteins and nucleic acids are linear macromolecules) of molecule differs from protein to protein. At a given pH, therefore, and under non-denaturing conditions, the electrophoretic separation (electrophoresis) of proteins is determined by both the size and charge of the molecules.

Proteins can be resolved either in their native conformation or in their denatured conformation. Sodium dodecyl sulfate (SDS) can denature proteins by 'wrapping around' the polypeptide backbone and binding to proteins specifically in a mass ratio of 1.4:1, thus conferring a negative charge to the polypeptide in proportion to its length (Figure 15.12).

15.5.2 Determination of Pore Size for Polyacrylamide Gel

Gel pores are created by the cross-linking of polyacrylamide with bis-acrylamide (bis) to create a network of pores. This structure allows the molecular sieving of molecules through the gel matrix. Gel pore size is a function of the acrylamide monomer concentration.

Gels can be made as a single continuous percentage throughout the gel or can be cast as a gradient %T through the gel. Typical compositions are from 5% up to 15% for single percentage gels or gradients ranging from 4–15% to 10–20%.

The total monomer concentration for optimal separation is referred to as optimal %T. Optimal %T will vary depending on the molecular weight of the molecule of interest. Empirically, the pore size providing optimum resolution for proteins is that which results in a relative mobility (Rf) value of 0.55-0.6.

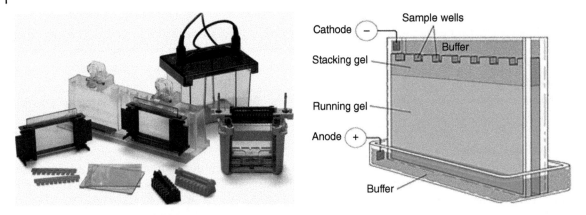

Figure 15.12 SDS-PAGE apparatus. *Source:* Bio-Rad Laboratories Inc.

Rf values for specific proteins are calculated as follows:

$$Rf = \frac{\text{Distance migrated by the protein of interest}}{\text{Distance migrated by the ion front}}$$

A linear relationship exists between the logarithm of the molecular weight of an SDS-denatured polypeptide, or native nucleic acid, and its Rf. A simple way of determining relative molecular weight (M_r) by electrophoresis is to plot a standard curve of distance migrated vs $\log_{10}$ MW for known samples and read off the log M_r of the sample after measuring distance migrated on the same gel.

15.5.3 Preparing Polyacrylamide Gel: Separation of the Proteins

Two types of gel/buffer systems are used in SDS-PAGE: continuous and discontinuous. A continuous system has only a single separating gel and uses the same buffer in the tanks and the gel. In a discontinuous system, a non-restrictive large-pore gel, called a stacking gel, is layered on top of a separating gel (running/resolving gel).

Each gel is made with a different buffer, and the tank buffers are different from the gel buffers. The resolution obtained in a discontinuous system is much greater than that obtained with a continuous system.

The following steps are used to prepare a discontinuous gel/buffer system.

1) Prepare the running gel by mixing the ingredients in a glass measuring cylinder. Add the ingredients sequentially as shown in the table, ensuring no air bubbles form.
2) Pour the mixture into the glass plate assembly.
3) Overlay gel with isopropanol to ensure a flat surface and exclude air.
4) Wash off isopropanol with water after gel is set (+15 minutes).
5) Once the running gel is set, mix the ingredients for the stacking gel into a measuring cylinder and pour on top of the running gel.
6) Adjust the comb on top of the stacking gel layer before it is solidified.
7) Load the samples into the wells that were formed due to the presence of the comb.
8) Carry out the electrophoresis at a constant current (25 mA) electrophoresis using Tris-glycine buffer (25 mM Tris, 190 mM glycine, 0.1% (w/v) SDS).
9) Now the gels are ready for detection (staining) of the proteins in gels.

15.5.4 Detection of the Separated Proteins in the Gel

Staining of proteins in gels is done using the standard Coomassie brilliant blue (or PAGE blue), Amido black and, more recently, silver stain reagents of different kinds. All these protocols are relatively long; silver staining requires a number of fiddly treatment and washing steps and takes at least a couple of hours, while other stains are two-step stain/destain procedures, but require hours (sometimes days) for satisfactory destaining.

Silver staining is (or can be) extremely sensitive – to +1 ng/band – while of the other commonly used stains, Coomassie brilliant blue G-250 is probably the best, but detects only to about 0.3 µg/band. None of these stains are easily reversible, and most often the protein cannot be recovered intact for other procedures.

However, it is possible to reversibly stain gels prior to blotting by a couple of methods. The simplest is soaking them in ice-cold 1 M potassium chloride. SDS precipitates as potassium dodecyl sulfate (KDS), and proteins are visible as whiter zones in an opaque-to-translucent white background.

15.5.5 Troubleshooting in Electrophoresis

- *Failure of the samples to stay in the well*: density of the sample solution is lower than that of the electrode buffer, which is typically brought on by the accidental omission of glycerol from the sample buffer.
- *Yellow sample colour*: since bromophenol blue turns yellow at lower pH levels, a yellow sample colour denotes an acidic pH for the sample. pH adjustment is therefore advised until the sample turns blue.
- *Tracking dye is unable to enter the gel*: make sure that current is flowing. If the electrodes are not forming any bubbles, there may not be a good electrical connection between the electrode and power source. If the current reading is normal, be certain that the electrode polarities have not been reversed accidentally.
- *Inability of protein to enter the resolving gel*: some proteins are highly sensitive to increased concentration and aggregate as a result of concentration effect of the stacking gel, preventing them from entering the resolving gel. If so, it might be wise to employ a continuous buffer system with less concentrated samples. In the presence of SDS, other proteins could precipitate. In that case, substitute with a different kind of detergent.
- *Appearance of protein in unloaded tracks*: usually caused by (i) overloading of wells, which cause sample overflow to adjacent wells, (ii) poorly polymerised stacking gel resulting in partial teeth formation causing the leakage in between wells, or (iii) contaminated running buffer. While unexpected bands in (i) and (ii) have the same size as the adjacent sample, protein staining is often visible in all tracks in (iii).
- *Appearance of unexpected bands only in loaded tracks*: this could have been due to sample buffer contamination.
- *Protein smears*: again accidental omission of SDS in the running buffer results in significant protein smearing and complete loss of resolution possibly due to gradual release of SDS from proteins.

15.6 Flow Cytometry

15.6.1 Basic Concept of Flow Cytometry and Fluorescence-activated Cell Sorting

Flow cytometry is used to count, sort and profile cells in a heterogeneous sample expected to have more than one type of cell that can be characterised by immunogenicity, size and shape. In a flow cytometer, a suspension of cells is passed through a laser beam in single flow fashion. While passing through, the interaction between the laser and the cells is measured in terms of light scatter and fluorescence intensity. If a fluorescent label, or fluorochrome, is specifically and stoichiometrically bound to a cell or cellular component, usually through a fluorescent conjugated Ab, the fluorescence intensity will ideally represent the amount of that cell component. The data are generated in the form of forward-scatter, side-scatter and fluorescent signal, which are subsequently utilised for characterisation, sorting and other purposes.

Fluorescence-activated cell sorting (FACS) is a flow cytometry technique that allows sorting of particles of different sizes, including live cells, by a nearly limitless number of different cell parameters. In a FACS analyser, the user defines the parameters for sorting the cells and based on that, the analyser imposes an electrical charge on each cell for sorting (using electromagnets) upon exiting the flow chamber. Flow cytometry and FACS (the terms are often used interchangeably) are useful for a wide range of scientific fields from research to clinical diagnosis (Figure 15.13).

A flow cytometer performs the given task based on two phenomena of light (laser) scattering upon interacting with the fluorescent marker: (i) forward light scatter (FS) and side light scatter (SS), and (ii) fluorescence emission signals. Forward scattered light beams are those which are refracted by a cell in the forward direction and continue in the same direction (typically <20° offset from the axis of the laser beam). Forward light scattering is commonly used to determine particle (cell) size. Usually, bigger particles will produce more forward scattered light than smaller ones, and larger cells will have a stronger forward scatter signal.

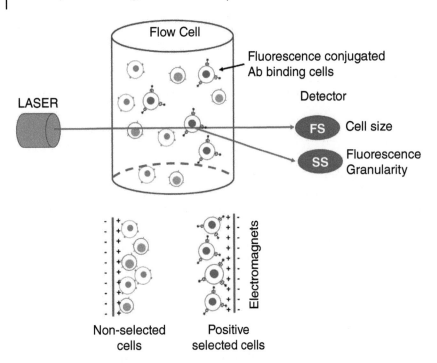

Figure 15.13   Principles of fluorescence-activated cell sorting.

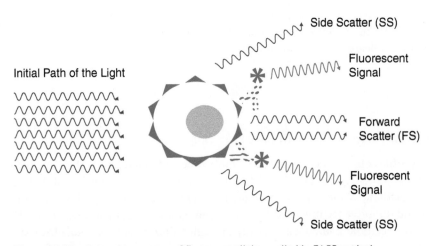

Figure 15.14   Scattering pattern of fluorescent light applied in FACS analysis.

Side-scattered (SS) beams are those which are refracted upon interacting with the cells and travel in a different direction from their original path (typically measured at a 90° angle to the excitation line). This usually provides information about the granularity and complexity of the cells. Cells with low granularity and complexity will produce less side scattered light, while highly granular cells with a high degree of internal complexity (such as neutrophils) will result in a higher side scatter signal (Figure 15.14).

15.6.2   The Flow Cytometer

The flow cytometer consists of three core components: (i) fluidics – a flow cell, where the sample fluid is injected; (ii) optics – various filters, light detectors and the light source (laser) producing a single wavelength of light at a specific frequency; and (iii) electronics – to decode the fluorescent signals and present them in a readable form.

While passing through the flow cell, the cells or particles encounter at least one laser beam. The laser beam excites fluorescent probes that are conjugated to Ab, resulting in emission of fluorescent light. Fluorescence detectors measure the fluorescence intensity emitted from cells or particles that are bound to the fluorescent conjugated Ab. Within the flow cytometer, all these different light signals are split into defined wavelengths and channelled by a set of filters and mirrors so that each sensor will detect fluorescence only at a specified wavelength. These sensors are called photo-multiplying tubes (PMTs).

As the fluorescing cell (or particle) interacts with the laser beam, the resulting fluorescent light or pulse of photon emission is detected by the PMTs and converted by the electronics system to a voltage pulse, typically called an 'event'. These events are assigned channel numbers based on measured intensity (pulse area). The higher the fluorescence intensity, the higher the channel number the event is assigned. This signal can be amplified by increasing the voltage running through the PMT.

Each PMT will also detect any other fluorophores emitting at a similar wavelength to the fluorophore it is detecting. These light signals are converted by the electronics system to data that can be visualised and interpreted by software.

15.6.3 Selection of Fluorescence and Fluorophore

A wide selection of fluorophores (fluorochromes) is available for flow cytometry. A good number of fluorophores (including, but not limited to, FITC, PerCP, APC, PE, Cy5.5, and Alexa Fluors) can be conjugated to an Ab that binds a specific Ag, and hence can label a specific structure of the cell.

Fluorophores used for the detection of target Ag (proteins) emit light after excitation by a laser of compatible wavelength. Each type of fluorescent dye or label has its own characteristic excitation and emission spectrum which is important for designing flow cytometry experiments.

It is important to note that fluorescent signals also occur from naturally fluorescing substances in the cell such as reduced pyridine nucleotides (NAD(P)H) and oxidised flavins (FAD). These are called intrinsic fluors. Upon interacting with the laser beam, these naturally occurring compounds also give rise to fluorescent signals, which is named 'autofluorescence'. In general, larger and more granular cells have higher levels of autofluorescence as they contain a higher number of fluorescent compounds.

The background signal, also called noise or autofluorescence, is determined using unlabelled samples, i.e. samples not incubated with the fluorescent conjugated target Ab. The noise needs to be subtracted from the resulting test fluorescence signals.

Some key features to know about fluorescent conjugate tags are listed here.

- *Maximum excitation wavelength (λex)*: the peak wavelength in the excitation (absorption) spectra, measured in nanometers (nm).
- *Maximum emission wavelength (λem)*: the peak wavelength in the emission spectra, measured in nanometers (nm).
- *Extinction coefficient or molar absorptivity ($\varepsilon\ max$)*: the capacity for the fluorochrome to absorb light at a given wavelength, usually measured at the maximum excitation wavelength with the units $M^{-1}\,cm^{-1}$.
- *Fluorescence quantum yield*: the number of photons emitted per absorbed photon. A high quantum yield is important, and this number ranges between 0 and 1.
- *Fluorescence decay time*: the time interval (measured in nanoseconds) after which the number of excited fluorescent molecules is reduced to $1/e$ (~37%) via the loss of energy.
- *Stokes shift*: the difference (in nm) between the λex and λem.

15.6.4 Basic Steps in Flow Cytometry or FACS Analysis

The primary requirement for all types of flow cytometric analysis is that the cells under analysis must be in a single-cell suspension. In other words, cells in the suspension should not form any clumps, which might clog the flow system. To achieve a single-cell suspension, the source materials, such as peripheral blood mononuclear cells, adherent cultured cells or cells present from tissue, need to be treated by enzymatic digestion or mechanical dissociation. The cells are then incubated in test tubes or microtitre plates with unlabelled (to have background or autofluorescence) or fluorescently conjugated Ab and analysed through the flow cytometer.

Labelling of target cells or particles through surface Ags can be done following the approach of direct or indirect labelling. However, for the labelling of intracellular components (antigens) such as cytokines or transcription factors, fixation and permeabilisation of cells are required. Fixing cells will retain the target protein in its original cellular location, while permeabilisation allows the Abs to enter the cells.

15.6.5 Data Analysis for Flow Cytometry or FACS

In a flow cytometry experiment, every cell that passes through the interrogation point and is detected because of the fluorescent label is counted as a distinct event. Each type of light that is detected (forward scatter, side scatter, fluorescence emission) also has its own unique channel. The data for each event are plotted independently to represent the signal intensity of light detected in each channel for every event.

Gating is an important procedure in flow cytometric data analysis used to selectively visualise the cells of interest and eliminate results from unwanted particles such as dead cells and debris.

These data a visually represented in one or more of following ways: histograms, dot plots, density plots and contour diagrams. More informative multiparametric analysis may also produce higher order plots such as 3-D plots and SPADE trees.

Univariate histogram plots measure the number of events, i.e. the number of cells or particles showing a given fluorescence, which is typically plotted on the y-axis. The x-axis shows the relative fluorescence intensity detected in a single channel. A large number of events detected at one particular intensity is represented as a peak (or spike) and interpreted as a positive dataset on the histogram (Figure 15.15).

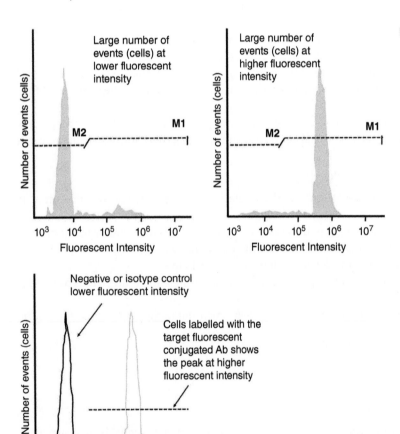

Figure 15.15 Histogram plotting of FACS analysis.

Figure 15.16 Dot plot of forward-scatter light vs side-scatter light. Each dot represents an individual cell analysed by the flow cytometer.

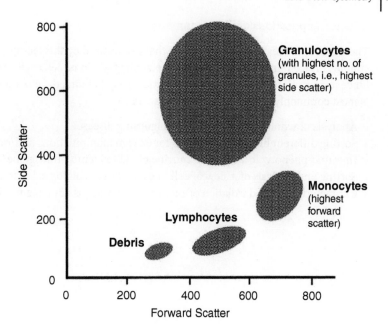

However, generally, flow cytometry analysis involves a mixed population of cells that might result in multiple peaks. In these situations, the experiment must include an appropriate negative control (without addition of the fluorescent conjugated Ab) to distinguish the positive dataset. Generally, there is a shift in fluorescent intensity between the negative control and positive samples while the positive control shows higher intensity.

When multiple parameters are analysed (also called bivariate analysis), data are represented as dot plots or density plots, and contour diagrams. These representations show the relationship between two different markers, allowing for more complex phenotypes to be identified and important populations of interest to be isolated via gating.

Dot plots and density plots compare two or three parameters simultaneously on a scatter plot where each event is represented as a single point (or dot). In the dot plot, parameters are presented in any combination of scatter and fluorescence signals such as: (i) forward scatter vs side scatter; (ii) single colour vs side scatter; and (iii) two-colour fluorescence plot.

On the density plot, each dot or point represents a single cell. Intensity measurements of different channels are represented along the different axes so that events with similar intensities will cluster together in the same region on the scatter plot. Density plots are useful for viewing the frequency, i.e. the number of subpopulations.

In the example of a dot plot shown in Figure 15.16, cell populations in a peripheral blood sample can be identified based on forward- and side-scatter light signals. Cell populations are marked by their probable identities.

The characteristic position of different cell populations is determined by different physical properties such as cell size and granularity, as explained below.

- *Debris*: very small items (such as cellular contaminants) with low forward and side scatter.
- *Leucocytes/monocytes*: small to medium cells with low internal granularity. These cells produce a medium forward-scatter and low side-scatter signal intensity.
- *Granulocytes*: large cells with high internal granularity. These cells produce high forward- and side-scatter signal intensities.

Some cell identities can be confirmed by forward- and side-scatter profiles, but fluorescent labelling with a cell type-specific marker will provide greater resolution and certainty when profiling complex heterogeneous cell populations. In the example plot in Figure 15.16, one may be able to distinguish between lymphocytes and granulocytes using forward- and side-scattered light measurements. However, among the granulocytes, there are three different classes (eosinophils, basophils, neutrophils) which are difficult to distinguish using light-scattering properties alone because of their similar cell size and structure. In order to identify the basophils, for example, we could selectively label them with fluorescently conjugated antibodies which target basophil-specific markers.

15.6.6 Applications of Flow Cytometry

The number of measurable parameters that can be used by this technology to separate cell populations is immense – from simple surface immune-phenotype to metabolic functions, cell cycle status, redox state and DNA content, to name a few. Since its inception, FACS has been used extensively in biomedical research and clinical diagnostics and therapeutics. FACS is most commonly used in the following areas.

- Analysis of whole human blood for diagnosing disease.
- Sorting different blood cell fractions for ex vivo manipulations and/or transplantations.
- Immuno-phenotypic analysis of murine blood to identify transgenic/knockout animals.
- Sorting and analysis of a slew of cell lines for various biological assays.
- Characterisation and isolation of rare cell types such as adult stem cells and cancer-initiating cells.

16

Control Selection and Statistical Analyses in Immunological Research

Mohammad Tariqur Rahman[1] *and Noor Lide Abu Kassim*[2]

[1] *Faculty of Dentistry, University of Malaya, Kuala Lumpur, Malaysia*
[2] *International Islamic University, Kuala Lumpur, Malaysia*

16.1 Control Selection

A simple study design is typically based on a research objective to investigate the possible influence of an independent variable on a dependent variable. Such research would require data collected from samples representing at least two different groups or conditions: (i) a sample under a condition (which will be referred as the typical condition) which is not subjected to the influence of the independent variable being investigated, and (ii) an experimental (test) condition where the dependent variable is subjected to the influence of the independent variable. The samples that are in their typical condition are often represented as a 'control' group. And the samples taken from the group that is being tested or treated to evaluate the influence of the independent variable are commonly referred to as the 'experimental' group.

It is important to note that the term 'typical' condition might be confusing in certain experimental settings. For example, if the influence of a drug (independent variable) on a disease (dependent variable) is being investigated, the diseased condition literally cannot reflect a 'typical' condition. However, in that experimental setting, the given diseased condition reflects the condition that needs to be studied and so is called a typical condition under that given circumstance.

However, contrary to common belief, using the right chemicals, reagents and tools, and performing the experiment or assay according to a given protocol using only those two groups, i.e. control and experimental groups of samples, do not necessarily enable one to make the right interpretation from the data obtained from the experiment.

It is important to ensure the technical validity of the data so that one can arrive at the correct interpretation of the results. Having control and experimental groups often is not enough to ensure the technical validity of the data. At the same time, the data obtained from those two groups of samples may need to be compared with other groups which are known to give either a positive or negative outcome or results.

Therefore, including different groups of samples in addition to the control and experimental groups is often required for a valid research design. Practically, those groups of samples also would serve as one or another kind of control measure for the data analysis and subsequent interpretation.

This chapter briefly explains the fundamentals of using different groups of appropriate controls that might vary in terms of types and nature, and according to the purpose or objectives of a given research design involving immunological techniques. Additionally, we also highlight the fundamentals of choosing appropriate statistical tools that can be used for data analysis and interpretation of results.

16.1.1 Example of a Simple Immunohistochemical-based Research Design

To describe the types, nature and purpose of appropriate controls, this chapter presents a simple research design based on immunohistochemical (IHC) staining (see Chapter 15). Let us assume that the research is aimed at investigating the influence of a toxic element (M) on the expression of a metal-inducible protein (Pr) in rat skin. Hence, in this research design, M is the independent variable and Pr is the dependent variable.

Immunology for Dentistry, First Edition. Edited by Mohammad Tariqur Rahman, Wim Teughels and Richard J. Lamont.
© 2023 John Wiley & Sons Ltd. Published 2023 by John Wiley & Sons Ltd.

At its minimum or basic level, the research design typically includes two different groups of rats. One group is kept in the typical condition, i.e. not exposed (such as through foods or drinks) to the toxic element M, hence representing the 'control' group. Since in practice there are different types of control groups, let us name such a control group the 'objective control' (OC) as this control group of samples fundamentally helps to achieve the main objective of the research. The other group is treated with a given amount of M (such as in diets or drinking water); hence, it is referred to as the 'experimental' (EX) group.

In an optimum research design set-up, the other conditions and potential variables which might influence the expression of Pr, such as age, sex, body weight, diet composition, days of treatment and consumption of total food and water of the animals being used, would be kept consistent between the two groups. For convenience, let us restrict the number of animals to five per group (n = 5 per group), assuming this is sufficient for statistical analyses to reach a reliable conclusion. However, the total number of animals (generally expressed using a capital '**N**') will vary depending on the number of other control groups that will be needed for an appropriate experimental design.

Please note that each animal from which a particular tissue sample is harvested represents a *biological* replicate of a given group, while more than one sample of the target (same) tissue of the same animal is referred to as a *technical* replicate. Depending on the purpose of the analyses, samples from different tissues or organs of the same animal also can be used, mainly as different types of control groups.

16.1.2 Possible Results and Their Interpretation

There are numerous possibilities for obtaining immune reactivity after IHC staining for Pr showing its expression level in the samples (tissues) from the OC and EX groups.

Based on the likelihood that the stained tissue sections could be either positive (+) or negative (−) for Pr immune reactivity, it is probable that skin samples from all animals of both groups (OC and EX) are either Pr negative (possibility 1, Table 16.1) or Pr positive (possibility 2, Table 16.1). It is also probable that skin samples of all animals of the OC group are either Pr negative (possibility 3, Table 16.1) or Pr positive (possibility 4, Table 16.1). It is also likely to have Pr positive and Pr negative sections in both groups (possibility 5, Table 16.1). However, the degree of Pr immune reactivity that could be inferred either by the intensity of the Pr staining or by counting the number of Pr-positive cells might vary from one section to another, as represented by different numbers of '+'.

According to possibility 1, there was no staining in any of the skin samples analysed from the OC and EX groups. Given this result, there are three probable interpretations that could be made using the outcome of possibility 1 (Table 16.1).

Interpretation 1.1 is linked to any potential technical error(s) that might have occurred during the staining. Determination of whether interpretation 1.1 is valid can be achieved by including two different types of control samples, one of which must be positive and the other negative for the target antigen i.e., Pr. These kinds of controls are commonly regarded as positive (P) or negative (N) controls respectively. Since this group of controls would aid in resolving any technical error(s) which might have occurred during staining, let us call them technical controls (TC) for convenience. Examples of these technical positive (TC-P1 and TC-P2) and technical negative (TC-N1 and TC-N2) controls that can be used for this given research are given in Table 16.2.

Having any of the combinations of TC-P and TC-N would validate interpretation 1.1 (Table 16.1 and Table 16.2). However, as far as interpretations 1.2 and 1.3 are concerned, specific sets of control groups such as TC-P2 and TC-N2 would be more useful (Table 16.2) since these control groups involve the same or similar types of tissue samples as the OC and EX groups.

Contrary to possibility 1, in possibility 2 all the samples from either the OC or the EX groups could be Pr positive. Hence, the likely interpretations for possibility 2 would be different from those of possibility 1 (Table 16.1). However, one of the interpretations, i.e. 2.1 which is linked to any potential technical error(s) that might have occurred during staining, could be resolved by using any one pair of the TC-P and TC-N as mentioned earlier. However, to validate interpretation 2.2, specific sets of control groups such as TC-P2 and TC-N2 would be more meaningful (Table 16.2). Furthermore, an additional group of parallel controls (PC) such as PC1 and PC2 will be useful to validate interpretation 2.2. The term 'parallel' refers to the fact that such a control is treated with an additional inducible independent variable such as M2 or an inhibitory independent variable on the dependent variable (Pr) respectively.

Unlike possibilities 1 and 2, possibilities 3 and 4 demonstrate different scenarios where each tissue section from one of the two groups (OC and EX) is Pr positive and the other group is Pr negative (Table 16.1). Hence, the occurrence of a technical error is unlikely. Therefore, neither TC-P nor TC-N would contribute to analysing any probable interpretations, i.e. interpretations 3.1 and 4.1 (Table 16.1). Yet one might still consider keeping TCs to endorse the technical validity of the

Table 16.1 Possible outcomes and interpretations of IHC staining for the target protein (Pr) expression[a] in the skin in response to the metal (M).

Animal no.	OC	EX	Interpretations
	Possibility 1		
1	−	−	1.1: Due to technical error(s), all the skin was Pr negative
2	−	−	1.2: Pr is not constitutively expressed in skin
3	−	−	1.3: M does not induce Pr expression in skin
4	−	−	
5	−	−	
	Possibility 2		
1	+	+	2.1: Due to technical errors such as non-specific binding of the Abs against Pr or incomplete washing might have caused false-positive reactions of all skin samples
2	++	+	
3	+	++	2.2: In skin, Pr is constitutively expressed, and its expression is not influenced by M
4	++	+	
5	+	++	
	Possibility 3		
1	−	++	3.1: Pr is not constitutively expressed in skin. However, its expression in skin is induced by M
2	−	+	
3	−	++	
4	−	+	
5	−	+	
	Possibility 4		
1	+	−	4.1. In skin, Pr is constitutively expressed. However, its expression in skin is inhibited by M
2	+++	−	
3	+	−	
4	++	−	
5	+	−	
	Possibility 5		
1	+	+++	5.1: Pr is constitutively expressed in skin. However, its expression in skin is upregulated by M
2	−	+	
3	++	−	
4	+	+++	
5	+	+++	

Abs, antibodies; EX, experimental group; OC, objective control group.

[a] Based on a score calculated either by measuring the intensity of the staining or by counting the number of Pr-positive cells.

staining, although in a real-world scenario such results could be questioned as they are 'too good to be true'. However, keeping different sets of inducible or inhibitory PCs is required to validate such a result (possibilities 3 and 4) (Table 16.2).

In reality, the most probable outcome of any IHC staining is what is presented in possibility 5 where different sections reveal different levels of staining (Table 16.1). The average level of staining for P in the samples from the OC group might be less than that from the EX group. This represents a positive influence of M (independent variable) on Pr expression (dependent variable). However, it could be the other way around. In other words, the independent variable might show negative influence on the dependent variable. Since there was both positive and negative staining for Pr in such possibilities, any technical error during the staining is unlikely. Nevertheless, the rationale for keeping different TCs will remain the same. However, to validate interpretation 5.1, one might need to add further PC groups, i.e. any combination of inducible and inhibitory PCs (Table 16.2).

Table 16.2 Validation of probable interpretations derived from the outcome of the experiment conducted or tool used.

Example of samples (tissues) to be used as control[a] and rationale	Pr expression		Tech. validity	Interpretations[b]					
	Expected	Detected		1.2	1.3	2.2	3.1	4.1	5.1
TC-P1: A tissue of the same animal of both OC and EX groups that will naturally synthesise Pr (e.g. kidney)	+	+	√	NA	N	N	N	R	N
		−	×	×	×	×	×	×	×
TC-P2: Skin from Pr transgenic rats (another group) that will express (synthesise) Pr	+	+	√	N	N	N	R	R	R
		−	×	×	×	×	×	×	×
TC-N1: A tissue of the same animal of both OC and EX groups that will not naturally synthesise the target antigen Pr (e.g. cornea)	−	+	×	×	×	×	×	×	×
		−	√	N	N	N	R	R	N
TC-N2: Skin from Pr-knockout (KO) rats (another group) that will not express (synthesise) the target antigen Pr	−	+	×	×	×	×	×	×	×
		−	√	N	N	N	R	R	R
NSC-1: Any positive signal after staining without 1°Ab from the skin sample of the OC group can be used for baseline correction of the group	+	+	NA	Use for baseline correction					
		−	NA	NA	NA	NA	NA	NA	NA
NSC-2: Any positive signal after staining without 1°Ab from the skin sample of the EX group can be used for baseline correction of the group	+	+	NA	Use for baseline correction					
		−	NA	NA	NA	NA	NA	NA	NA
PC1: Skin from M2 (a known Pr inducer)-treated rats[c]	+	+	√	√	N	N	N	N	N
		−	×	×	×	×	×	×	×
PC2: Skin from M + M2-treated rats where the combined effect of M and M2 might alter[d] inducible Pr	U	+	√	N	N	N	N	N	N
		−	U	U	U	U	U	U	N
PC3: Kidney from M2 (a known Pr inducer)-treated rats[c] since kidney (TC-P1) naturally synthesises Pr; hence M2 is expected to upregulate Pr in kidney	+	+	√	U	U	U	U	U	U
		−	×	×	×	×	×	×	U
PC4: Kidney from M + M2-treated rats where the combined effect of M and M2 might alter[d] M2-inducible Pr	U	+	U	U	U	U	U	U	U
		−	U	U	U	U	U	U	U
PC5: Skin from rats (another group) given Pr inhibitor that should stop the synthesis of Pr in the skin	−	+	×	×	×	×	×	×	×
		−	√	N	N	N	N	N	R

+, present/positive; −, absent/negative; √, valid; ×, invalid; N, need this control to validate; U, uncertain; NA, not applicable; R, redundant.
[a] Examples are given based on the objective of analysing the influence of M on Pr expression in rat skin.
[b] The interpretations (taken from Table 16.1) are validated based on Pr expression in response to M2 and/or M.
[c] Same samples also could be used as positive technical control (TC-P).
[d] Reduce, neutralise or enhance (upregulate).

Note that in any antigen–antibody (Ag–Ab) interaction-based technique, non-specific signals might be produced due to non-specific binding of the Ab which is conjugated with the detection marker. It is important to rule out the influence of such non-specific signals to interpret the data more accurately. In reality, non-specific binding of the marker conjugated Ab will always produce some positive (or baseline) signals. Therefore, it is important to have control samples that can be used for baseline corrections or to evaluate the non-specific signals. For convenience, let us call these non-specific signal controls (NSC). In principle, the tissue samples which are being evaluated for the target antigen, i.e. Pr, can be used for such NSCs (Table 16.2). There are, of course, different possible ways to analyse the presence or absence of any non-specific signal, depending on the research design and tools used for analysis. In the case of indirect IHC staining for Pr, omitting the 1°Ab during staining will allow evaluation of whether the 2°Ab that is conjugated with the detection marker binds non-specifically (Table 16.2).

In the given research design, the different groups of controls discussed so far, namely TC-P, TC-N, PC, NC and NSC (Table 16.2), would confirm inducible or inhibitory Pr expression in the skin in response to M. Therefore, having samples from groups OC, EX, TC-P, TC-N and NSC might be sufficient to make appropriate interpretations as well as to ensure the technical validity of the results.

However, a more insightful research design may have additional research objectives such as investigating whether the influence (which could be positive or negative) of M on Pr expression is higher or lower compared to a known independent variable. To answer this objective, additional groups of samples must be analysed to demonstrate the specified influence of the known independent variable on the dependent variable. For example, M2 (a well-known inducer of Pr) could be used to treat a similar EX group in the given research design to answer the additional objective. In other words, in parallel to the M-treated EX group, an M2-treated EX group must be analysed.

Depending on the additional, more specific objective(s) of the research, different kinds of PC can be used (Table 16.2). At the same time, different tissues can be used to evaluate the influence of the independent variable (M) on PCs. For example, one can use a known inducer (such as M2) of the dependent variable (Pr) which is expected to induce (or upregulate) the expression of Pr. Similarly, one can also use a known inhibitor to evaluate the inhibitory (downregulatory) effect of M – the independent variable.

16.1.3 Types and Number of Control Samples

With the above explanation, it is now possible to deduce several fundamental principles for selecting different types of controls for a given experimental design (Table 16.3).

16.1.3.1 Objective Control
The objective control (OC) group serves to evaluate the background status (level of expression) of the dependent variable (Pr in the given example) under natural or typical conditions. The OC group must be selected based on a certain theoretical rationale to observe the influence of an independent variable on the dependent variable. The number of animals (or samples) of the OC group must be calculated based on a given theoretical framework. Often this refers to sample size calculation.

16.1.3.2 Experimental Control
In principle, the samples from the experimental control (EX) group are treated with a given independent variable to observe the changes in the dependent variable. The samples from the EX group must share similar properties or characteristics for all other possible variables as those in the OC group. Therefore, the nature and source of the samples from the OC and the EX groups must be the same. The number of samples from the EX group also must match that of the OC group as decided based on a given theoretical framework.

16.1.3.3 Technical Control
In principle, the samples from the technical control (TC) group must demonstrate either positive (TC-P) or negative (TC-N) results for the dependent variable under investigation. Generally, these are called positive or negative controls. However,

Table 16.3 Principles of selecting different groups of controls for IHC staining-based research design.

Control type	Principles of selecting the control type
Objective control (OC)	Samples of the OC group serve to evaluate the background status (level of expression) of the dependent variable (Pr in the given example) under natural or typical conditions
Experimental control (EX)	Samples from the EX group are expected to show changes in the expression of the target marker (i.e. a given independent variable) under the influence of the dependent variable
Technical control-positive (TC-P)	Samples from the same/similar source where the target-dependent variable occurs naturally
Technical control-negative (TC-N)	Samples from a same/similar source where the target-dependent variable is absent/inhibited
Parallel control (PC)	Samples from a similar source that are treated with an independent variable (different from the target-independent variable) that is known (or expected) to have an influence on the target-dependent variable. The measured influence might be useful to evaluate the level of influence of the independent variable under investigation by comparing that of the known independent variable
Non-specific control (NSC)	Samples from OC/EX groups to check background signals therein, that might have occurred due to a non-specific response or reaction

using the terms positive or negative might lead to confusion, especially if the research design involves parallel control groups (see below) either for positive or negative responses. Ideally, the main purpose of having TC-P or TC-N samples is to evaluate any possible technical error in conducting the experiment or using a tool that might lead to a false-positive or false-negative result.

In an ideal set-up, the nature and source of the TC would be similar to those of the OC and EX samples. However, this might not be possible in many research designs. Since TCs are not involved in the analysis of data obtained from the OC and EX groups and subsequent interpretations of the results, the selection of samples for the TC group can be compromised as long as it demonstrates the positive and/or negative response with regard to the dependent variable. However, the steps involved in conducting the experiment or in using the tool and subsequent standard of analysis must match the steps used for the samples from the OC and EX groups.

The number of samples from the TC group does not necessarily have to match the number of samples from the OC and EX groups, as the TC samples are used essentially to evaluate the technical validity of the experiment or tool.

16.1.3.4 Non-specific Signal Control

Non-specific signal control (NSC) is meant to evaluate any signal that could be confused as a signal (or response) that is otherwise expected due to the influence of the independent variable on the dependent variable. In many experimental outcomes, there might be some signals or responses that are not linked with the occurrence of the independent variable under investigation. The NSC aids in the identification of such signals (responses). In actual analysis, a non-specific signal must be considered to minimise over- or underestimation of the signal due to the actual changes in the independent variable. This is also known as baseline correction. Furthermore, NSC will also allow a semi-quantitative analysis to evaluate relative changes of the independent variables between the OC and EX groups.

Preferably, NSC comprises samples with similar sources and types as the OC and EX groups. If additional samples other than those of the OC are not necessary, this needs to be stated when the interpretations are made. However, this may not be the case in all research designs. If the results from the NSC are used for data analysis, the number of samples in the OC and EX groups must be calculated based on a required theoretical framework.

16.1.3.5 Parallel Control

A parallel control (PC) allows evaluation of the relative efficiency of the independent variable in influencing the dependent variable. In any given research, an independent variable is expected to cause certain changes in the dependent variable. To evaluate the efficiency of a given independent variable in influencing a given dependent variable, a different independent variable that is known to influence the dependent variable can be analysed using similar sets of samples as the EX group. Depending on the nature of the expected influence, samples of the PC group might be treated either for a positive or inducible (e.g. PC1–PC3) response or for a negative inhibitory (PC5) response, which of course is different from a TC-P or TC-N. The PC group comprises samples similar to the EX group but treated with a different independent variable that has a known effect/influence on the dependent variable.

To minimise any potential confusion between technical positive control and parallel positive control or between technical negative control and parallel negative control, these controls are best defined separately. However, unlike TC, the number of samples in the PC group needs to be determined according to a required theoretical framework. This is because the results of the PC group are meant to be used to make appropriate interpretations of the data obtained from the samples of the OC and EX groups.

16.2 Statistical Analyses in Immunological Research

To support claims that particular treatments provide particular solutions, statistical tests are typically carried out to define the statistical significance of the experimental outcomes, i.e. the data collected. Each statistical test generates a set of numerical values which indicates the differences or relatedness of the data that are used to analyse two or more variables in one or more samples representing a population.

Statistical tests can be used to compare treatment (experimental) and control (objective control) groups, or to find the relationships (correlation) between given groups such as whether smoking is related to lung cancer or obesity is related to cardiovascular diseases. Statistical tests can further be used to identify the strength of a causal (cause and effect) relationship between variables using regression analysis, such as whether smoking can cause lung cancer.

Statistical tests are often concluded as statistically significant if the calculated results fall outside the range of values predicted by the null hypothesis. Significance is usually denoted by a probability value (p-value). When this probability value falls below a certain alpha (α) value, then we can conclude that the result of the test is statistically significant. The alpha value is often set at 0.05 – that is, when there is a less than 5% probability that the result could have happened by chance.

16.2.1 Considerations for Choosing the Right Statistical Test

When choosing the most appropriate statistical analysis or test, there are several things to consider. Naturally, the first of these would be the experiment and study design. And of course, most studies related to the use of immunoassays are experimental in nature at the cellular level.

The study or experiment design is important as it tells us whether we are comparing the observed effect of the manipulation of an independent variable (treatment) on preassigned groups, investigating changes in the dependent variable over particular time periods or predicting and estimating the amount of change as a result of the influence of the independent variable on the dependent variable.

The second aspect for consideration would be the type of variable investigated and the type of data collected. The type of data indicates the level of measurement and the appropriate statistical test that we can use.

The third aspect is sample size, which is crucial as some statistical tests require a minimum sample number apart from the assumptions that must be met for the use of these statistical tests. Equal sample size is an important consideration for an experimental study as it can compensate for a small sample size when using parametric tests.

Why is choosing the right statistical analysis important? It is necessary for us to make a correct interpretation of the data for whether (i) it accurately represents the population, (ii) a given hypothesis on the change of a variable is valid, and last but not least, (iii) the change of a variable in a given condition is reproducible.

All these are important so that valid interpretation of the data and results of the statistical tests can be made.

16.2.2 Assumptions for Statistical Tests

To choose the right statistical test for a valid observation, one must look at the basic criteria of the data in terms of (i) type of data, (ii) sample size, and (iii) distribution pattern of the data representing the population being studied. In other words, choosing a statistical test will depend on whether these criteria and other statistical assumptions are met.

16.2.2.1 Independence of Observations
According to this assumption, observations should be independent. Observations are not considered independent if they are related in some sense. For example, multiple measurements of a single test subject are considered as observations that are not independent, as in the counting of the number of cells in a 'single' cell culture over two or three time periods. Following the same principle, (single) measurements of multiple or different test subjects which are unrelated are considered independent. However, if the measurements are not independent of each other (i.e. they are dependent), this assumption is violated.

For data that do not meet the assumption of independence of observations, a statistical test that accounts for the interrelatedness in the data (such as paired sample t-test or repeated-measures [within-subjects] ANOVA) or other relevant tests that can remove the influences of co-variates (continuous 'noise' variable as in ANCOVA) or blocking variables (categorical noise variables) should be used.

16.2.2.2 Data Variation or Variability of Data Distribution is Comparable or Similar Across Groups
In statistical terms, this is called homogeneity of variance. The variance basically represents the variation in the data obtained from the groups (two or more) involved in the statistical test. If one group has much greater variation than others, it will limit the test's effectiveness, if this assumption is required such as in the case of parametric tests such as t-tests and analysis of variance (ANOVA).

16.2.2.3 Normality of Data
Normality of the data relates to the shape of the data distribution. Normally distributed data have the shape of a bell curve. This assumption applies only to quantitative data. If the data do not meet the assumptions of normality, a non-parametric statistical test should be selected as it allows for valid comparisons without requiring any assumptions about the data distribution that parametric statistical tests require.

16.2.3 Variables: The Core of Statistical Testing

In a statistical test, the data represent the values of a variable or variables. For example, in a research design analysing the occurrence of obesity among males or females, both obesity and sex are variables. The number of males and females with obesity are the data representing the variables. Notably, the number of males and females without obesity are also part of the data and essential for the statistical analysis. Without this group, the relationship or association between gender and obesity cannot be determined.

Therefore, if a given parameter is analysed for its effect or influence on another (one or more) parameter, then both these parameters are regarded as variables in statistical terms.

For example, if we want to analyse how obesity is connected with cardiovascular disease (CVD), then both obesity and CVD are variables. If occurrence of CVD is a possible outcome of obesity, then CVD is the *dependent variable* and obesity is the *independent variable.*

In an experimental set-up, if we want to know whether Zn intake can affect or influence the expression of a protein, such as metallothionein (P), then Zn intake is the independent variable and P expression is the dependent variable. Hence, the independent variable is the cause (which is typically manipulated in the experiment) and the dependent variable is the effect as a result of the manipulation of the independent variable. In other words, changing or manipulating the independent variable will affect the dependent variable.

It is important to remember that all other variables that may influence or affect the dependent variable (i.e. intervening or confounding variables) have to be kept constant. In reality, this may not always be possible so a number of strategies need to be used. The most common way is through *randomisation*, which helps to control for extraneous variables that may have an effect on the results of an experiment. It prevents selection bias as well as accidental bias in an experiment, thus producing comparable groups in the experiment and providing accurate results.

Another strategy would be to identify the possible intervening or confounding variables – either mediating or moderating variables – and incorporate them into the study design. Mediating variables are typically continuous-level variables that can be used as co-variates in statistical tests such as analysis of co-variance (ANCOVA) or multivariate analysis of co-variance (MANCOVA). Moderating variables are categorical blocking variables.

16.2.3.1 Confounding Variable

A variable, other than the target independent and dependent variables being analysed, that can affect or influence the dependent variable is a confounding variable. In the previous example, where the occurrence of CVD (dependent variable) is tested in relation to obesity (independent variable), smoking and alcohol consumption could be confounding variables as these are known to cause CVD. If the population being analysed for a link between obesity and CVD is also known to include smokers and/or alcohol consumers, then the influence of these known factors must be partialled out before a correct interpretation of the results can be made.

16.2.3.2 Latent Variable

A variable that cannot be measured directly is regarded as a latent variable. For example, if a research question demands the analysis of stress level for which there is no direct measure, then a different variable such as level of acetylcholine can be used to measure the stress level. Here the stress level is a latent variable.

16.2.3.3 Surrogate Endpoint

A surrogate endpoint is one that can be used as a substitute for a clinical endpoint (Aronson 2005). For example, in demonstrating the effectiveness of a treatment, lower biomarker levels can be used as an indicator in place of clinical indicators, such as survival rate. Although these surrogate endpoints may not be true indicators of clinical or laboratory measurements, they are useful alternatives.

16.2.3.4 Composite Variable

A composite variable is made by combining multiple variables in an experiment. These variables are created during analysis of the data, but not during collection of the data. For example, the influence of Zn supplementation on the in vitro growth and multiplication of a given cell population can be measured by combining two sets of data: (i) the number of cells and (ii) the size of the cells. Combining these two datasets can give rise to a composite variable.

16.2.3.5 Predictor Variable

In regression analyses, an independent variable is commonly called a *predictor variable*. Predictor variables are also called input variables and x-variables. A predictor variable explains changes in the response of a dependent variable which is also known as an *outcome variable*. Typically, changes in one or more predictors are associated with changes in the response or dependent variable. Therefore, in regression analysis, the dependent variables or response variables are also known as outcome variables and y-variables.

For example, in the analysis to find the causal link between a disease such as lung cancer and risk factors such as smoking and air pollution, the predictors might be the number of cigarettes smoked per day or air pollution index respectively. Therefore, a predictor variable provides information on an associated dependent variable regarding a particular outcome in the analysis. At the most fundamental level, predictor variables are variables that are linked with particular outcomes.

16.2.4 Understanding the Relationship between Variables and Data

As mentioned earlier, a variable is represented by a number of values. If Y is a variable that represents family size, then it can have values such as (3, 2, 4, 3, 5. . .) for a given population. These values are the *data* or values for the variable Y (i.e. family size).

Broadly there are two types of data: *quantitative* data and *categorical* data. A quantitative (i.e. numerical) datum is a number that gives a count or numerical value to represent a variable. For example, in a given experiment, the number of apoptotic cells and the number of positively stained cells are quantitative data. If the intensity of the staining is presented using a continuous numerical value, then it can also be considered as quantitative data.

Quantitative variables can be of two types: (i) *discrete* data (also known as integer variables) that represent counts that cannot be divided into units smaller than one, and (ii) *continuous* data which represent numerical values which can be divided into units smaller than one (e.g. 0.75). In the examples given above, the number of apoptotic cells or number of P-positive cells are practically discrete variables because we cannot have 0.5 or 0.75 of cells. However, when the numbers of cells from different samples are averaged, we often get a number with decimal values; conventionally that allows a researcher to use the number of cells as a continuous variable. Volume, weight, height and also intensity of a staining (if presented using a numerical value) are examples of continuous variables.

Categorical data represent grouped or categorised data. Broadly, categorical variables are of three types: (i) *ordinal* data – represented by data presented in an order or rank, (ii) *nominal* data – represented by data in terms of identifications such as names or brands of groups that are not ranked, (iii) *binary* data – represented by data that have only two categories and can be presented with a yes or no, present or absent, male or female, 1 or 0, and/or win or lose.

In biomedical research, whether it involves in vitro, in vivo or ex vivo experiments, the number of parameters or variables involved can be more than those which are aimed to be analysed.

It is important to highlight that variables such as intensity of staining are sometimes classified as either quantitative or categorical. As mentioned earlier, if such a variable is presented using continuous numerical values, it is considered as quantitative data. However, if intensity of staining is presented as 'high' 'moderate' or 'less', the data are considered as categorical data, which is ordinal, although these categories may be assigned corresponding numerical values.

It is also important to highlight that the terms 'variable' and 'data' are sometimes used synonymously. However, as mentioned earlier, data are values of a variable.

16.2.5 Choosing a Parametric Test

Parametric tests can be conducted only if the data adhere to the common statistical assumptions of independence, normality and homogeneity of variance; hence, are able to make stronger inferences from the data. The most common parametric tests used in experimental research are comparison tests, correlation tests and regression.

16.2.5.1 Comparison Tests

Comparison tests look for differences between or among group means. They can be used to test the effect of a categorical independent variable on the mean value of a dependent variable. The common comparison parametric tests are shown in Table 16.4.

Table 16.4 Comparison parametric tests.

Name of the test	Independent variable	Dependent variable	Example research design
One sample t-test	One categorical variable	One quantitative variable	• Single group statistic compared to a known value (e.g. sample mean of diastolic blood pressure compared with the population mean)
Paired samples t-test	One categorical variable	One quantitative variable	• Single group pre- and post-test design (the group is its own control) • Related samples (e.g. twins) Two related groups from the same population (where one of the related groups serves as the control)
Independent samples t-test	One categorical variable	One quantitative variable	• Two groups from different populations (typically treatment and control groups)
One-way ANOVA	One categorical variable	One quantitative variable	• Usually more than two groups from different populations (multiple groups)
Repeated measures ANOVA	One or more categorical variable	One quantitative variable	• Single group over time periods (within-subjects design) • Multiple groups over time periods (within- and between-subjects design)
MANOVA	Multiple categorical variables	Two or more quantitative variables	• Usually when multiple dependent variables are indicators of one single composite variable

16.2.5.2 Correlation Tests

Correlation tests check whether two variables are related without assuming cause-and-effect (causal) relationships (Table 16.5).

16.2.5.3 Regression Tests

Regression tests are used to test cause-and-effect relationships (Table 16.6). They look for the effect of one or more variables on another variable.

Table 16.5 Correlation tests.

Name of the test	Variable 1	Variable 2	Example research design
Pearson *r*	Continuous	Continuous	Correlational
Chi-square test of independence	Categorical	Categorical	Association between nominal or ordinal level variables

Table 16.6 Regression tests.

Name of the test	Predictor variable	Outcome variable
Simple linear regression	• Quantitative/categorical/dichotomous • One predictor	• Quantitative • One outcome
Multiple linear regression	• Quantitative/categorical/dichotomous • Two or more predictors	• Quantitative • One outcome
Logistic regression	• Quantitative	• Binary

Table 16.7 Non-parametric tests.

Name of the test	Independent variable	Dependent variable	Alternative/similar to
Spearman rho (bivariate)	• Ordinal	• Ordinal	Pearson *r*
Sign test	• Categorical	• Quantitative	One sample t-test
Kruskal–Wallis H test	• Categorical • Three or more groups	• Quantitative	ANOVA
ANOSIM	• Categorical • Three or more groups	• Quantitative • Two or more outcome variables	MANOVA
Mann–Whitney U test (aka Wilcoxon rank-sum test)	• Categorical • Two groups	• Quantitative • groups from different populations	Independent samples t-test
Wilcoxon signed-rank test	• Categorical • Two groups	• Quantitative • groups from the same population	Paired samples t-test

16.2.6 Choosing a Non-parametric Test

Non-parametric tests do not make as many assumptions about the data as parametric tests. They are useful when one or more of the statistical assumptions for parametric tests are violated. However, the inferences they make are not as strong as those derived from parametric tests (Table 16.7).

16.2.7 Interpretation of Statistical Tests

The interpretation of statistical tests to accept or reject a null hypothesis usually focuses on three aspects: the significance level, the confidence interval and the practical importance.

A *hypothesis* is a well-informed guess about a population reached by examining a sample of that population. Statistical hypotheses are usually stated in a way that they may be evaluated using statistical tests. Below are examples of the null hypothesis and the alternative hypothesis.

- H_0: There is *no association* between smoking and lung cancer.
- H_1: There is *an association* between smoking and lung cancer.

16.2.7.1 Elements of Hypothesis Testing

1) State the null hypothesis and the alternative hypothesis.
2) Identify whether or not to use a two-tailed or one-tailed test.
3) State the level of significance, i.e. alpha value.
4) Select an appropriate test statistic such as z, t, F or χ^2.
5) Compute the value of the test statistic and find its probability value (p-value).
6) Make statistical decisions based on the p-value, i.e. reject or fail to reject the null hypothesis (H_0).

16.2.7.2 Significance Level

Significant in everyday speech means important; however, in statistics, it means probably true and not due to chance. When we say that the results of our experiment are statistically significant, it means that they are almost certainly true.

The significance level, denoted as alpha (α), helps to determine which hypothesis is supported by the data. In other words, based on the strength of the significance level, a null hypothesis can be rejected to conclude that the effect is statistically significant and not due to chance.

The researcher determines the significance level before conducting the experiment. For example, a significance level of 0.05 indicates a 5% risk of concluding that a difference exists when there is no actual difference. Lower significance levels indicate that you require stronger evidence before you will reject the null hypothesis.

The p-value and the α-level are related concepts, but there are important differences between them. The *α-level* should be determined as a part of the process of setting up the hypothesis test. It should be set before the test is actually conducted. Setting the α-level at, say, α = 0.05 is the way we implement the decision as to how willing we are to reject the null hypothesis as being true when it is actually true.

The p-value, on the other hand, can be determined only *after* the test statistic is calculated. If the p-value from the statistical test is less than the significance level that you have set, you can reject the null hypothesis and conclude that the effect is statistically significant. In other words, the evidence in your sample is strong enough to be able to reject the null hypothesis at the population level. For example, if α = 0.05, then we will reject the null hypothesis as being true if the value we calculate for p is <0.05.

16.2.7.3 Statistical Power

In hypothesis testing, statistical power has tremendous influence as it provides the ability to detect the presence of a true effect if it actually exists. Statistical power is related to the probability of avoiding a type II error, which is not rejecting the null hypothesis when it is actually false. A high statistical power provides a low risk of making this type of error and drawing an incorrect conclusion. Hence, it is important to calculate statistical power to detect a true effect in an experiment.

Power analyses help researchers to estimate the minimum sample size required to detect a true effect and subsequently to draw accurate conclusions. Statistical power depends on the chosen significance level, sample size and effect size (i.e. magnitude of the effect of the treatment) for any given experiment.

Power is typically set at 80%, although higher power is sometimes set to ensure that the probability of making a type II error is avoided. When sample size increases, power typically increases, making a small difference (i.e effect size) become statistically significant. Hence, when interpreting the results of statistical tests, it is important to also consider a meaningful difference or *practical significance* and not just statistical significance.

16.2.7.4 Confidence Interval

When reporting the results of experiments, it is important that confidence intervals are stated. Confidence intervals are a plausible range of values for a population parameter. For example, the confidence interval for the population mean is the mean of the sample in our experiment ± the confidence intervals. Hence, the true mean for the population will be within this range of values.

A 95% confidence interval means that the true mean of the population from which our sample comes will be within this range of values 95% of the time.

16.2.8 Technical Replicates and Biological Replicates

Technical replicates (for example, assaying your samples in triplicate) are used when measurements are taken from the same sample multiple times. The primary purpose of this is to test the variability or reliability of the testing protocol. In other words, technical replicates can tell you if there are any errors in your experimental technique or if you have made any pipetting error in the experiment.

A biological replicate, on the other hand, is when the same test is performed on different samples drawn from the same population. Biological replicates provide evidence of random variation within subjects.

Technical replicates are important as they can reduce the effect of measurement errors but having more biological replicates is 'preferable for improving the efficiency of statistical testing' (Blainey et al. 2014).

16.2.9 Repeating Experiments

It is often recommended that experiments are repeated to ensure reliability or consistency of results by reducing the effect of random errors. Repeated experiments that produce similar results give confidence and trustworthiness to the results.

Repeating experiments helps with increasing reliability, but it does not improve the validity of the results. The validity of an experiment can be increased by controlling for more variables (such as possible confounders), improving measurement technique, utilising randomisation to reduce sample selection bias and having suitable controls.

In other words, reliability indicates the consistency of measurements or results whereas validity demonstrates the accuracy of measurements or results. Both are necessary for our results to be accepted as valid.

Further Reading

Aronson, J.K. (2005). Biomarkers and surrogate endpoints. *Br. J. Clin. Pharmacol.* 59 (5): 491–494.

Blainey, P., Krzywinski, M. and Altman, N. (2014). Replication. *Nat. Methods* 11 (9): 879–880.

Crowther, J.R. (1995). ELISA: theory and practice. *Methods Mol. Biol.* 42: 1–218.

de la Rica, R. and Stevens, M.M. (2012). Plasmonic ELISA for the ultrasensitive detection of disease biomarkers with the naked eye. *Nat. Nanotechnol.* 7 (12): 821–824.

Elgert, K.D. (2009). *Immunology: Understanding the Immune System*. Hoboken: John Wiley & Sons.

Leng, S.X., McElhaney, J.E., Walston, J.D., Xie, D., Fedarko, N.S. and Kuchel, G.A. (2008). ELISA and multiplex technologies for cytokine measurement in inflammation and aging research. *J. Geront. A Biol. Sci. Med. Sci.* 63 (8): 879–884.

Lequin, R.M. (2005). Enzyme immunoassay (EIA)/enzyme-linked immunosorbent assay (ELISA). *Clin. Chem.* 51 (12): 2415–2418.

Msagati, T.A. (2017). *Food Forensics and Toxicology*. Hoboken: John Wiley & Sons.

Sonntag, O. (1993). Introduction to dry chemistry. In: *Dry Chemistry: Analysis with Carrier-Bound Reagents* (ed. P.C. van der Vliet, P.C.). Philadelphia: Elsevier.

Van Weemen, B.K. and Schuurs, A.H.W.M. (1971). Immunoassay using antigen–enzyme conjugates. *FEBS Lett.* 15 (3): 232–236.

Wide, L. and Porath, J. (1966). Radioimmunoassay of proteins with the use of Sephadex-coupled antibodies. *Biochim. Biophys. Acta* 130 (1): 257–260.

Yalow, R.S. and Berson, S.A. (1960). Immunoassay of endogenous plasma insulin in man. *J. Clin. Invest.* 39 (7): 1157–1175.

Index